In A Page
Emergency Medicine

In A Page
Emergency Medicine

Jeffrey M. Caterino, MD
Chief Resident
Emergency Medicine/Internal Medicine Residency Program
Allegheny General Hospital
Pittsburgh, Pennsylvania

Scott Kahan, MD
Class of 2002
MCP-Hahnemann University
Philadelphia, Pennsylvania

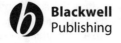
Blackwell
Publishing

Blackwell Publishing, Inc., 350 Main Street, Malden, Massachusetts 02148-5018, USA
Blackwell Publishing Ltd, 9600 Garsington Road, Oxford OX4 2DQ, UK
Blackwell Science Asia Pty Ltd, 550 Swanston Street, Carlton South, Victoria 3053, Australia
Blackwell Verlag GmbH, Kurfürstendamm 57, 10707 Berlin, Germany

03 04 05 06 5 4 3 2 1

ISBN: 1-4051-0357-4

Library of Congress Cataloging-in-Publication Data

In a page emergency medicine / [edited by] Jeffrey M. Caterino, Scott Kahan.
    p. ; cm.
Includes index.
ISBN 1-4051-0357-4
    1. Emergency medicine–Handbook, manuals, etc.   I. Caterino, Jeffrey M.
II. Kahan, Scott.
    [DNLM: 1. Emergencies–Handbooks.   2. Emergency Treatment–Handbooks. WB
39 I35 2003]
    RC86.8.I5 2003
    616.02´5—dc21   2002043911

A catalogue record for this title is available from the British Library

Acquisitions: Beverly Copland
Development: Julia Casson
Production: Debra Lally
Cover design: Gary Ragaglia
Interior design: Meral Dabcovich
Typesetter: TechBooks in York, PA
Printed and bound by Sheridan Books in Ann Arbor, MI

For further information on Blackwell Publishing, visit our website:
www.blackwellpublishing.com

Notice: The indications and dosages of all drugs in this book have been recommended in the
medical literature and conform to the practices of the general community. The medications
described and treatment prescriptions suggested do not necessarily have specific approval by
the Food and Drug Administration for use in the diseases and dosages for which they are recommended. The package insert for each drug should be consulted for use and dosage as
approved by the FDA. Because standards for usage change, it is advisable to keep abreast of
revised recommendations, particularly those concerning new drugs. This book is intended solely
as a review book for medical students and residents. It is not written as a guide for the intricate
clinical management of medical patients. The publisher and editor cannot accept any legal
responsibility for the content contained within this book nor any omitted information.

Table of Contents

Table of Contents

Table of Contents

Table of Contents

Table of Contents

Table of Contents

Section Sixteen: Environmental Emergencies   185

Jeffrey M. Caterino, MD
H. William Zimmerman, MD
Robert Driver, MD
Lorone C. Washington, MD

Section Seventeen: Terrorism and Disaster Medicine   199

Christopher R. Carpenter, MD
Scott Kahan, MD

Section Eighteen: Psychiatric Emergencies   205

Amy Smookler, MD

Abbreviations

α_1-AT	α-1 Antitrypsin Deficiency	CA	Carcinoma
AAA	Abdominal Aortic Aneurysm	CABG	Coronary Artery Bypass Graft
ABG	Arterial Blood Gas	CAD	Coronary Artery Disease
AC	Alternating Current	CAH	Congenital Adrenal Hyperplasia
ACE	Angiotensin Converting Enzyme	cANCA	cytoplasmic Anti-Neutrophilic
ACh	Acetylcholine		Cytoplasm Antibody
ACL	Anterior Cruciate Ligament	CBC	Complete Blood Count
ACLS	Advanced Cardiac Life Support	CCHB	Congenital Compete Heart Block
ACTH	Adrenocorticotropic Hormone	CD	Crohn's Disease
ADH	Antidiuretic Hormone	CDC	Centers for Disease Control
	(vasopressin)	CFL	Calcaneo-Fibular Ligament
Afib	Atrial Fibrillation	CHF	Congestive Heart Failure
AG	Anion Gap	CK	Creatine Kinase
AH	Aqueous Humor	CM	Cardiomyopathy
AICD	Automated Implantable	CML	Chronic Myelogenous Leukemia
	Cardioverter-Defibrillator	CMV	Cytomegalovirus
AIDS	Acquired Immunodeficiency	CN	Cranial Nerve
	Syndrome	CNS	Central Nervous System
ALL	Acute Lymphocytic Leukemia	CO	Cardiac Output
ALT	Alanine Aminotransferase	COPD	Chronic Obstructive Pulmonary
ALTE	Apparent Life-Threatening Event		Disease
AML	Acute Myelogenous Leukemia	COX	Cyclo-Oxygenase Inhibitor
AMS	Acute Mountain Sickness	CP	Chest Pain
ANA	Antinuclear Antibody	CPAP	Continuous Positive Airway
AP	Anteroposterior		Pressure
AR	Aortic Regurgitation	CPM	Central Pontine Myelinolysis
ARF	Acute Renal Failure	CPR	Cardiopulmonary Resuscitation
ARDS	Acute Respiratory Distress	Cr	Creatinine
	Syndrome	CRAO	Central Retinal Artery Occlusion
AS	Aortic Stenosis	CRVO	Central Retinal Vein Occlusion
ASA	Aspirin	CRP	C-Reactive Protein
ASD	Atrial Septal Defect	CSF	Colony Stimulating Factor
ASMA	Anti-Smooth Muscle Antibody	CSF	Cerebrospinal Fluid
AST	Aspartate Aminotransferase	CT	Computerized Tomography
ATFL	Anterior Talo-Fibular Ligament	CVA	Cerebrovascular Accident
ATN	Acute Tubular Necrosis	CVP	Central Venous Pressure
ATP	Adenosine triphosphate	CAVH	Continuous Arteriovenous
AV	Arteriovenous		Hemofiltration
AV	Atrioventricular	CVVH	Continuous Venovenous
AVM	Arteriovenous Malformation		Hemofiltration
AVRT	AV Reentrant Tachycardia	CXR	Chest X-Ray
AVNRT	AV Nodal Reentrant Tachycardia	D50	50% Dextrose Solution
β-hCG	β Human Chorionic Gonadotropin	D5W	5% Dextrose in Water
BiPAP	Bilevel Positive Airway Pressure	DBP	Diastolic Blood Pressure
BMI	Body Mass Index	DC	Direct Current
BNP	B-type Natriuretic Peptide	DDD	Degenerative Disk Disease
BOOP	Bronchiolitis Obliterans Organizing	DDx	Differential Diagnosis
	Pneumonia	DGI	Disseminated Gonococcal
BP	Blood Pressure		Infection
BP	Bullous Pemphigoid	DH	Dermatitis Herpetiformis
BPH	Benign Prostatic Hypertrophy	DHEA	Dehydroepiandrosterone sulfate
BPV	Benign Paroxysmal Vertigo	DI	Diabetes Insipidus
BSA	Body Surface Area	DIC	Disseminated Intravascular
BUN	Blood Urea Nitrogen		Coagulation

Abbreviations

DIP	Distal Interphalangeal joint	HCV	Hepatitis C Virus
DJD	Degenerative Joint Disease	HCT	Hematocrit
DKA	Diabetic Ketoacidosis	HCTZ	Hydrochlorothiazide
DM	Diabetes Mellitus	HDV	Hepatitis D Virus
DMV	Department of Motor Vehicles	HELLP	Hemolysis, Elevated LFTs, Low
DPL	Diagnostic Peritoneal Lavage		Platelets
DPT	Diphtheria, Pertussis, Tetanus	HEV	Hepatitis E Virus
	vaccine	HHNKC	Hyperglycemic Hyperosmolar
DTs	Delirium Tremens		Non-Ketotic Coma
DTR	Deep Tendon Reflex	HIV	Human Immunodeficiency Virus
DVT	Deep Venus Thrombosis	HLA	Human Leukocyte Antigen
EBV	Epstein-Barr Virus	HPF	High Power Field
ECHO	Echocardiogram	HPV	Human Papillomavirus
ED	Emergency Department	HR	Heart Rate
EEG	Electroencephalogram	HSM	Hepatosplenomegaly
EGD	Esophagogastroduodenoscopy	HSP	Henoch-Schönlein Purpura
ECG	Electrocardiogram	HSV	Herpes Simplex Virus
EMG	Electromyogram	HTN	Hypertension
ERCP	Endoscopic Retrograde	HUS	Hemolytic-Uremic Syndrome
	Cholangiopancreatography	IBD	Inflammatory Bowel Disease
ESR	Erythrocyte Sedimentation Rate	ICH	Intracranial Hemorrhage
ESRD	End Stage Renal Disease	ICP	Intracranial Pressure
ET	Endotracheal Tube	ICU	Intensive Care Unit
EtOH	Alcohol	IFN	Interferon
FAST	Focused Abdominal Sonography	IgA	Immunoglobulin A
	in Trauma	IgE	Immunoglobulin E
FENa	Fractional Excretion of Sodium	IgG	Immunoglobulin G
FEV_1	Forced Expiratory Volume	IgM	Immunoglobulin M
FFP	Fresh Frozen Plasma	IM	Intramuscular
F_iO_2	Fractional Inspiration of Oxygen	IMA	Inferior Mesenteric Artery
FOOSH	Fall On an Out-Stretched Hand	INH	Isoniazid
FRC	Forced Residual Capacity	INR	International Normalization Ratio
FSH	Follicle Stimulating Hormone	IOP	Intraocular Pressure
FVC	Forced Ventilatory Capacity	ITP	Idiopathic Thrombocytopenic
GBS	Guillain-Barré Syndrome		Purpura
GCS	Glasgow Coma Scale	IUGR	Intrauterine Growth Retardation
GERD	Gastroesophageal Reflux Disease	IUP	Intrauterine Pregnancy
GFR	Glomerular Filtration Rate	IVC	Inferior Vena Cava
GH	Growth Hormone	IVF	Intravenous Fluids
GHRH	Growth Hormone Releasing	IVH	Intraventricular Hemorrhage
	Hormone	IVIG	Intravenous Immunoglobulin
GI	Gastrointestinal Tract	JVD	Jugular Venous Distension
GnRH	Gonadotropin Releasing Hormone	KS	Keratoconjunctivitis Sicca
GSW	Gunshot Wound	LA	Left Atrium
HA	Headache	LAD	Left Axis Deviation
HACE	High Altitude Cerebral Edema	LBBB	Left Bundle Branch Block
HACEK	Haemophilus, Actinobacillus,	LDH	Lactate Dehydrogenase
	Cardiobacterium, Eikenella,	LES	Lower Esophageal Sphincter
	Kingella	LFT	Liver Function Test
HAPE	High Altitude Pulmonary Edema	LLQ	Left Lower Quadrant
HAV	Hepatitis A Virus	LMWH	Low Molecular Weight Heparin
Hb	Hemoglobin	LOC	Loss of Consciousness
HBV	Hepatitis B Virus	LP	Lumbar Puncture
HCG	Human Chorionic Gonadotropin	LR	Lactated Ringer's Solution

Abbreviations

LSB	Left Sternal Border	PaO$_2$	Partial Pressure of Oxygen
LUQ	Left Upper Quadrant	PBC	Primary Biliary Sclerosis
LV	Left Ventricle	PCA	Patient Controlled Analgesia
LV	Lymphogranuloma Venereum	PCL	Posterior Cruciate Ligament
LVH	Left Ventricular Hypertrophy	PCN	Penicillin
MAC	Mycobacterium Avium Complex	PCP	Primary Care Physician
MAI	Mycobacterium Avium Intracellulare	PCP	*Pneumocystis Carinii* Pneumonia
		PCOS	Polycystic Ovarian Syndrome
MAST	Military Anti-Shock Trousers	PCT	Porphyria Cutanea Tarda
MAT	Multifocal Atrial Tachycardia	PDA	Patent Ductus Arteriosus
MCH	Mean Corpuscular Hemoglobin	PE	Pulmonary Embolism
MCL	Medial Collateral Ligament	PEEP	Positive End Expiratory Pressure
MCV	Mean Corpuscular Volume	PEFR	Peak Expiratory Flow Rate
MDRTB	Multi-Drug Resistant Tuberculosis	PEP	Post-Exposure Prophylaxis
MEN	Multiple Endocrine Neoplasia	PET	Positron Emission Tomography
MG	Myasthenia Gravis	PFT	Pulmonary Function Test
MI	Myocardial Infarction	PICU	Pediatric Intensive Care Unit
MICU	Medical Intensive Care Unit	PID	Pelvic Inflammatory Disease
MMR	Measles, Mumps, Rubella	PMI	Point of Maximal Impulse
MPGN	Membranoproliferative Glomerulonephritis	PMN	Polymorphonuclear cell
		PMR	Polymyalgia Rheumatica
MR	Mitral Regurgitation	PND	Paroxysmal Nocturnal Dyspnea
MRA	Magnetic Resonance Angiography	PPC	Postpartum Cardiomyopathy
MRCP	Magnetic Retrograde Cholangiopancreatography	PPD	Purified Protein Derivative
		PPI	Proton Pump Inhibitor
MRI	Magnetic Resonance Imaging	PS	Pulmonic Stenosis
MRSA	Methicillin-Resistant *Staphylococcus Aureus*	PSC	Primary Sclerosing Cholangitis
		PSGN	Post-Strep Glomerulonephritis
MS	Mitral Stenosis	PSI	Pneumonia Severity Index
MVA	Motor Vehicle Accident	PT	Prothrombin Time
MVC	Motor Vehicle Collision	PT(S)	Patient(s)
MVP	Mitral Valve Prolapse	PTCA	Percutaneous Transluminal Coronary Angioplasty
N/V	Nausea/Vomiting		
NAC	N-acetylcysteine	PTH	Parathyroid Hormone
NaHCO$_3$	Sodium bicarbonate	PTFL	Posterior Talo-Fibular Ligament
NF	Neurofibromatosis	PTT	Partial Thromboplastin Time
NG	Nasogastric	PTU	Propothiouracil
NHL	Non Hodgkin's Lymphoma	PTX	Pneumothorax
NMBA	Neuromuscular Blocking Agent	PUD	Peptic Ulcer Disease
NPO	Nulla Per Os (nothing by mouth)	PV	Pemphigus Vulgaris
NS	Normal Saline	PVC	Premature Ventricular Contraction
NSS	Normal Saline Solution	PVR	Pulmonary Venous Resistance
NSAID	Non-steroidal Anti-Inflammatory Drug	RA	Rheumatoid Arthritis
		RA	Right Atrium
OA	Osteoarthritis	RAD	Right Axis Deviation
OCP	Oral Contraceptive Pill	RAS	Renal Artery Stenosis
OMFS	Oral and Maxillofacial Surgery	RBBB	Right Bundle Branch Block
ORIF	Open Reduction with Internal Fixation	RBC	Red Blood Cell
		RDW	Red Cell Distribution Width
P$_{Cr}$	Plasma creatinine concentration	RF	Rheumatoid Factor
P$_{Na}$	Plasma sodium concentration	RF	Risk Factor
PALS	Pediatric Advanced Life Support	RHD	Rheumatic Heart Disease
pANCA	perinuclear Antineutrophilic Cytoplasmic Antibody	RLL	Right Lower Lobe
		RLQ	Right Lower Quadrant

Abbreviations

RMSF	Rocky Mountain Spotted Fever	TIA	Transient Ischemic Attack
ROM	Range of Motion	TIBC	Transferrin Iron Binding Capacity
RPR	Rapid Plasma Reagin	TLC	Total Lung Capacity
RS	Reed-Sternberg cell	TM	Tympanic Membrane
RSI	Rapid Sequence Intubation	TMJ	Temporal-Mandibular Joint
RSV	Respiratory Syncytial Virus	TMP	Trimethoprim
RTA	Renal Tubular Acidosis	TNF	Tissue Necrosis Factor
RUQ	Right Upper Quadrant	TOF	Tetralogy of Fallot
RV	Right Ventricle	TORCH	Toxoplasmosis, Other, Rubella virus, Cytomegalovirus, Herpes Simplex virus
RVH	Right Ventricular Hypertrophy		
SA	Sinoatrial node		
S/S	Signs & Symptoms	tPA	Tissue Plasminogen Activator
S_1	First heart sound	TPN	Total Parenteral Nutrition
S_2	Second heart sound	TR	Tricuspid Regurgitation
S_3	Third heart sound	TRH	Thyroglobulin Releasing Hormone
S_4	Fourth heart sound	TS	Tricuspid Stenosis
SAH	Subarachnoid Hemorrhage	TSH	Thyroid Stimulating Hormone
SBE	Subacute Bacterial Endocarditis	TSS	Toxic Shock Syndrome
SBP	Systolic Blood Pressure	TTE	Transthoracic Echocardiogram
SIADH	Syndrome of Inappropriate Antidiuretic Hormone	TTP	Thrombotic Thrombocytic Purpura
		U/A	Urinalysis
SIDS	Sudden Infant Death Syndrome	U/S	Ultrasound
SIRS	Systemic Inflammatory Response Syndrome	UC	Ulcerative Colitis
		UCL	Ulnar Collateral Ligament
SLE	Systemic Lupus Erythematosis	U_{Cr}	Urine creatinine concentration
SMA	Superior Mesenteric Artery	U_{Na}	Urine sodium concentration
SMX	Sulfamethoxazole	UGI	Upper GI series
SOB	Shortness of Breath	URI	Upper Respiratory Infection
SQ	Subcutaneous	UTI	Urinary Tract Infection
SSRI	Selective Serotonin Reuptake Inhibitor	Vfib	Ventricular Fibrillation
		V/Q	Ventilation-Perfusion Ratio
SSSS	Staphylococcal Scalded Skin Syndrome	VBAC	Vaginal Birth After Cesarean section
SubQ	Subcutaneous	VCUG	Voiding Cystourethrogram
SV	Stroke Volume	VDRL	Venereal Disease Research Laboratory
SVC	Superior Vena Cava		
SVR	Systemic Venous Resistance	VSD	Ventricular Septal Defect
SVT	Supraventricular Tachycardia	Vtach	Ventricular Tachycardia
SX(S)	Symptom(s)	VWD	Von Willebrand's Disease
TB	Tuberculosis	VWF	Von Willebrand's Factor
TBSA	Total Body Surface Area	VZV	Varicella Zoster Virus
TCA	Tricyclic Antidepressant	WBC	White Blood Cell
TEE	Transesophageal Echocardiogram	WPW	Wolff-Parkinson-White syndrome
TEF	Tracheo-Esophageal Fistula		

Contributors

Ademola O. Adewale, MD
Chief Resident, Emergency Medicine
Allegheny General Hospital
Pittsburgh, Pennsylvania

Nihar Bhakta, MD
Staff, Children's Hospital
Medical Center of Akron
Akron, Ohio

Michael C. Bond, MD
Resident, Emergency Medicine and Internal Medicine
Allegheny General Hospital
Pittsburgh, Pennsylvania

Christopher R. Carpenter, MD
Chief Resident, Emergency Medicine and Internal Medicine
Allegheny General Hospital
Pittsburgh, Pennsylvania

Adam Cohen, MD
Resident, Emergency Medicine and Internal Medicine
Allegheny General Hospital
Pittsburgh, Pennsylvania

Mary Davis, DO
Resident, Emergency Medicine and Internal Medicine
Allegheny General Hospital
Pittsburgh, Pennsylvania

Robert Driver, MD
Resident, Emergency Medicine
Allegheny General Hospital
Pittsburgh, Pennsylvania

Carolyn S. Dutton, MD
Resident, Emergency Medicine and Internal Medicine
Allegheny General Hospital
Pittsburgh, Pennsylvania

Salima Kassab, MD
Resident, Neurology
Allegheny General Hospital
Pittsburgh, Pennsylvania

Kevin Mace, MD
Resident, Emergency Medicine
Allegheny General Hospital
Pittsburgh, Pennsylvania

Contributors

Tom Malinich, MD
Resident, Emergency Medicine
Allegheny General Hospital
Pittsburgh, Pennsylvania

Melissa L. McLane, DO
Fellow, Sports Medicine
Brigham Young University
Salt Lake City, Utah

Nathan W. Mick, MD
Clinical Fellow, Emergency Medicine
Brigham and Women's Hospital
Boston, Massachusetts

Mehul M. Patel, MD
Fellow, Gastroenterology
Allegheny General Hospital
Pittsburgh, Pennsylvania

Jack Perkins, MD
Resident, Emergency Medicine and Internal Medicine
University of Maryland Medical System
Baltimore, Maryland

Dave Saloum, MD
Resident, Emergency Medicine
Newark Beth Israel Hospital
Newark, New Jersey

Amar J. Shah, MD, MPH
Resident, Emergency Medicine
St. Luke's-Roosevelt Hospital Center
Columbia University College of Physicians and Surgeons
New York, New York

George Small, MD
Assistant Professor of Neurology
Drexel University College of Medicine
Director, Neuromuscular Division
Allegheny General Hospital
Pittsburgh, Pennsylvania

Amy Smookler, MD
Resident, Emergency Medicine
Allegheny General Hospital
Pittsburgh, Pennsylvania

Josef Stehlik, MD
Fellow, Cardiology
Allegheny General Hospital
Pittsburgh, Pennsylvania

Contributors

Mark Summers, MD
Resident, Emergency Medicine
Allegheny General Hospital
Pittsburgh, Pennsylvania

Matthew Stupple, MD
Resident, Emergency Medicine
Allegheny General Hospital
Pittsburgh, Pennsylvania

Melora J. Trotter, MD
Resident, Emergency Medicine
Allegheny General Hospital
Pittsburgh, Pennsylvania

Serv Wahan, MD, DMD
Resident, Oral and Maxillofacial Surgery
Allegheny General Hospital
Pittsburgh, Pennsylvania

Lorone C. Washington, MD
Resident, Emergency Medicine
Allegheny General Hospital
Pittsburgh, Pennsylvania

Svetlana Williams, MD
Resident, Psychiatry
Allegheny General Hospital
Pittsburgh, Pennsylvania

Richard R. Watkins, MD, MS
Resident, Internal Medicine
Allegheny General Hospital
Pittsburgh, Pennsylvania

H. William Zimmerman, MD
Resident, Emergency Medicine
Allegheny General Hospital
Pittsburgh, Pennsylvania

Consultants

Mara Aloi, MD
Assistant Director, Emergency Medicine Residency Program
Allegheny General Hospital, Pittsburgh, PA
Assistant Professor of Emergency Medicine
Drexel University College of Medicine

Jon Brillman, MD
Chairman of Neurology
Allegheny General Hospital, Pittsburgh, PA
Professor of Neurology
Drexel University College of Medicine

David M. Chuirazzi, MD, FACEP
Vice-Chair of Operations, Department of Emergency Medicine
Allegheny General Hospital, Pittsburgh, PA
Assistant Professor of Emergency Medicine
Drexel University College of Medicine

Nick E. Colovos, MD, FAAEM
Assistant Director of Emergency Medical Services
Department of Emergency Medicine
Allegheny General Hospital, Pittsburgh, PA
Assistant Professor of Emergency Medicine
Drexel University College of Medicine

Christopher Deflitch, MD, FACEP
Assistant Professor of Emergency Medicine
Clinical Director, Department of Emergency Medicine
The Pennsylvania State University College of Medicine
Milton S. Hershey Medical Center, Hershey, PA

Michael R. Dunn, MD
Attending Physician, Department of Emergency Medicine
Allegheny General Hospital, Pittsburgh, PA

Michael L. Forbes, MD
Pediatric Intensivist
Medical Director of Inpatient Pediatrics
Allegheny General Hospital, Pittsburgh, PA
Associate Professor of Pediatrics
Drexel University College of Medicine

Earlie H. Francis, MD
Attending Physician, Department of Emergency Medicine
Allegheny General Hospital, Pittsburgh, PA

Peter Grondziowski, MD
Director, Center for Diabetes and Endocrine Health
Allegheny General Hospital, Pittsburgh, PA

Consultants

Dennis P. Hanlon, MD, FAAEM
Director, Emergency Medicine Residency Program
Allegheny General Hospital, Pittsburgh, PA
Assistant Professor of Emergency Medicine
Drexel University College of Medicine

Fred P. Harchelroad, Jr., MD, FACEP, FAAEM, FACMT
Chairman, Department of Emergency Medicine
Allegheny General Hospital, Pittsburgh, PA
Associate Professor of Emergency Medicine
Drexel University College of Medicine

Janene Hecker-Kline, MD
Attending Physician, Department of Emergency Medicine
Sewickley Valley Hospital
Sewickley, PA

Lucian L. Kahan, DDS
Central Jersey Periodontics & Implants
East Brunswick, NJ

Pankaj Mohan, MD
Department of Medicine, Division of Cardiology
Allegheny General Hospital, Pittsburgh, PA
Assistant Professor of Medicine
Drexel University College of Medicine

Laurel Omert, MD
Associate Professor of Surgery
Drexel University College of Medicine
Attending Physician, Trauma Surgery
Allegheny General Hospital, Pittsburgh, PA

Peter S. Martin, MD
Assistant Director of Emergency Medical Services
Allegheny General Hospital, Pittsburgh, PA
Clinical Instructor
Drexel University College of Medicine

David Rottinghaus, MD
Attending Physician, Department of Emergency Medicine
Allegheny General Hospital, Pittsburgh, PA
Clinical Instructor
Drexel University College of Medicine

Mark Scheatzle, MD, MPH
Assistant Director, Emergency Medicine Residency Program
Resident Research Director
Allegheny General Hospital, Pittsburgh, PA
Assistant Professor of Emergency Medicine
Drexel University College of Medicine

Consultants

Daniel A. Shade, Jr., MD, FCCP, ABSMD
Attending Physician, Department of Medicine, Division of Respiratory Diseases
Allegheny General Hospital, Pittsburgh, PA

Joel Spero, MD
Associate Professor of Medicine
Drexel University College of Medicine
Coagulation Specialist, Division of Hematology/Medical Oncology
Allegheny General Hospital, Pittsburgh, PA

Robert Volosky, MD
Clinical Assistant Professor of Medicine, Temple University
Division of Infectious Diseases
Allegheny General Hospital, Pittsburgh, PA

Ralph J. Miller, MD
Department of Urology
Allegheny General Hospital, Pittsburgh, PA
Associate Professor of Surgery
Drexel University College of Medicine

Preface

The *In A Page* series was designed to streamline the vast amount of material that saturates the study of medicine, providing students, residents, and health professionals a high-yield, big picture overview of the most important clinical medical topics.

In A Page Emergency Medicine is the third book of this series. The format we use is especially effective for use in the emergency setting, where the high volume of patients and short time allotted per patient dictate the need for a quick-access, "no nonsense" handbook. It is so essential in this setting to be able to retrieve the most important information about your patients' conditions in as little time as possible. We selected the most appropriate emergent conditions and organized them efficiently for quick retrieval and study. Wherever appropriate, we have included the latest, evidenced-based data.

As in the initial books of the series, we were constrained by the size of the template and the need to keep each disease within a single page. We had to be quite succinct in our explanations and descriptions and we sacrificed details in some cases, such as drug dosages. Furthermore, we abbreviated liberally.

Since emergency medicine is not a clinical rotation for 3rd year medical students, we aimed the content at the level of 4th year medical students and interns. We are certain that the final product will be an effective resource. Reviews from medical students, residents, and other health professionals have been very positive. We anticipate that this book will be a valuable tool in the emergency room, as board review, and for independent study. We welcome any comments, questions, or suggestions. Please address correspondence to drkahan@yahoo.com.

Acknowledgments

We sincerely thank the residents, fellows, and attendings who contributed to the writing of this text. Special thanks to the faculty of Allegheny General Hospital emergency department, who have provided the knowledge and clinical skills upon which the book is based.

We are grateful to the staff at Blackwell Publishing, especially Julia Casson, Bev Copland, and Debra Lally. Their help during the course of this project was invaluable.

Assembling this book would not have been possible without the support of Jeff's wife, Stephanie Caterino. We also must thank Guy and Joanne Caterino and Lucian and Roberta Kahan for all the love, support, and guidance they have offered throughout the years and continue to provide today.

Resuscitation

JACK PERKINS, MD
SCOTT KAHAN, MD
JEFFREY M. CATERINO, MD

1. Cardiac Arrest

Etiology & Pathophysiology

- Cessation of circulation due to ineffective cardiac function (either asystole, ventricular fibrillation, pulseless ventricular tachycardia, or pulseless electrical activity)
- Results in absent pulses, blood pressure, respirations, and cerebral function
- Rapid restoration of organized cardiac activity and peripheral perfusion is essential
- Ventricular arrhythmias are the most common cause of arrest in patients with heart disease—early defibrillation is the key to survival
- Recommended management of cardiac arrest is contained in the protocols of the Advanced Cardiac Life Support (ACLS) course—an organized approach directed by established algorithms based on the clinical presentation

Differential Dx

- Myocardial infarction
- Structural heart disease
- Hypoxia
- Acidosis
- Metabolic (e.g., hyperkalemia)
- Hypovolemia/hemorrhage
- Drugs (e.g., anti-arrhythmics, Ca-channel/β-blockers, TCAs)
- Cardiac tamponade
- Tension pneumothorax
- Pulmonary embolism
- Stroke/cerebral hemorrhage
- Hypothermia
- Trauma
- Electrocution

Presentation

- Patient may be unresponsive (or minimally responsive if arrest is impending)
- Assess airway patency and ability to protect airway
- Assess breathing (spontaneous respirations, agonal respirations, tachypnea, adequate or shallow breaths, oxygenation, breath sounds)
- Assess circulation for pulses, blood pressure, and signs of poor peripheral perfusion and oxygenation (e.g., pallor, cold extremities)

Diagnosis

- If pulses and respirations are absent, immediately institute basic life support (chest compressions and breaths)
- Cardiac monitoring
- Assess pulse and rhythm first—defibrillate immediately if Vfib or pulseless Vtach is present
- Perform primary and secondary surveys
- Airway/breathing: Look for obstructions, initiate airway adjuncts if necessary (e.g., oral airways, bag-valve mask), and intubate early if necessary (based on presentation and any future expected decompensation)
- Circulation: Institute chest compressions if no pulse is palpated and obtain IV access
- Administer cardiovascular medications (by IV or endotracheal tube) according to ACLS algorithms
- Potentially reversible conditions (e.g., hyperkalemia, hypocalcemia) must be considered and treated

Treatment

- Treat potential causes (e.g., hyperkalemia requires IV calcium)
- Vfib/pulseless Vtach
  - Defibrillate × 3 (shock at 200J, 300J, then 360J)
  - Check rhythm and pulse after each defibrillation attempt
  - Persistent arrhythmias require drug therapy alternating with shocks (epinephrine every 3–5 minutes, vasopressin bolus, amiodarone, lidocaine, and/or procainamide; consider bicarbonate in prolonged resuscitation)
- Stable Vtach (wide-complex tachycardia): Amiodarone or lidocaine if monomorphic; magnesium if torsades de pointes
- Pulseless electrical activity: Epinephrine every 3–5 minutes alternating with atropine; aggressively identify and treat potential causes
- Asystole: Transcutaneous pacing (especially during the first few minutes) and alternating epinephrine and atropine
- Symptomatic bradycardia: Atropine, dopamine, epinephrine, transcutaneous pacing, with or without transvenous pacing
- Narrow-complex tachycardia: Cardioversion for severe symptoms; otherwise, administer medical therapy based on rhythm and co-morbidities

Disposition

- Wide-complex tachycardia should be considered Vtach until proven otherwise
- Early defibrillation of Vfib and pulseless Vtach is the most effective intervention
- Proceed as rapidly as possible to definitive care (e.g., PTCA for MI, correction of electrolytes)
- Prognosis is generally poor
  - Witnessed arrest and immediate CPR by a bystander slightly improves outcomes
  - Reversible causes have better outcomes
  - Many who survive have permanent neurologic sequelae
- Complications include death (in the majority), hypoxic brain injury, shock liver, MI, and acute renal failure

2. Overview of Shock

Etiology & Pathophysiology

- A physiologic state of inadequate circulation, resulting in insufficient tissue perfusion and oxygenation
- Organ dysfunction and damage (may be reversible or irreversible) occurs with prolonged lack of perfusion
- Hypovolemic shock: Decreased intravascular volume
- Cardiogenic shock: Decreased cardiac output
- Distributive shock: Loss of vasomotor tone results in inappropriate vasodilatation despite hypotension
  - Septic (infectious) shock: Bacterial toxins cause decreased vascular tone
  - Neurogenic shock: Head or spinal cord injury causes decreased vascular tone

Differential Dx

- Hypovolemic shock
  - Hemorrhage
  - Dehydration (e.g., diarrhea)
  - Extravascular fluid sequestration (3rd spacing)
- Cardiogenic shock
  - Intrinsic (e.g., ischemia, LV dysfunction, valve disease)
  - Extrinsic (e.g., tamponade, PE, pneumothorax)
- Distributive shock
  - Septic shock
  - Neurogenic shock
- Hypoadrenal shock
- Anaphylaxis

Presentation

- Early signs include orthostatic hypotension, mild tachycardia, diaphoresis
- Late signs include hypotension, significant tachycardia and tachypnea, altered mental status
- Vasoconstriction (resulting in narrow pulse pressure and cool extremities) in hypovolemic and cardiogenic shock
- Vasodilatation (wide pulse pressure and warm extremities) in distributive shock
- Signs and symptoms of underlying disease may be apparent (e.g., fever due to infection, chest pain due to MI, pallor due to blood loss)

Diagnosis

- Emergent diagnosis, supportive care, and treatment are essential
- Clinical recognition of inadequate organ perfusion (e.g., hypotension, tachycardia, decreased urine output, altered mental status)
- Initial studies may include CBC, electrolytes, renal function, lactate level (elevated in tissue hypoperfusion), PT/PTT, ABG (measures degree of acidosis), ECG, blood type and cross
- Workup as necessary depending on the type of shock (see individual entries)
- Swan-Ganz catheter placement may help identify the type of shock and guide management

	Cardiac Output	CVP/wedge pressure	SVR
Hypovolemic	↓	↓	↑
Cardiogenic	↓	↑	↑
Neurogenic	↓	↓	↓
Septic	↑	↓	↓

Treatment

- Airway, Breathing, and Circulation—secure airway, administer supplemental O_2, and establish two large-bore IVs (and possibly a central line)
- Intubation with mechanical ventilation eases cardiac workload significantly and helps to stabilize most patients with shock
- Re-establish adequate tissue perfusion
  - IV fluid administration is the initial treatment for all forms of shock (be careful in cases of cardiogenic shock as pulmonary edema can occur from fluid overload)
  - Choice of vasoactive agents depends on the type of shock (e.g., dobutamine or dopamine in cardiogenic shock, dopamine or norepinephrine in distributive shock)
- Determine the specific type of shock and treat underlying causes appropriately (see individual entries)
  - Blood transfusion and surgery for hemorrhagic shock
  - Antibiotics and vasopressors for septic shock
  - IV fluids and vasopressors for neurogenic shock
  - Inotropes and treatment of underlying cause for cardiogenic shock

Disposition

- Outcome depends on etiology and rapid restoration of adequate perfusion
- Continuously monitor for adequacy of resuscitation (e.g., stabilization of blood pressure, improvement of tachycardia, good perfusion on exam, resolution of acidosis, adequate urine output)
- Admit all patients to an ICU
- Persistent oxygen deprivation quickly causes irreversible cellular injury
- Sequelae include ARDS, cardiac ischemia, shock liver, DIC, neurologic damage, and acute renal failure due to ATN

3. Hypovolemic Shock

Etiology & Pathophysiology

- Blood or fluid loss that overwhelms the body's compensatory mechanisms to maintain perfusion and oxygenation
- Hypovolemic shock includes hemorrhage and volume loss from vomiting, diarrhea, third spacing of intravascular fluid, or burns
- Hemorrhage
    - Trauma: Pelvic fracture, long bone injury (especially femur), vascular injury, retroperitoneal hemorrhage, solid organ injury
    - GI bleeds: Esophageal varices, Mallory-Weiss tears, esophagitis, peptic ulcers, IBD, malignancy
    - Vascular: Aneurysm (e.g., ruptured AAA), AVM
    - Reproductive tract losses: Miscarriage, ectopic pregnancy, placenta previa, malignancy
- Dehydration/fluid loss (e.g., vomiting, diarrhea, inadequate intake)
- 3rd spacing (e.g., pancreatitis, nephrotic syndrome, liver failure, bowel infarction)

Differential Dx

- Cardiogenic shock
    - Intrinsic (e.g., ischemia, valvular disease, LV dysfunction)
    - Extrinsic (e.g., tamponade, PE, pneumothorax)
- Hypovolemic shock
    - Hemorrhage
    - Dehydration
    - 3rd spacing
- Distributive shock
    - Septic shock
    - Neurogenic shock
- Anaphylaxis
- Hypoadrenal shock

Presentation

- Based on degree of blood loss (decompensation occurs after 40% of blood volume is lost)
- Mild (<20% of blood volume lost): Cool extremities, poor capillary refill, diaphoresis (BP and urine output will be normal)
- Moderate (20–40%): Tachycardia, tachypnea, orthostasis, oliguria, anxiety
- Severe (>40%): Hypotension, narrow pulse pressure, weak distal pulses, severe tachycardia, tachypnea, impending cardiovascular collapse, absent bowel sounds, altered mental status (ranges from confusion to lethargy)

Diagnosis

- Initial studies include CBC, electrolytes, renal function, lactate level (elevated in tissue hypoperfusion), PT/PTT, ABG (measures degree of acidosis), ECG, blood type and cross
- Increased BUN/creatinine ratio and hypernatremia
- Identify sources of bleeding via ultrasound (aneurysm, organ injury) or CT scan (aneurysm, retroperitoneal hemorrhage)
- Swan-Ganz catheter placement may help distinguish from other types of shock and guide management:

	Cardiac Output	CVP/wedge pressure	SVR
Hypovolemic	↓	↓	↑
Cardiogenic	↓	↑	↑
Neurogenic	↓	↓	↓
Septic	↑	↓	↓

Treatment

- Secure airway, establish two large-bore IVs (and possibly a central line), and administer supplemental O_2
- Volume resuscitation
    - Rapid infusion of IV fluids (normal saline or LR)—infuse 2 liters or 3 times the amount of estimated blood loss (no evidence has proven albumin/colloid solutions to be beneficial)
    - Emergent RBC transfusion for hemorrhage (O^- blood)
- Inotropic support (only used after replacing volume)
    - Dopamine if hypotensive (inotropy plus vasoconstriction)
    - Dobutamine if normotensive (inotropy plus vasodilatation)
    - In general, avoid vasoconstrictors as they will increase BP via vasoconstriction but may not improve perfusion
- Replace electrolytes as necessary
- Clotting factors: Give fresh frozen plasma and platelets for every 5 units of blood infused
- Surgery to identify and repair the sites of uncontrolled bleeding

Disposition

- Outcome depends on etiology and rapid restoration of adequate perfusion
- Continuously monitor for adequacy of resuscitation (e.g., stable blood pressure, improvement of tachycardia, adequate perfusion on exam, resolution of acidosis, and adequate urine output)
- Admit all patients with shock to an ICU
- Persistent oxygen deprivation quickly causes irreversible cellular injury
- Sequelae include ARDS, cardiac ischemia, shock liver, DIC, neurologic damage, and acute renal failure due to ATN

4. Cardiogenic Shock

Etiology & Pathophysiology

- Cardiac output insufficient to meet metabolic demands, resulting in tissue hypoxia, despite *adequate* intravascular volume
- Hemodynamic criteria include hypotension, decreased cardiac index, and elevated pulmonary capillary occlusion pressure
- Three-quarters of patients diagnosed with cardiogenic shock have evidence of left ventricular dysfunction
- Intrinsic etiologies include MI (most common cause), valvular disease (e.g., acute mitral regurgitation), decompensated CHF, arrhythmias (e.g., due to electrolyte abnormalities), myocarditis, myocardial contusion, ventricular free wall or septal rupture, and dilated or hypertrophic cardiomyopathy
- Extrinsic etiologies (compressive, obstructive) include tension pneumothorax, pneumomediastinum, pericardial tamponade, mediastinal hematoma, diaphragmatic hernia, and positive pressure ventilation

Differential Dx

- Hypovolemic shock
  - Hemorrhage
  - Dehydration (e.g., diarrhea)
  - Extravascular fluid seques-tration (3rd spacing)
- Cardiogenic shock
  - Intrinsic (e.g., ischemia, LV dysfunction, valve disease)
  - Extrinsic (e.g., tamponade, PE, pneumothorax)
- Distributive shock
  - Septic shock
  - Neurogenic shock
- Hypoadrenal shock
- Anaphylaxis

Presentation

- Systolic BP <90 mmHg
- Pulse pressure (SBP - DBP) <20
- Cyanosis, ashen skin color, diaphoresis, mottled extremities
- Altered mental status
- Tachycardia
- Tachypnea
- Dyspnea
- Weak distal pulses, cool extremities
- JVD
- Crackles in lungs
- Cardiac exam may reveal distant heart sounds, precordial heave, S_3, S_4, murmurs (e.g., mitral regurgitation, VSD)
- Oliguria

Diagnosis

- ECG may reveal arrhythmias or acute myocardial infarction
- CXR often shows signs of CHF (e.g., vascular congestion, cephalization, Kerley B lines); may show evidence of the underlying etiology (e.g., wide mediastinum in aortic dissection)
- Anion gap metabolic acidosis due to poor tissue perfusion
- Cardiac enzymes may be elevated in acute MI
- ED echocardiogram to identify pericardial tamponade/effusion
- Complete echocardiogram may be performed at bedside to assess ejection fraction, LV function, valvular function/regurgitation, pericardium for tamponade, free wall rupture, and VSD
- Pulmonary artery catheterization reveals decreased cardiac output/index (<2.2 $L/min/m^2$), increased wedge pressure (>18 mmHg), increased systemic vascular resistance, and increased peripheral O_2 extraction
- Arterial line is recommended for blood pressure monitoring
- Cardiac catheterization is often diagnostic and may be therapeutic

Treatment

- Airway control with intubation or CPAP as necessary
- Fluid resuscitation as necessary to maximize cardiac filling and output
- IV inotrope administration
  - Dopamine (β- and α-agonist) for hypotensive patients to cause increased inotropy and vasoconstriction
  - Dobutamine (β-agonist only) for normotensive patients to cause increased inotropy and vasodilatation
- Avoid vasopressors (e.g., neosynephrine, norepinephrine) as they may improve blood pressure, but may diminish tissue perfusion
- Correct arrhythmias immediately with cardioversion, external pacing, and medications
- PTCA is the preferred method for reperfusion in cases of cardiogenic shock following MI; thrombolytics are much less effective in shock states
- Correct electrolyte abnormalities as necessary
- Intra-aortic balloon pump placement may be used as a temporizing measure to decrease afterload, thereby improving perfusion and cardiac output

Disposition

- Admit all patients to an ICU
- Overall mortality approaches 80%
- Mortality in the setting of an MI may exceed 80% with medical treatment alone, approaches 70% in patients who are administered fibrinolytics, and is 30% in patients treated with PTCA
- In general, the goal of initial therapy is to stabilize patients so that revascularization can be attempted
- Risk factors for the development of cardiogenic shock after an MI include increasing age, diabetes, decreased ejection fraction, large myocardial infarctions, female gender, multivessel disease, anterior wall MI, and history of a previous MI
- Shock most often occurs 6–7 hours after an acute MI

5. Distributive Shock

Etiology & Pathophysiology

- Hypoperfusion due to a loss of vasomotor tone, resulting in inappropriate vasodilatation despite hypotension
- Vasodilatation increases the intravascular space; thus, the normally adequate intravascular volume is distributed throughout a much greater space, resulting in inadequate effective circulating volume
- Neurogenic shock is caused by blunt or penetrating trauma to the brain and/or spinal cord—CNS injury impairs sympathetic output, resulting in bradycardia, arterial and venous dilatation, and hypotension
- Septic shock is caused by overwhelming microbial infection that results in hypotension and hypoperfusion despite adequate fluid resuscitation
- See related Sepsis entry (99)

Differential Dx

- Cardiogenic shock
  - Intrinsic (e.g., ischemia, LV dysfunction, valve disease)
  - Extrinsic (e.g., tamponade, PE, pneumothorax)
- Hypovolemic shock
  - Hemorrhage
  - Dehydration
  - 3rd spacing
- Distributive shock
  - Septic shock
  - Neurogenic shock
- Anaphylaxis
- Hypoadrenal shock

Presentation

- Hypotension
- Wide pulse pressure
- Warm extremities (due to vasodilatation)
- Mental status changes
- Decreased urine output
- Septic shock: Hyper- or hyperthermia, tachypnea, tachycardia
- Neurogenic shock: Hypothermia, bradycardia
- Evidence of underlying infection (e.g., fever, sputum production, urinary symptoms) or CNS injury (e.g., history of trauma, focal neurologic deficits)

Diagnosis

- Initial studies include CBC, electrolytes, renal function, lactate level (elevated in tissue hypoperfusion), PT/PTT, ABG to measures degree of acidosis (sepsis often has a respiratory alkalosis due to hyperventilation), ECG
- Additional tests in cases of sepsis should include blood cultures, urinalysis with culture, CXR, CT of potentially infectious areas, cultures of infected lines or indwelling devices, DIC panel, and lumbar puncture
- Additional tests in cases of neurogenic shock include head CT and spinal X-ray/CT
- Swan-Ganz catheter placement may help identify the type of shock and guide management:

	Cardiac Output	CVP/wedge pressure	SVR
Hypovolemic	↓	↓	↑
Neurogenic	↓	↓	↓
Septic	↑	↓	↓
Cardiogenic	↓	↑	↑

Treatment

- Secure airway, establish two large-bore IVs (and possibly a central line), and administer supplemental O_2
- Administer large fluid volumes of normal saline or lactated Ringer's solution to compensate for the increased intravascular space
- Vasopressor drips (norepinephrine, dopamine, or phenylephrine)
- Neurogenic shock
  - Maintain C-spine protection
  - Rapid fluid administration is generally successful in the absence of other interventions
  - Atropine and/or cardiac pacing for significant bradycardia
  - Methylprednisolone IV bolus and infusion in cases of blunt spinal cord injury
- Septic shock (refer to the Sepsis entry)
  - Obtain blood, urine, and sputum cultures
  - Begin IV empiric antibiotics to cover likely pathogens based on the presenting clinical picture

Disposition

- Outcome depends on etiology and rapid restoration of adequate perfusion
- Continuously monitor for adequacy of resuscitation (e.g., stabilization of blood pressure, improvement of tachycardia, good perfusion on exam, resolution of acidosis, adequate urine output)
- Admit all patients with shock to an ICU
- Persistent oxygen deprivation quickly causes irreversible cellular injury
- Sequelae include ARDS, cardiac ischemia, shock liver, DIC, neurologic damage, and acute renal failure due to ATN

6. Pediatric Resuscitation

Etiology & Pathophysiology

- Differentiate respiratory arrest (much more common in pediatric populations) from cardiac arrest
  - Respiratory arrest: Inadequate respirations or cessation of breathing with preserved pulse and blood pressure
  - Cardiac arrest: Absence of organized cardiac activity and lack of blood pressure (most commonly secondary to respiratory failure with prolonged hypoxia and acidosis)
- Respiratory arrest alone has a much better outcome than cardiac arrest—prompt recognition and treatment of impending respiratory failure is necessary to prevent subsequent cardiac arrest
- 50% of pediatric cardiopulmonary arrests occur in infants (children <1 year old)
- SIDS is the most common cause of cardiopulmonary arrest in infants; trauma is the most common cause in children >1 year old

Differential Dx

- Respiratory failure (e.g., infection)
- Respiratory obstruction/foreign body
- Sudden Infant Death Syndrome
- Sepsis
- Toxic ingestion
- Congenital cardiac disease
- Trauma
- Drowning/near-drowning
- Anaphylaxis

Presentation

- Assess airway patency
- Assess breathing for respiratory distress (e.g., tachypnea, retractions), check pulse oximetry, and monitor for progressive respiratory decompensation
- Assess perfusion—blood pressure, peripheral pulses, cyanosis of fingers or lips, extremities (cool in cardiogenic shock, warm in septic shock), capillary refill, brady- or tachycardia, and mental status changes
- Assess heart rhythm (the most common initial rhythm is asystole or bradysystole)

Diagnosis

- Airway/breathing
  - Note differences in child airway anatomy (smaller size, larger tongue, and more anterior airway than in adults)
  - A child lying supine will have a flexed neck (due to the prominent occiput) that may result in airway obstruction; hyperextended neck may also result in airway obstruction
  - Straight laryngoscope (i.e., Miller blade) is generally preferred since it better elevates the large epiglottis
  - Uncuffed endotracheal tube is used until age 8
- Circulation
  - Technique for external compressions depends on child size
  - Cardiac monitoring is used to guide drug treatment of arrhythmias and asystole (see below)
  - Multiple IV fluid boluses if hypovolemia is suspected
- Check glucose in all pediatric arrests
- Broselow emergency tape is used to determine equipment sizes and drug dosages for pediatric arrest situations

Treatment

- Immediately ensure oxygenation to prevent impending cardiac arrest—emergent intubation if necessary
- Fluid administration with multiple boluses of 20 cc/kg of normal saline in cases of suspected hypovolemia
- Manage dysrhythmias per PALS protocols
  - Bradycardia/asystole is the most common presenting rhythm (often due to severe hypoxia, drug ingestion, or structural heart disease)—treat with atropine (contraindicated in neonates) or epinephrine
  - Distinguish ventricular from supraventricular tachycardias
  - Cardioversion or defibrillation of unstable rhythms
  - Trial of adenosine for SVT
  - Lidocaine or bretylium for persistent ventricular arrhythmias
- Sodium bicarbonate for children with profound acidosis and persistent hypotension
- Epinephrine, dopamine, or dobutamine infusions for persistent hypotension or bradycardia

Disposition

- If there is no response beyond 20–30 minutes, continued resuscitation will generally not be of benefit
- Isolated respiratory arrest (pulse and blood pressure are maintained) has a 75% survival to discharge
- Survival in pediatric cardiac arrests is much worse than in adults
  - 2–13% survive to hospital discharge; the vast majority of survivors are neurologically devastated
  - Survival is especially poor if the patient is pulseless on arrival at the ED

7. Neonatal Resuscitation

Etiology & Pathophysiology

- Infants delivered in ED require resuscitation until proven otherwise
- Resuscitation is more likely needed following precipitous delivery, prematurity, meconium aspiration, extremes of maternal age, maternal HTN or diabetes, maternal substance abuse, maternal sepsis, recent maternal analgesic/sedative use, multiple gestations
- Newborn pathophysiology
  - The infant has two tasks: Clear the alveoli of fluid and redirect cardiac blood flow to the pulmonary circulation
  - Alveolar fluid is removed and alveoli expanded by the first few breaths following delivery
  - Pulmonary vascular resistance decreases upon exposure of the lungs to oxygen, resulting in increased pulmonary blood flow; however, persistent hypoxia causes a right-to-left shunt through the ductus arteriosus and persistent fetal circulation
- Survival of all premature infants is 30% at 24 wks, rare at <22 wks

Differential Dx

- Prematurity
- Infection
- Meconium aspiration
- Narcotic depression of respiratory drive
- Hypoglycemia
- Hemorrhage (placental abruption or previa)
- Seizures
- Shock (e.g., sepsis)
- Congenital heart lesions
- Diaphragmatic hernia
- Gastroschisis

Presentation

- Symptoms indicative of neonatal distress include bradycardia (heart rate <80), poor respiratory effort, cyanosis, lethargy, and weak cry
- Bradycardia is due to hypoxia until proven otherwise
- Note any presence of meconium
- Other possible presentations
  - Shock: Tachycardia, hypotension, poor respirations, poor capillary refill, cyanosis
  - Seizure activity: Tonic, clonic, tonic-clonic, or localized
  - Hypoglycemia: Apnea, cyanosis, lethargy, seizures, acidosis, shock, or jitteriness

Diagnosis

- Immediately check glucose in all patients—stressed neonates become hypoglycemic rapidly
- Maintain temperature by drying and keeping under a warmer
- Maintain airway by suctioning nose and mouth with bulb syringe
- Maintain breathing as necessary
  - 100% supplemental oxygen for all infants
  - Aid breathing with bag-valve mask at 40 breaths/minute if infant is apneic, cyanotic, or heart rate <100
  - Intubate if infant does not quickly improve
- Maintain circulation—treat bradycardia with adequate oxygenation, cardiac massage (encircle chest with hands, place thumbs over sternum, and compress at 120 bpm), and epinephrine (if manual stimulation fails to elicit response)
- APGAR score (based on heart rate, respiratory effort, presence/absence of cyanosis, muscle tone, reflex response) is calculated at 1 and 5 minutes post-delivery to evaluate the condition of the newborn

Treatment

- ABCs and resuscitation steps as above
- Observe for the presence of meconium
  - If thick meconium is present, suction nose, mouth, and pharynx immediately after delivery of the head
  - After delivery, immediately intubate the neonate, attach a meconium aspirator to the endotracheal tube, and apply suction as the tube is withdrawn; repeat this procedure until no further meconium is aspirated
  - Clear airway before beginning assisted respirations
- Glucose to treat hypoglycemia (avoid D50 in neonates as its osmolarity is too high)
- Epinephrine (IV or via ET tube) to treat bradycardia or asystole if ventilation and compressions are ineffective
- Naloxone administration for symptomatic neonates (apnea, respiratory distress, or lethargy) who have been exposed to therapeutic or illegal narcotics prior to delivery
- Bicarbonate is used to correct acidosis during prolonged resuscitations
- Fluid replacement and blood products for hemorrhage
- Dopamine for persistent hypotension

Disposition

- Hypoxia is the most common cause of bradycardia
- All resuscitated neonates should be admitted to an ICU
- Outcomes depend on etiology as well as speed and effectiveness of resuscitation
- Complications from hypoxia and shock include hypoxic brain damage, seizure disorders, SIADH, renal failure, cardiac damage, and necrotizing enterocolitis

Cardiovascular Emergencies

JOSEF STEHLIK, MD

8. Chest Pain

Etiology & Pathophysiology

- Chest pain is the chief complaint in 5–10% of ED patients—etiology may be of cardiac or non-cardiac origin
  - Cardiac sources include the myocardium (ischemic pain) and pericardium
  - Non-cardiac sources include the intrathoracic organs (aorta, pulmonary artery, bronchopulmonary tree, pleura, diaphragm, and esophagus), thoracic wall (bony structures, muscles, breasts, and skin), extrathoracic structures (stomach, duodenum, gallbladder, and pancreas), or psychogenic pain
- Acute life-threatening causes of chest pain include myocardial infarction, aortic dissection, esophageal rupture, tension pneumothorax, and pulmonary embolus
- A thorough history is the cornerstone of diagnosis to recognize and treat serious pathology while minimizing unnecessary testing and hospitalization

Differential Dx

- Cardiac: Myocardial ischemia, pericarditis, pericardial effusion, aortic dissection
- Pulmonary embolus
- Pulmonary: Pneumothorax, tracheitis, bronchitis, pleuritis, pneumonia, pleurisy, COPD
- GI: Esophagitis, esophageal spasm or perforation, GERD, PUD, gastritis, duodenitis, cholecystitis, pancreatitis
- Musculoskeletal: Rib fracture, costochondritis, herpes zoster, muscle strain, contusion
- Anxiety/psychogenic chest pain

Presentation

- Myocardial ischemia: Pain or pressure with exertion
- Pericarditis: Pain is notably decreased by leaning forward; friction rub is present on exam
- Aortic dissection: Sudden, tearing pain radiating to the back; unequal extremity blood pressures
- PE: Pleuritic pain, tachypnea, tachycardia, dyspnea
- Pneumonia: Fever, dyspnea, tachypnea, sputum production
- Tension pneumothorax: Tracheal deviation, JVD, hypotension, decreased breath sounds
- Zoster: Vesicular rash
- GI: Pain at night; related to food

Diagnosis

- History should include characteristics of the pain (e.g., dull, tight, pressure-like, burning, sharp, stabbing), location, radiation, duration and frequency, aggravating factors (e.g., exertion, deep respiration, supine position, palpation), alleviating factors (e.g., immobility, leaning forward, nitroglycerin), cardiac risk factors, family and medical history, and associated symptoms (e.g., diaphoresis, lightheadedness, nausea/vomiting, dyspnea)
- ECG may show ischemia or arrhythmias
- CBC may reveal leukocytosis if infection is present
- Cardiac enzymes may be elevated in MI
- LFTs, amylase/lipase, and U/S may rule out GI pathology
- Chest X-ray may show aortic dissection (mediastinal widening), pneumothorax, pneumonia, PE, pericardial effusion, or CHF
- Chest CT will evaluate for aortic dissection, pulmonary embolus, pneumothorax, and pneumonia
- V/Q scan (PE), echocardiogram (pericardial effusion), angiography or transesophageal echocardiogram (dissection) are also used

Treatment

- History, physical exam, and a limited diagnostic workup should be used to categorize patient risk
  - Patients likely experiencing an acute coronary event
  - Patient with a non-coronary, but potentially life-threatening event (e.g., aortic dissection, pulmonary embolism, pneumothorax, GI viscus perforation)
  - Patients with benign, non-coronary pain (GI, muscular)
- Cardiac etiologies require emergent, aggressive therapy
  - Nitrates and morphine for initial pain relief
  - Thrombolysis or emergent PTCA for ST elevation MI
  - Treat unstable angina/non-ST elevation MI per protocol (e.g., heparin, glycoprotein IIb/IIIa inhibitors, β-blockers)
- Treat pneumonia with appropriate antibiotics
- Treat pulmonary embolus with IV heparin or LMWH
- Insert chest tube to relieve pneumothorax (needle decompression followed by chest tube for tension PTX)
- GI cocktail (donnatol, viscous lidocaine, Mylanta) and anti-acid therapy for GERD or esophageal disease; however, symptom resolution does not rule out cardiac disease

Disposition

- No single sign, symptom, or test is definitive for the diagnosis of any of these conditions
- Admit patients with acute coronary syndromes, aortic dissection, pulmonary embolus, pneumothorax, esophageal rupture, serious pneumonia, or serious pericarditis
- Patients in whom serious disease cannot be ruled out (e.g., those with multiple risk factors for cardiac disease) should be admitted for observation
- Other patients may be discharged with appropriate follow-up

9. ST-Elevation MI

Etiology & Pathophysiology

- Previously called "transmural" or "Q-wave" MI
- Usually caused by rupture of an atherosclerotic plaque in an epicardial coronary artery, resulting in a highly thrombogenic surface; subsequent formation of an occlusive thrombus obstructs blood flow to the associated myocardium
- Results in transmural (i.e., full-thickness) infarction of myocardium
- Less frequent causes include thrombus formation in the absence of athero-sclerotic disease, vasospasm (e.g., Prinzmetal's angina, cocaine use), coro-nary dissection, and coronary thromboembolism
- Risk factors for coronary atherosclerosis include increasing age, tobacco use, hyperlipidemia, diabetes mellitus, hypertension, elevated homocys-teine levels, male gender, and family history
- Rapid reperfusion by thrombolytic agents or percutaneous transluminal coronary angioplasty (PTCA) is the mainstay of definitive therapy and should be performed ASAP

Differential Dx

- Unstable angina
- Non ST-elevation MI
- Pericarditis
- Aortic dissection
- Pulmonary embolus
- Pneumothorax
- Pleurisy
- Costochondritis
- GERD
- Esophageal spasm
- Stress/anxiety
- Pancreatitis
- Biliary colic
- Herpes zoster

Presentation

- Chest pain: Dull, substernal pain or pressure, often radiating to the jaw, left arm, and shoulders
- May be associated with nausea, vomiting, and diaphoresis
- Unremitting symptoms for >20 min
- Other frequent symptoms include dyspnea, lightheadedness, loss of consciousness, and hypotension
- Sinus tachycardia, ventricular ectopy, ventricular tachycardia, or ventricular fibrillation may occur
- In some cases, pain may be repro-ducible by palpation
- Physical exam is generally not help-ful (may have S_3, systolic murmur, or signs of CHF)

Diagnosis

- Obtain ECG within 10 minutes arrival to the ED
  - Criteria for emergent revascularization therapy includes ST-eleva-tion of 1 mm or more in at least 2 contiguous leads or new LBBB in the setting of typical symptoms
  - Leads with ST elevation may identify the infarcted vessel(s)
  - Ischemia may also cause hyperacute (peaked) T waves, inverted T waves, or reciprocal changes (i.e., ST depression)
  - LBBB or paced rhythm often confounds interpretation—acute infarction should be suspected with concordant ST elevation >1 mm (ST elevation in the same direction as the QRS complex), discor-dant ST elevation >5 mm (ST elevation in opposite direction of QRS), or ST depression >1 mm in V1–V3
  - Right-sided ECG leads may be used in the presence of inferior ischemia to rule out RV infarct (ST elevation in rV4)
- Cardiac enzymes (troponin, CK, CK-MB) become elevated within 6–12 hours—serial measurements are required
- CXR may rule out other potential sources of CP

Treatment

- Administer aspirin (160–325 mg) as soon as possible; clopidogrel or dipyridamole for patients intolerant to aspirin
- Revascularization is the definitive therapy
  - Primary PTCA is preferred as the initial revascularization ther-apy if available in a timely fashion (<2 hrs); indicated within 12 hrs of symptom onset in the presence of the above ECG criteria or with persisting symptoms >12 hrs
  - Thrombolysis is indicated if timely PTCA is not available; indicated within 12 hours of symptom onset in patients with ECG criteria and no contraindications
- IV heparin or enoxaparin (LMWH); enoxaparin may be superior
- Clopidogrel and/or glycoprotein IIb/IIIa inhibitors should be administered if PTCA is planned
- IV β-blockers given within 12 hours have been shown to improve mortality (avoid in patients with hypotension, bradycardia, or severe lung disease)
- Nitroglycerin and morphine
- ACE inhibitors are indicated within the first 24 hrs to improve post-MI left ventricular function

Disposition

- Continuous ECG monitoring is manda-tory given the risk of developing ven-tricular arrhythmias
- All patients are admitted
- If thrombolytics are administered, admit to an ICU
- Rescue PTCA is indicated for failed thrombolysis (i.e., lack of resolution of chest pain, persistent ST elevation, or reperfusion arrhythmias after 1–2 hrs), recurrent pain following successful thrombolysis, and cardiogenic shock
- Complications include arrhythmias, acute mitral insufficiency due to papil-lary muscle rupture, myocardial wall rupture, pericarditis, and cardiogenic shock

10. Unstable Angina and Non ST-Elevation MI

Etiology & Pathophysiology

- Formerly called "subendocardial" or "non Q-wave" MI
- Acute coronary syndromes: A spectrum of disorders ranging from unstable angina (myocardium at risk) to ST elevation MI (transmural infarction), resulting from decreased coronary blood flow (e.g., thrombus formation, vasospasm, or coronary artery dissection)
- Unstable angina: Angina at rest (lasting >20 minutes) within the previous week, angina presenting with increasing frequency, angina with lower level of exertion in a patient with chronic anginal symptoms, or new-onset exertional angina (during the past 2 months)
- Non ST-elevation MI: Infarction of the subendocardial myocardium
  - Diagnosed by symptoms of cardiac ischemia with elevated serum cardiac enzymes, but lack of transmural injury on ECG (no ST elevations)
  - Non ST-elevation MI can only be ruled out after serial cardiac enzymes have been obtained (i.e., 2–3 sets at 6–8 hour intervals)

Differential Dx

- ST-elevation MI
- Pericarditis
- Aortic dissection
- Pulmonary embolus
- Pneumothorax
- Pleurisy
- Costochondritis
- GERD
- Esophageal spasm
- Stress/anxiety
- Pancreatitis
- Biliary colic
- Herpes zoster
- Trauma

Presentation

- Chest pain: Dull, substernal pain or pressure, often radiating to the jaw, left arm, and shoulders
- May be associated with nausea, vomiting, and diaphoresis
- Other frequent symptoms include dyspnea, lightheadedness, loss of consciousness, and hypotension
- In some cases, pain may be reproducible by palpation
- Physical exam is generally not helpful (may have S_3, systolic murmur, or signs of CHF)

Diagnosis

- Obtain ECG within 10 minutes of presentation to ED—ischemia may be inferred by ST-segment depression and/or T-wave flattening (may be normal even if ischemia is present)
- Cardiac enzymes (troponin, CK, CK-MB, LDH) become elevated 6–12 hrs after the onset of chest pain; by definition, enzymes are elevated in non ST-elevation MI but normal in unstable angina
- CXR should be ordered to rule out other potential sources of CP
- Echocardiogram may be used to evaluate for wall motion abnormalities consistent with ischemia
- Resting nuclear perfusion scan may be used immediately to assess for ischemia at rest
- High-risk patients generally undergo diagnostic catheterization even if an acute MI has been ruled out (negative enzymes after 6–12 hours) and symptoms have resolved
- Low- or intermediate-risk patients with resolution of pain, no ECG changes, and negative serial enzymes generally undergo stress testing with imaging to evaluate for evidence of ischemia

Treatment

- Supplemental O_2 to maintain saturation >92%
- Administer aspirin (160–325 mg) as soon as possible (clopidogrel or dipyridamole for patients allergic to aspirin)
- IV unfractioned heparin or subcutaneous LMW heparin have been shown to decrease mortality and thrombus progression
- IV β-blockers have been shown to improve mortality (avoid in hypotension, bradycardia, or severe lung disease)
- IV morphine or IV/topical nitroglycerin should be administered in patients with continued chest pain
- IV glycoprotein IIb/IIIa receptor inhibitors (e.g., tirofiban, eptifibatide, abciximab) should be used in patients with elevated enzymes, ischemic ECG changes, at high risk for ischemia, or if percutaneous intervention is planned—they have been shown to decrease mortality, recurrent pain, and need for emergent revascularization
- ACE inhibitors are indicated if hypertension persists or in the presence of poor LV function or diabetes
- Catheterization with PTCA is indicated within 5 days for patients with elevated enzymes or at high risk for ischemia; patients with persistent pain require emergent intervention

Disposition

- Patients require at least two sets of cardiac enzymes 6–8 hours apart to rule out acute infarction (either obtained in the ED or as an inpatient)
- Low-risk or intermediate risk patients should undergo cardiac stress test with imaging after enzymes are negative
- Admit high-risk patients (i.e., resting angina >20 minutes, S_3 gallop, CHF symptoms, hypotension, dynamic ECG changes, elevated enzymes, or history of MI) for aggressive medical treatment and stress testing or catheterization

11. Atrial Fibrillation/Flutter

Etiology & Pathophysiology

- Atrial fibrillation is a disorganized electrical activation of the atria, resulting in irregular conduction through the AV node to the ventricles
- Atrial flutter is a regular, rapid depolarization of the atria, usually at a rate of 300 bpm; conduction to the ventricles is often regular, with every second or third atrial contraction being conducted
- Risk factors include hypertension, alcohol use, sick sinus syndrome, thyrotoxicosis, valvular disease (MS, MR), cardiomyopathy, myocarditis, CAD/MI, cardiac surgery, digoxin toxicity, and pulmonary disease (asthma, COPD)
- Persistent atrial fibrillation/flutter may allow clots to form in the atria, which can embolize to cause CVAs (approximate risk is 6%/year)—risk of clot formation and CVA increase after 48 hours of sustained arrhythmia

Differential Dx

- Marked sinus arrhythmia
- Sinus rhythm with frequent premature atrial complexes
- Multifocal atrial tachycardia
- Ventricular tachycardia
- Supraventricular tachycardia (AVNRT, AVRT)
- "Noisy" baseline on ECG

Presentation

- Patients may be asymptomatic, especially if the ventricular rate is controlled
- Palpitations
- Dyspnea
- Lightheadedness/presyncope
- Chest pain
- Signs and symptoms of CHF may be present
- Heart rate is often tachycardic but may be normal or even bradycardic
- Atrial fibrillation: Irregularly irregular rhythm, variable intensity of S_1
- Atrial flutter: Rapid regular rhythm

Diagnosis

- ECG is diagnostic in most cases
  - Atrial fibrillation: p waves are absent, ECG baseline has fine irregular fibrillation waves at 300–600/min, and QRS complexes are irregularly irregular
  - Atrial flutter: p waves are absent, ECG baseline shows regular "sawtooth" flutter waves at about 300/min, and QRS conduction is usually 1:2 (150/min and regular); however, conducted p waves may slow to 1:3 or less and this slowed conduction may be intermittent
  - Atrial fibrillation (i.e., no p waves) with a regularly occurring QRS complex (regular RR interval) is pathognomonic for digitalis toxicity
- Continuous ECG monitoring may detect paroxysms of arrhythmia
- If rate is so rapid such that atrial activity is difficult to see and the diagnosis is unclear, a dose of IV adenosine may be administered to transiently slow AV conduction to aid rhythm interpretation

Treatment

- If rapid ventricular response is causing hemodynamic compromise or serious symptoms, emergent DC cardioversion is indicated
- There are three major treatment considerations: Rate control, anticoagulation, and/or rhythm control
- Rate control using AV node blocking agents
  - β-blockers (e.g., metoprolol, atenolol, propranolol)
  - Calcium-channel blockers (e.g., diltiazem, verapamil)
  - Digoxin (several hours to take effect)
- Anticoagulation to reduce the risk of cardioembolic CVA; full anticoagulation with IV heparin is indicated if Afib/flutter lasts >48 hrs
- Rhythm control using antiarrhythmic therapy
  - DC cardioversion emergently as needed; IV ibutilide may be used to attempt rapid pharmacologic cardioversion
  - Non-emergent electrical or pharmacological (e.g., amiodarone) cardioversion should not be done in the ED until the risk of thromboembolic events is assessed (conversion in the presence of atrial clot may cause CVA)
- CHF symptoms usually improve with rate control

Disposition

- Cardiology or Internal Medicine consultation should be obtained for most patients with newly diagnosed or recurrent atrial fibrillation/flutter with rapid ventricular response
- Most of these patients will need to be admitted for further workup and treatment decisions
- Procainamide should be used if Wolff-Parkinson-White syndrome cannot be ruled out; avoid β-blockers, Ca-channel blockers and digoxin in these cases
- Elective cardioversion may be attempted in patients with <48 hours of atrial fibrillation/flutter

12. Supraventricular Tachycardia

Etiology & Pathophysiology

- Tachycardia that originates above the ventricles
- Sinus tachycardia is a SVT not caused by a primarily cardiac process; may be due to drugs, hypovolemia, hypotension, sepsis, LV dysfunction, or stress
- Multifocal atrial tachycardia (MAT) occurs when at least 3 atrial foci exist; causes include pulmonary disease, structural heart disease, and digoxin
- Atrial fibrillation/flutter: See associated entry
- Nonparoxysmal junctional tachycardia is caused by an impulse originating at the AV node; due to myocarditis, digoxin, inferior MI
- AV Nodal Reentrant Tachycardia (AVNRT) is caused by a reentrant circuit within the AV node
- AV Reentrant Tachycardia (AVRT) is caused by a reentrant circuit with accessory pathway outside the AV node (Wolff-Parkinson-White syndrome refers to the direct atrial-ventricular connection)

Differential Dx

- Ventricular tachycardia (treat all wide-complex tachycardias as ventricular tachycardia until proven otherwise)
- SVT with aberrancy (wide QRS tachycardia despite supraventricular origin)

Presentation

- Palpitations (in >90%)
- Dizziness (in >70%)
- Presyncope
- Syncope
- Shortness of breath
- Chest pain
- Fatigue
- Tachycardia
- Hypotension
- CHF may occur

Diagnosis

- ECG reveals a narrow QRS complex (<0.12 sec) tachycardia
- Regular rhythm SVTs
  - Sinus tachycardia: Rate 100–180; p wave for each QRS
  - Junctional: Narrow QRS; p wave absent or follows QRS
  - Atrial flutter: Atrial rate 250–350 with "sawtooth" flutter waves; ventricular conduction is often 150 bpm
  - AV Nodal Reentrant: Rate >150, narrow and regular QRS, may see retrograde p waves after each QRS
  - AV Reentrant Tachycardia: Rate >150, QRS may be narrow or wide, may see retrograde p waves after each QRS; WPW is seen (short PR, wide QRS, delta wave) when rate slows
- Irregular rhythm SVTs
  - MAT: 3 or more discrete p waves are present
  - Atrial fib: Rate 75–200; irregularly irregular; no p waves
  - Atrial flutter with variable conduction: "Sawtooth" p waves, variable ventricular response (2:1, 3:1, or 4:1 are common)
- Adenosine will briefly slow the rate to aid rhythm identification

Treatment

- Immediate cardioversion for hemodynamically unstable patients (unless the rhythm is sinus tachycardia)
- Sinus tachycardia: Treat the underlying disorder
- Atrial tachycardia or MAT: Treat underlying pulmonary disease; use Ca-channel or β-blockers for rate control
- AV Nodal Reentrant/AV Reentrant Tachycardia
  - Vagal maneuvers (increase parasympathetic tone): Ocular or carotid massage, Valsalva, immerse face in cold H_2O
  - Adenosine: Causes complete AV blockade for seconds, and converts majority of AVNRT and AVRT to sinus
  - AV node blockers: IV β-blockers or Ca-channel blockers should be used for rate control if adenosine fails to convert the rhythm
  - Caution: Ca-channel or β-blockers can induce ventricular fibrillation in a wide complex AVRT (i.e., antidromic WPW syndrome) and are contraindicated in these patients
  - Chronic treatment is with AV nodal blocking agents or by catheter ablation of the accessory pathway
  - Other agents for rate control include digoxin, amiodarone, procainamide, and sotalol

Disposition

- Sinus tachycardia: Disposition depends on the underlying disorder
- Atrial tachycardia and MAT usually do not require admission unless associated with hemodynamic compromise
- AVNRT and AVRT patients are not at risk of sudden cardiac death
- Admit patients presenting with a first episode of AVNRT or AVRT or if there is associated hemodynamic instability
- Patients with known history of bypass tract, rare paroxysms of SVT without hemodynamic compromise, and swift response to medical therapy can usually be discharged home with AV nodal blocking drugs

13. Ventricular Tachycardia

Etiology & Pathophysiology

- Any wide-QRS complex tachycardia (QRS >0.12 sec) is considered ventricular tachycardia (Vtach) until proven otherwise
  - Nonsustained Vtach lasts <30 sec and is asymptomatic
  - Sustained Vtach lasts >30 sec or results in hemodynamic compromise
  - Monomorphic Vtach: Single stable QRS complex
  - Polymorphic Vtach: Changing QRS morphology and axis—may have normal or prolonged QT interval (e.g., torsades de pointes)
- Etiologies/risk factors include acute or past MI, decreased LV function, any cardiomyopathy, myocarditis, sarcoidosis, electrolyte abnormalities, pro-arrhythmic medications, congenital long QT syndrome, right ventricular dysplasia, family history of sudden cardiac death
  - The majority of ventricular tachycardias are caused by ischemic heart disease

Differential Dx

- SVT with aberrant conduction through nodal fibers (i.e., bundle-branch block)
- Preexcitation tachycardia (e.g., AVNRT, Afib/flutter, antidromic AVRT)
- Ventricular fibrillation
- Ventricular escape rhythm (ventricle depolarizes at 30–60 bpm without stimulation from the atria or AV node)
- Accelerated idioventricular rhythm (rapid ventricular escape rhythm at 60–100 bpm)
- Monitor artifact

Presentation

- Older age and a history of MI/CAD, CHF, and angina are often present
- Symptoms may include dyspnea, dizziness, presyncope or syncope, angina, palpitations
- Tachycardia, hypotension, cardiorespiratory arrest, cannon A waves (AV dissociation), and cardiomegaly (on CXR) may be seen

Diagnosis

- 12-lead ECG shows wide QRS tachycardia (QRS >0.12 seconds)
  - Rate does not reliably distinguish Vtach from other ventricular arrhythmias (Vtach is usually >130)
  - Vtach and SVT are regular; atrial fibrillation is irregular
  - AV dissociation occurs in Vtach (p waves not related to QRS)
  - Fusion beats occur only in Vtach (p wave partially activates a QRS at the same time as the ectopic circuit, resulting in a hybrid QRS complex)
  - Capture beats are only seen in Vtach (occasionally, the p wave will conduct a normal, narrow QRS complex)
  - Extreme left axis deviation usually indicates Vtach
  - QRS duration >0.16 seconds likely indicates Vtach
  - Precordial (V_1–V_6) concordance (QRS waves all in the same direction) strongly suggests Vtach
  - Look for bundle branch blocks (e.g., R-S-R_1 in VI for RBBB)
  - Note polymorphic versus monomorphic complexes

Treatment

- Patients with ventricular escape or accelerated idioventricular rhythms are dependent on these ventricular beats to maintain cardiac output—they should not be treated with anti-arrhythmics as this may terminate the ventricular rhythm, resulting in asystole
- Unstable Vtach with hypotension or cardiac ischemia requires immediate electrical intervention
  - Vfib and pulseless Vtach should be defibrillated per ACLS protocols; if defibrillation fails, then IV epinephrine, amiodarone, and/or lidocaine may be attempted
  - Patients with hemodynamic instability must be treated with synchronized cardioversion; if cardioversion fails, IV amiodarone or lidocaine should be used
- Stable monomorphic Vtach should be treated initially with anti-arrhythmic medications (e.g., IV amiodarone, lidocaine, procainamide); cardiovert if there is no response
- Stable polymorphic Vtach with long QT requires correction of electrolyte abnormalities and IV magnesium for torsades de pointes

Disposition

- Most patients with Vtach require admission to a cardiology or electrophysiology service for further therapy and risk stratification
- Be sure to rule out ongoing myocardial ischemia
- Patients with Vtach are at increased risk of sudden cardiac death; definitive long-term therapy is usually required
- Long-term treatment options include revascularization of ischemic myocardium, automated implantable cardioverter-defibrillator (AICD), long-term anti-arrhythmic therapy, and radiofrequency ablation of the focus of ventricular tachycardia

14. Bradycardia and Heart Block

Etiology & Pathophysiology

- A resting heart rate <60 beats per minute
- Classified based on presence of p waves and their relation to the QRS
- Sinus bradycardia: Normal p waves with a slowed sinus node rate
- Junctional escape rhythm: Originates from either the AV node or bundle of His following a long period without SA nodal stimulation
- Idioventricular rhythm: Originates from the ventricle after a lack of stimulation from the SA node, AV node, and bundle of His
- AV conduction block: Slowed conduction through the AV node
    - 1st degree: Slowed AV conduction without dropped beats
    - 2nd degree (Mobitz type I or II): Intermittent dropped beats
    - 3rd degree (complete heart block): No electrical communication between atria and ventricles
- Atrial fibrillation/flutter with slow ventricular conduction
- Causes of bradyarrhythmias include medications, vagal stimulation, and degeneration or structural abnormality of the conduction system

Differential Dx

- Acute MI
- Electrolyte abnormalities
- Meds (e.g., β-blockers, digoxin, calcium blockers, TCAs)
- Vagal stimulation (e.g., nausea, vomiting, vasovagal reaction)
- Sick-sinus syndrome
- Paravalvular abscess
- Infiltrative disease (e.g., sarcoidosis, amyloidosis)
- Congenital heart block
- Increased ICP (Cushing's reflex): ICH, CVA, SAH
- Myocarditis
- Hypothyroid
- Lyme disease
- Chagas disease

Presentation

- May be asymptomatic
- Symptoms may include palpitations, dyspnea, dizziness, presyncope or syncope, chest pain, and mental status changes
- Physical exam may reveal irregular heartbeat, jugular venous distension, cannon jugular waves (in 3rd degree AV block), hypotension, or signs of heart failure
- Atrial fibrillation with complete heart block (i.e., regular junctional or ventricular escape rhythm) is pathognomonic for digitalis toxicity

Diagnosis

- Sinus bradycardia: Rate <60 with normal p waves, PR interval, and PP interval
- Junctional rhythm: Rate 40–60 with narrow QRS and absent or retrograde p waves
- Idioventricular rhythm: Rate 30–40 with wide QRS and no p waves
- 1st degree AV block: Prolonged but constant PR interval (>0.2 sec); each p wave is followed by a QRS
- 2nd degree AV block: Irregular rhythms
    - Mobitz I (Wenkebach): Progressively prolonged PR resulting in a p wave that fails to conduct to the ventricles (dropped beat); PP interval remains constant; RR shortens progressively
    - Mobitz II: Intermittent nonconducted p waves; PR interval remains fixed (does not prolong); PP and RR interval constant
- 3rd degree AV block (complete heart block): P waves unrelated to the QRS; escape rhythm is regular and originates from the AV junction (narrow QRS) or the ventricle (wide QRS)

Treatment

- Asymptomatic bradycardia does not require immediate therapy—monitor for onset of symptoms or asystole
- Emergent treatment is indicated for symptomatic bradycardia
    - Atropine: Increases SA and AV nodal conduction; indicated for asystole, symptomatic bradycardia, or symptomatic AV block
    - Epinephrine: Indicated for asystole and refractory symptomatic bradycardia
    - Emergency cardiac pacing (transcutaneous or transvenous): Indicated for asystole, symptomatic bradycardia, and patients at high risk of progression to asystole (e.g., Mobitz II or 3rd degree heart block)
    - Dopamine infusion may also increase the heart rate
- Bradycardia induced by β-blockers or Ca-channel blockers should be treated with IV calcium and IV or IM glucagon, which increases chronotropy and inotropy by a non-adrenergic mechanism
- Bradycardia due to digoxin toxicity may be treated with Digibind (digoxin specific antibody fragments) in cases of life-threatening toxicity

Disposition

- Sinus bradycardia or a junctional escape rhythm may be normal in well-trained athletes and do not require treatment if asymptomatic
- Asymptomatic 1st degree and 2nd degree Mobitz I AV-block without other conduction abnormalities do not require specific treatment
- Admission depends on comorbid conditions, etiology of bradycardia (e.g., overdose or MI), and chance of progression to asystole
- Patients with 2nd degree Mobitz II AV block and 3rd degree AV block should be admitted as they may progress to asystole—these patients will likely require permanent pacemaker implantation

15. Heart Failure

Etiology & Pathophysiology

- Inability of the heart to maintain adequate cardiac output
  - Pericardial etiologies: Pericardial constriction or tamponade
  - Endocardial etiologies: Valvular stenosis, insufficiency, or rupture
  - Myocardial: Ischemia/infarction, cardiomyopathy, arrhythmias
- Myocardial failure may be classified as systolic (inability to eject blood) or diastolic (inability to adequately fill with blood)
  - Systolic dysfunction (more common): Decreased myocardial contractility and ejection fraction
  - Diastolic dysfunction: Impaired myocardial relaxation, resulting in decreased ventricular filling (ejection fraction may be normal)
- Left-sided heart failure results in pulmonary symptoms
- Right-sided heart failure results in peripheral symptoms—commonly secondary to left heart failure, but may occur alone (e.g., RV infarct)
- High output failure: Inability to meet abnormally high tissue demands (e.g., thyrotoxicosis, sepsis, anemia) despite a normal heart

Differential Dx

- Cardiovascular: Ischemia, valve disease or rupture, aortic dissection, arrhythmia, endocarditis, myocarditis, hypertensive emergency
- Pulmonary: COPD, pneumonia, pulmonary embolus, other lung disease, ARDS
- Renal failure with fluid overload
- Hepatic insufficiency
- Hypoalbuminemia
- Anemia
- Sepsis
- Thyrotoxicosis

Presentation

- Dyspnea (ranges from exertional dyspnea to severe dyspnea at rest)
- Orthopnea
- Paroxysmal nocturnal dyspnea
- Fatigue, weakness, decreased exercise tolerance
- Abdominal fullness, weight gain
- Tachypnea, tachycardia
- S_3
- Rales (crackles)
- Jugular venous distention
- Laterally displaced apical impulse
- Hepatomegaly, hepatojugular reflux
- Ascites, peripheral edema

Diagnosis

- Chest X-ray shows cardiomegaly, increased pulmonary vasculature (e.g., cephalization, hilar fullness, Kerley B lines), interstitial edema, and possibly a pleural effusion
- ECG may show evidence of coronary artery disease, arrhythmias, or changes suggestive of acute ischemia
- Cardiac enzymes are positive in 30% of patients with acute CHF
- Check CBC (for anemia), electrolytes, and renal function
- ABG may show signs of respiratory failure (hypoxemia or elevated pCO_2)
- Serum B-type natriuretic peptide (BNP) is a fairly accurate marker of heart failure (released by ventricles in response to stretch): Differentiates dyspnea due to heart failure (BNP >100) from dyspnea due to other causes (BNP <100)
- Echocardiography defines systolic function, wall motion abnormalities, valvular function, and evaluates the pericardium
- Right or left heart catheterization may be done as an inpatient

Treatment

- Mainstay of therapy is to decrease preload (by venodilation) and afterload (by arteriodilation and volume removal) to improve forward blood flow and decrease symptoms
- Supplemental O_2 via nasal cannula or face mask as needed
- Treat refractory respiratory distress with CPAP or intubation
- Nitrates (sublingual and IV) are first line treatment for rapid relief of symptoms (act as vasodilators to decrease preload and afterload); however, they may cause hypotension
- Loop diuretics are used to remove volume and decrease preload (via mild venodilation)
- IV morphine for anxiety/discomfort and to decrease preload
- ACE inhibitors will decrease both preload and afterload
- Systolic dysfunction may require inotropic support
  - Dobutamine will increase inotropy and cause vasodilation (use only if SBP >90 as it may cause hypotension)
  - Dopamine increases inotropy and causes vasoconstriction (use if SBP <90 as it will not worsen hypotension)
- Diastolic dysfunction may require negative inotropes (e.g., β- or Ca-channel blockers)
- Cardiac ischemia may require revascularization

Disposition

- CHF results in >1 million ED visits per year
- Most patients are admitted for further therapy and/or workup
- In-hospital mortality is 7%
- Even "low risk" patients (mild symptoms and no recent MI, arrhythmia, or electrolyte abnormality) may have poor outcomes
- Some criteria for admission include moderate-severe symptoms, ischemia, hypoxia, severe medical disease, hypotension, no obvious precipitating cause for decompensation, new-onset CHF, or poor outpatient support
- Patients to be discharged should first be observed in the ED for clinical improvement and have close follow-up arranged

16. Cardiomyopathy

Etiology & Pathophysiology

- Abnormal myocardium, resulting in impaired function and CHF
- Dilated cardiomyopathy: Impaired systolic ventricular function with dilation of the ventricles; etiologies include CAD (ischemic cardiomyopathy), HTN, infection (e.g., myocarditis, Lyme, Chagas disease), valvular insufficiency, pregnancy, toxins (e.g., alcohol, cocaine, heroin, doxarubicin, lead, arsenic), sepsis, congenital heart disease, rheumatic fever, persistent tachycardia, thyroid disease, obesity, or nutritional deficiencies
- Hypertrophic cardiomyopathy: Asymmetric ventricular hypertrophy with diastolic dysfunction (i.e., abnormal diastolic relaxation), resulting in decreased ventricular filling, stroke volume, and cardiac output; 50% are familial; carries an increased risk of sudden death
- Restrictive cardiomyopathy: Diastolic dysfunction caused by infiltrative diseases (e.g., amyloid, sarcoid, hemochromatosis), scleroderma, hypereosinophilia

Differential Dx

- Ischemic cardiomyopathy
- Diastolic heart failure (impaired LV relaxation due to HTN, DM, or constrictive pericarditis)
- Valvular disease
- Myocarditis
- COPD
- Asthma
- Pulmonary embolus
- Non-cardiogenic pulm edema
- Renal failure
- Hepatic insufficiency
- Hypoalbuminemia
- Hypothyroidism

Presentation

- Symptoms of heart failure (e.g., fatigue, dyspnea on exertion, orthopnea, PND)
- Left heart failure signs (e.g., respiratory distress, bilateral crackles)
- Right heart failure signs (e.g., JVD, enlarged liver, peripheral edema)
- Dilated CM: Laterally displaced PMI, S_3, arrhythmias, thrombus formation
- Hypertrophic CM: Increased magnitude of PMI, S_4, symptoms worsen with exertion (including syncope and chest pain)
- Restrictive CM: Primarily right sided symptoms, S_4

Diagnosis

- Dilated CM
  - CXR: Cardiomegaly, pulmonary edema, +/− pleural effusion
  - ECG: Non-specific ST-T wave changes, ischemic changes, abnormal conduction, or arrhythmias may be present
  - Echocardiogram: Dilated ventricles, systolic dysfunction
  - Serum B-type natriuretic peptide (BNP): Differentiates dyspnea due to heart failure (BNP>100) from dyspnea due to other causes (BNP<100)
- Hypertrophic CM
  - CXR: Normal or large heart size
  - ECG: LVH, small septal Q waves (pseudoinfarct pattern)
  - Echo: Asymmetric septal hypertrophy, diastolic dysfunction
- Restrictive CM
  - CXR: Signs of CHF, normal heart size
  - EKG: Nonspecific ST-T changes, low voltage QRS
  - Echo: Diastolic dysfunction, may show evidence of amyloid

Treatment

- Emergent treatment of acute CHF exacerbations
  - Intubation for severe respiratory distress
  - Loop diuretics decrease pulmonary edema by decreasing blood vessels and causing venodilation
  - Vasodilators for patients with volume overload and SBP >100 (nitroglycerin will cause preload reduction by venodilation; ACE inhibitors and hydralazine will decrease afterload to improve cardiac output)
  - Morphine will improve subjective sensation of SOB
  - Consider Swan-Ganz catheter or intra-aortic balloon pump in refractory cardiogenic shock
- Dilated CM (systolic dysfunction) requires positive inotropy
  - Dobutamine will increase inotropy and cause vasodilation (use only if SBP >90 as it may cause hypotension)
  - Dopamine increases inotropy and causes vasoconstriction (use if SBP <90 as it will not worsen hypotension)
- Hypertrophic and restrictive CM (diastolic dysfunction): Negative inotropes (β- or Ca-channel blockers) increase ventricular filling time and promote relaxation to increase ventricular filling and cardiac output

Disposition

- Recurrent exacerbations of heart failure and frequent ED visits are common
- Patients with newly diagnosed cardiomyopathy should be admitted for further workup and adjustment of medications
- Patients with severe acute CHF decompensation should be admitted to an ICU
- Less sick patients should be admitted to a monitored floor
- Patients with mild exacerbations of CHF with good clinical response to ED therapy can be discharged with close follow-up
- Rule out causes of the exacerbation (e.g., MI, pneumonia, PE) prior to discharge

17. Infective Endocarditis

Etiology & Pathophysiology

- Infection of the heart valves or other endocardial surfaces
- Seeding of valves most commonly occurs during transient bacteremia
- Classified as acute or subacute depending on the speed of onset and severity of symptoms
- Most cases involve abnormal valves (e.g., prosthetic valves, myxomatous changes, rheumatic valves, MV prolapse, bicuspid aortic valve, internal cardiac devices)
- Other cases occur in patients with increased risk of bacteremia (e.g., IV drug use, elderly, diabetes, poor dentition, recent instrumentation)
- Infecting organisms include *Streptococcus viridans* (50%), *S. aureus* (20%), *Enterococcus* (10%), gram-negative bacilli, HACEK group, and fungi (*Candida, Aspergillus*)
- Left-sided disease is much more common (mitral > aortic > tricuspid > pulmonic)—IV drug abuse predisposes to right-sided endocarditis
- Consider the diagnosis in all patients with fever of unknown origin

Differential Dx

- Septicemia without endocardial involvement (e.g., line sepsis)
- Systemic vasculitis
- Rheumatologic disease
- Non-infectious endocarditis (Libman-Saks disease in SLE, marasmic endocarditis in terminal diseases)
- Acute valvular dysfunction of non-infectious etiology (e.g., papillary muscle rupture, ischemic mitral regurgitation)

Presentation

- Fever, malaise, sweats, myalgias, arthralgias, weight loss, back pain
- Heart murmur (new or changing)
- Vascular phenomena: Conjunctival petechiae, splinter hemorrhages, Janeway lesions (painless hemorrhages on palms and soles)
- Arterial emboli: Stroke, septic pulmonary infarcts, mycotic aneurysm, renal failure or infarct, splenic infarct or splenomegaly
- Immunologic phenomena: Osler's nodes (painful nodular lesions on digits), Roth's spots (pale retinal lesions with hemorrhage)
- Signs of CHF (valve rupture or insufficiency) and/or heart block

Diagnosis

- Workup should include blood cultures (2 sets), ECG, and echo
- Duke criteria: Endocarditis is diagnosed if 2 major *or* 1 major and 2 minor *or* 5 minor criteria are present
- Major criteria
  - Positive blood culture for typical organisms from 2 different blood cultures or persistently positive blood cultures for other organisms
  - Evidence of endocardial involvement: New valvular regurgitation, echocardiogram positive for vegetation or abscess, or new dehiscence of prosthetic valve
- Minor criteria: Predisposing heart condition or IV drug abuse, fever ≥38°C, vascular phenomena, immunologic phenomena, or positive blood culture or echo that does not meet major criteria
- Echocardiogram: Transthoracic is 80% sensitive, 98% specific (worse sensitivity in prosthetic valves); transesophageal increases sensitivity to >98% (findings include vegetations, perivalvular extension/abscess, valvular dehiscence)

Treatment

- In patients with suspected acute endocarditis, obtain three sets of blood cultures within 1 hr and begin empiric therapy
- In patients with subacute endocarditis, obtain three sets of cultures over 24 hours and then begin antimicrobial therapy
- Empiric therapy (all IV):
  - Native valve: Penicillin plus nafcillin plus gentamycin; or vancomycin plus gentamycin
  - Prosthetic valve: Vancomycin, gentamicin, and rifampin
- Adjust initial antibiotic choice according to culture and sensitivity of the organism; course is usually 2–4 weeks
- Indications for surgical therapy
  - CHF and hemodynamic instability due to valvular dysfunction
  - Paravalvular infection or abscess
  - Persistent bacteremia despite antimicrobial therapy
  - Fungal, gram-negative, *Brucella*, or *Enterococcus* disease
  - *S. aureus* infection of a prosthetic valve
  - Recurrent arterial emboli
  - Large vegetations

Disposition

- Overall 20% mortality (increased with gram negative and *S. aureus* infection)
- 40–60% mortality for endocarditis of prosthetic valves
- All patients with suspected infective endocarditis should be admitted for IV antibiotics
- Complications include valvular insufficiency with CHF, perivalvular abscess, conduction defects from extension of infection, septic CVA, mycotic cerebral aneurysm, acute MI from embolism of vegetation fragment, renal or splenic infarct/abscess

18. Pericardial Disease

Etiology & Pathophysiology

- Acute pericarditis: Inflammation of the pericardium due to viruses (e.g., coxsackievirus, echovirus, adenovirus, HIV), TB, bacteria, fungi, connective tissue disease (e.g., SLE, scleroderma, RA), malignancy (e.g., lymphoma, leukemia, lung cancer, breast cancer), post-MI (Dressler's syndrome), postpericardiotomy, uremia, hypothyroidism, medications (hydralazine, procainamide), idiopathic
- Pericardial effusion: Collection of fluid in the pericardial space
- Pericardial tamponade: Pericardial fluid collection resulting in compression of cardiac chambers and hemodynamic compromise (amount of fluid needed to cause tamponade is just 50 cc if accumulation is rapid; but the pericardium can accommodate >1 L of fluid if accumulation is slow)
  - Etiologies include acute pericarditis, hemopericardium (increased risk with anticoagulant use), penetrating or blunt trauma, myocardial rupture, aortic dissection, post-cardiac surgery

Differential Dx

- Acute coronary syndrome
- Aortic dissection
- Restrictive cardiomyopathy (e.g., amyloid)
- Valvular disease
- Dilated cardiomyopathy
- Hypertrophic cardiomyopathy
- Constrictive pericarditis
- Pleuritis
- Pulmonary embolism
- Costochondritis
- Pneumothorax
- Esophageal spasm
- GERD
- Herpes zoster

Presentation

- Acute pericarditis
  - Sharp, stabbing, pleuritic pain, radiating to scapula, neck, back
  - Relieved by leaning forward
  - Dyspnea, dysphagia, fever, cough
  - Pericardial friction rub on exam
- Pericardial tamponade
  - SOB, tachycardia, palpitations, presyncope, and/or syncope
  - Hypoxia, pulsus paradoxus, hypotension, JVD, and decreased heart sounds on exam
  - Signs of left (CHF) and/or right heart failure (lower extremity edema, hepatomegaly, ascites) may be present

Diagnosis

- Acute pericarditis
  - ECG shows progressive changes: ST elevation and PR depression in precordial leads; followed by an isoelectric ST segment with T-wave flattening; followed by T-wave inversion (especially in leads I, V5, and V6)
  - Echocardiogram will show pericardial effusion and thickening
  - Rule out other etiologies with CBC (infection or leukemia), BUN/Cr (uremia), ANA and RF (connective tissue disease), TSH, and cardiac enzymes (slight increase with myocarditis)
  - Diagnostic pericardiocentesis is usually unnecessary
- Pericardial effusion/tamponade
  - CXR may show cardiomegaly in chronic effusions
  - ECG: Low voltage +/− electrical alternans (variable QRS size)
  - Echocardiogram identifies the size of effusion and presence of tamponade (i.e., RA/RV collapse, variation of transvalvular blood flow with respiration, or paradoxical septal movement)
  - CT scan will diagnose pericardial effusion but not tamponade

Treatment

- Acute pericarditis therapy depends on etiology
  - Viral, idiopathic, post-MI, and post-pericardiotomy require only NSAIDs; use steroids for recurrent pain
  - TB, bacterial, and fungal disease require IV antibiotics
  - Uremic pericarditis requires urgent hemodialysis
  - Discontinue offending drug if drug-induced
  - Avoid anticoagulation in patients with acute pericarditis due to possible hemorrhage into the inflamed pericardium
- Pericardial tamponade
  - Administer IV fluids to increase preload and counteract cardiac compression
  - Emergent therapeutic pericardiocentesis should resolve symptoms instantly; a pigtail catheter may be left in place
  - Surgery to create a pericardial window may be necessary
  - Send pericardial fluid for analysis of protein, LDH, cytology, cell count and differential, gram stain, bacterial and fungal cultures, and acid-fast bacilli stain
- Pericardial effusion: In the absence of tamponade, treat the underlying disorder; pericardiocentesis may also be done

Disposition

- Acute pericarditis: Admit most patients to rule out conditions requiring specific therapy and watch for signs of pericardial tamponade (develops in 15% of cases)
- Pericardial tamponade: All patients should be admitted for at least 24 hours to ensure the effusion does not recur
- Pericardial effusion: Most patients with newly diagnosed effusions without tamponade should be admitted for further workup
- Constrictive pericarditis is due to fibrous thickening of the pericardium after an injury; presents with a pericardial knock, CHF, and impaired ventricular filling; treat with pericardiotomy

19. Acute Aortic Dissection

Etiology & Pathophysiology

- A tear of the aortic intima that extends into the media and longitudinally separates the two layers
- 60% of cases are Stanford type A (proximal) dissections of the ascending aorta (may also involve transverse or descending aorta); 30% are type B (distal) dissections that only involve the descending aorta
- Incidence increases with age—nearly 90% of patients are age >60
- Predisposing factors include HTN (most common etiology), atherosclerosis, aortic coarctation, bicuspid aortic valve, pregnancy, tertiary syphilis (i.e., syphilitic aortitis), blunt chest trauma, connective tissue disorder (e.g., Marfan's), cocaine abuse, iatrogenic insult (e.g., cardiac catheterization, cardiac surgery), male gender
- Dissection may extend into other large vessels resulting in CVA, mesenteric ischemia, pericardial hemorrhage, myocardial infarction, renal failure, acute aortic insufficiency, or paraplegia

Differential Dx

- Myocardial infarction
- GERD
- Esophageal spasm
- Acute pericarditis
- Pulmonary embolus
- Pneumothorax
- Cholecystitis
- Peptic ulcer disease
- Extremity arterial occlusion
- CVA

Presentation

- Acute onset of severe, tearing chest pain that radiates to the back (10% are painless)
- Cardiac/coronary involvement may ensue (aortic regurgitation murmur, CHF, heart block, MI)
- Hypertension (however, hypotension may occur if a proximal dissection penetrates into the pericardial sac, resulting in hemopericardium and tamponade)
- Tachycardia
- Decreased right subclavian and carotid pulses

Diagnosis

- Chest X-ray is 90% sensitive for dissection: May see widened mediastinum, blurred aortic knob, an aortic double density, deviation of the trachea to the right, elevation of the right mainstem bronchus and depression of the left bronchus, apical cap (indicating apical hemothorax), or pleural effusion
- ECG may show non-specific changes (e.g., LVH, ischemia) and is used to rule out MI
- Transesophageal echocardiogram, chest CT, and MRI are the imaging tests of choice, with sensitivity and specificity near 100% (in low suspicion patients, one negative test is enough; in high suspicion patients, 2 negative tests are required to rule out the diagnosis)
    - Transesophageal echocardiogram is especially useful in unstable patients and can be done at bedside
    - MRI is difficult to administer in critically ill patients
- Aortography was previously the gold standard, but is now used less frequently as its sensitivity is only 80%

Treatment

- Control blood pressure in hypertensive patients to decrease the shear forces on the aorta—goal is systolic BP <120 mmHg
    - Begin therapy with negative inotropes (e.g., β-blocker, Ca-channel blocker), then add a vasodilator if necessary (e.g., nitroprusside, nitroglycerin)
    - Administering vasodilators prior to negative inotropes may increase shear forces (via reflex tachycardia/inotropy in response to the vasodilation) and worsen the dissection
- Administer IV fluids to hypotensive patients with suspected tamponade
- Further treatment depends on the type of dissection
    - Type A dissection requires emergent surgical repair (mortality increases by 1%/hr during the first 48 hrs)
    - Type B dissection usually only requires medical treatment (i.e., observation in an ICU with aggressive BP control); however, surgical repair is warranted if it is complicated by continued pain, aneurysm rupture, cardiac ischemia, renal or gut ischemia, or neurological deficits

Disposition

- Ascending dissections have a much worse prognosis
- Mortality without therapy is 50% at 48 hours
- Admit all patients to an ICU
- All patients must have lifelong blood pressure control
- Postoperative complications (5–10%) include paraplegia, MI, renal insufficiency, mesenteric ischemia, and impotence

20. Hypertensive Crisis

Etiology & Pathophysiology

- Hypertensive crises are seen in both primary and secondary hypertensive disease
- Hypertensive urgency: Severe hypertension (usually diastolic >115) *without* acute complications of end-organ damage (however, organs are at increased risk of damage); goal of therapy is gradual blood pressure reduction over 24 hours
- Hypertensive emergency (includes the newer terms "malignant HTN" and "accelerated HTN"): Severe hypertension (diastolic >115–130) *with* evidence of end-organ damage (absolute BP is irrelevant—the presence of ongoing organ damage is enough to make the diagnosis); goal of therapy is to reduce blood pressure within 1 hour
- Brain, retina, kidney, heart, and great vessels are at highest risk for acute damage as the high blood pressure overwhelms local autoregulatory mechanisms

Differential Dx

- Non-compliance with antihypertensive medications
- CVA
- Intracerebral or subarachnoid hemorrhage
- Brain tumor
- Cocaine/amphetamine use
- Narcotic withdrawal
- Pheochromocytoma
- Spinal cord injury
- Renal failure
- Aortic dissection
- Anxiety/panic attack
- Pre-eclampsia/eclampsia
- Cushing's syndrome

Presentation

- Signs and symptoms are due to end-organ damage (hypertensive urgency, by definition, has no symptoms related to the HTN)
- CNS: Headache, confusion, coma, focal deficits, seizure, intracerebral or subarachnoid hemorrhage
- Retina: Papilledema, exudates, retinal hemorrhage
- Cardiac: Angina, MI, CHF, aortic dissection; exam may reveal a right ventricular heave, S_4, or a prominent apical impulse
- Renal: Proteinuria, hematuria, oliguria, renal failure
- GI: Nausea, vomiting

Diagnosis

- Differentiate hypertensive urgency from emergency by evaluating symptoms, exam findings, and laboratory testing to identify end-organ damage
- BUN/creatinine may be elevated and urinalysis may reveal hematuria or proteinuria in renal injury
- ECG may reveal LV hypertrophy with strain and/or ischemia
- CK, CK-MB, and troponin may be elevated in cardiac injury
- CXR may show pulmonary congestion and cardiomegaly
- CBC may be normal or show microangiopathic hemolytic anemia
- Head CT may reveal ischemic or hemorrhagic changes
- Chest CT or transesophageal echo may reveal aortic dissection
- Urine drug screen should be obtained in suspected cocaine/amphetamine use
- Consider initiating an evaluation for secondary causes of hypertensive disease (e.g., pheochromocytoma, renovascular disease, aortic coarctation, pre-eclampsia/eclampsia)

Treatment

- Hypertensive urgency: Oral agents are generally administered to decrease BP over 24 hrs (e.g., clonidine, hydralazine, ACE-inhibitor, β-blocker, Ca-channel blocker)
- Hypertensive emergency: Intravenous agents should be used to rapidly decrease the mean BP by 20% or diastolic BP to 110 within 1 hour; then gradually decrease the diastolic BP to 90–100 mmHg over 24 hours (cerebral hypoperfusion may occur with more intensive BP lowering)
  - Establish arterial line and consider central venous access
  - BP goals vary based on co-morbidities (e.g., HTN secondary to cerebral hemorrhage and baseline BP
  - Nitroprusside is an easily-titratable (fast-on, fast-off) arterial and venous vasodilator; side effects may include hypotension, elevated ICP, cyanide toxicity, and coronary steal with ischemia
  - Labetalol (α- and β-blocker) and esmolol (short-acting β-blocker) are other commonly used agents
  - Enalaprilat (ACE-inhibitor), nitroglycerin (venodilator), hydralazine (arterial vasodilator), nicardipine (Ca-channel blocker), and fenoldopam (dopa-1 agonist) are also used

Disposition

- Close observation is warranted as a rapid reduction of blood pressure may result in a relative *hypo*tension, resulting in further end-organ dysfunction (especially neurologic deterioration)
- Hypertensive urgency: Admit to a telemetry floor if serious co-morbid conditions are present or potential for decompensation exists; other patients may be discharged on oral therapy if follow-up can be arranged within 24 hours
- Hypertensive emergency: Admit to ICU

21. Venous Thrombosis

Etiology & Pathophysiology

- Superficial venous thrombosis involves the superficial veins of upper or lower extremities (cephalic veins, basilic veins)
- Deep venous thrombosis (DVT) involves deep veins
- Virchow's triad describes the factors that predispose to thrombus formation—vascular damage, stasis, and hypercoagulability
  - Vascular damage: Surgery (especially orthopedic, thoracic, abdominal, and GU surgery), trauma (e.g., large bone fractures), indwelling central venous catheter
  - Stasis: Immobilization (e.g., travel, post-surgery), edema (e.g., CHF)
  - Hypercoagulability: Pregnancy, malignancy (e.g., pancreas, lung, breast), hypercoagulable states (e.g., estrogen use, factor V Leiden mutation antiphospholipid antibodies, protein C or S deficiency)

Differential Dx

- Cellulitis
- Muscle trauma/hemorrhage
- Ruptured popliteal cyst
- Lymphedema
- Arthritis, tendonitis
- Postphlebitic syndrome (swelling due to destruction of venous valves by a previous DVT—occurs after 60% of DVTs)
- CHF
- Nephrotic syndrome
- Cirrhosis
- Hypoalbuminemia

Presentation

- Superficial venous thrombosis: Swelling, erythema, and warmth localized to the site of thrombus; a tender cord may be palpated
- DVT
  - May be asymptomatic
  - Unilateral extremity edema, erythema, warmth, tenderness
  - Prominent venous collaterals
  - Phlegmasia cerulea dolens (cyanotic extremity due to deoxygenation of stagnant blood)
  - Phlegmasia alba dolens (pale extremity due to elevated interstitial tissue pressure)

Diagnosis

- Superficial venous thrombosis: Physical exam is usually sufficient for diagnosis; further studies may be used to rule out a DVT
- Deep venous thrombosis
  - Physical exam is insensitive
  - Duplex venous ultrasonography has high sensitivity/specificity for proximal veins but is less sensitive for DVT of calf veins (in patients with symptoms of DVT but negative ultrasound results, a repeat ultrasound should be done in 5–7 days)
  - ELISA D-dimer is 80% sensitive but nonspecific for DVT; not sufficient as a sole test to rule out DVT
  - MRI is used to evaluate for thrombosis of the SVC, IVC, and pelvic veins
  - Contrast venography is seldom used because it is invasive
  - Consider hypercoagulable workup in patients without obvious inciting events or risk factors

Treatment

- Superficial venous thrombosis
  - Extremity elevation, warm compresses, NSAIDs for pain
  - Consider anticoagulation if thrombosis is near deep veins
- Deep venous thrombosis—systemic anticoagulation is required to prevent clot extension or pulmonary embolism
  - Begin IV unfractionated heparin or SQ low-molecular-weight heparin
  - Warfarin may be started concurrently with heparin
  - Stop heparin 48 hours after INR reaches 2.0 (warfarin causes a transient hypercoagulable state so patients are not anticoagulated until 48 hours after the INR is therapeutic)
  - Continue warfarin for 3–6 months after a DVT with an identified cause or a first idiopathic DVT
  - Indefinite warfarin may be needed for recurrent idiopathic DVTs or if risk factors persist (e.g., hypercoagulability)
  - Inferior vena cava filter may be inserted to prevent PE; indications include contraindication to anticoagulation, failure of therapy (i.e., PE occurred while on anticoagulants), and severely compromised baseline pulmonary status

Disposition

- Superficial venous thrombosis is common and often self-limiting
- Discharge home with timely outpatient follow-up to make sure the thrombosis is not propagating
- DVT warrants admission for IV heparin therapy if significant co-morbidities exist, patient is unable to ambulate, has poor follow-up, or is unable to understand therapy
- Remainder of patients with uncomplicated DVTs can be started on SQ low-molecular-weight heparin and warfarin and discharged home with close follow-up
- Isolated calf DVT carries no risk of PE; thus, anticoagulation is not needed (recheck ultrasound in 5–7 days to detect propagation of DVT, which would require anticoagulation)

22. Syncope

Etiology & Pathophysiology

- A brief loss of consciousness and postural tone with spontaneous recovery due to decreased cerebral blood flow
- No cause is identified in nearly half of cases
- Orthostatic syncope (due to decreased relative intravascular volume): Due to drugs (e.g., antihypertensives), alcohol, hypovolemia, or autonomic dysfunction (e.g., diabetes)
- Reflex-mediated syncope
    - Vasovagal: Stress (e.g., pain, emotional upset) → strong ventricular contraction with stretching of LV mechanoreceptors → increased parasympathetic tone (vasodilatation, bradycardia) → syncope
    - Hypersensitive peripheral receptors: Carotid sinus-, cough-, micturition-, swallow-, or postprandial-induced syncope
- Cardiac syncope: Due to arrhythmia or decreased output (e.g., MI, valve disease, PE, cardiac hypertrophy, long QT, dissection)
- Neurologic syncope: Due to subclavian steal, migraine, seizure, CVA

Differential Dx

- Seizure
- Hypoglycemia
- Hyperventilation
- Vertigo
- Anxiety/panic attack

Presentation

- Loss of consciousness lasting seconds to minutes
- Prodromal symptoms are often present (e.g., lightheadedness, dizziness, nausea, weakness, vision changes, pallor, diaphoresis)
- Incontinence and brief clonic movements may occasionally occur
- Mental status is at baseline following the syncopal episode
- Symptoms due to specific etiologies may be present (e.g., palpitations, slow heart rate, headache, murmurs, carotid bruit)
- Syncope without prodrome or with associated trauma suggests a cardiac etiology

Diagnosis

- ECG should be evaluated in all patients (note any prolongation of the QT interval, arrhythmias, or acute ischemia patterns)
- Cardiac enzymes if ECG and history suggest ischemia
- β-hCG in all female patients to rule out ectopic pregnancy
- CBC and electrolytes are rarely useful
- Head CT is required only if focal neurologic deficits are present
- Holter monitor or event recorder may be used as an outpatient for recurrent syncope of unknown etiology
- Further inpatient tests may include echocardiogram (to diagnose structural abnormalities), electrophysiology studies (to diagnose arrhythmias), or a tilt table test (provides evidence of neural-mediated syncope)
- Red flags of serious underlying cardiac cause include syncope while supine, cardiac symptoms, old age, incontinence, prolonged LOC, tongue biting, trauma following the syncope (signifies lack of warning), headache or focal neurologic symptoms, or absence of prodromal symptoms

Treatment

- Hypovolemic states should be treated with IV fluids and blood, if necessary
- Treat any cardiac arrhythmias per established protocols
- Patients with orthostatic and reflex-mediated syncope should avoid the precipitating factors and may benefit from pharmacologic therapy, including β-blockers, SSRIs, midodrine, and fludrocortisone
- Other therapies are directed at specific identified causes of the syncope (e.g., heparin for pulmonary embolus)

Disposition

- Patients with cardiac syncope have a high mortality if specific treatment is not instituted
- Discharge patients with typical orthostatic or reflex-mediated syncope in whom the precipitating factor was identified and no cardiovascular disease or risk factors are present
- Admit patients with identified cardiac syncope, red flags for cardiac syncope, or history of CHF, ventricular arrhythmia, chest pain, valvular disease, or ischemia/arrhythmia on ECG
- Consider admission in patients >60, history of CAD, first episode of syncope with unknown cause, family history of sudden death, or in young patients with exertional syncope

Pulmonary Emergencies

DAVE SALOUM, MD

23. Dyspnea

Etiology & Pathophysiology

- Subjective sensation of difficulty breathing
- Caused by a variety of pathophysiologic mechanisms that cause a disparity between work of breathing and oxygen demand
- Majority of cases are of pulmonary or cardiac etiology
- Respiratory drive is controlled by areas of the cerebral cortex and medulla, with feedback from central and peripheral chemoreceptors
  - Central chemoreceptors respond primarily to increased levels of $PaCO_2$
  - Peripheral chemoreceptors (in the carotid bodies) respond primarily to decreased levels in PaO_2

Differential Dx

- Airway: Mass, foreign body
- Lung: Asthma, COPD, edema, bronchitis, pneumonia, interstitial disease, pleural effusion, pneumothorax
- Cardiac: CHF, MI, pericarditis, tamponade, arrhythmia, valve disease, cardiomyopathy
- Vascular: Pulmonary embolus, pulmonary HTN, vasculitis
- Neuromuscular: Guillain-Barré, myasthenia gravis, myopathy
- Other: Anemia, acidosis, sepsis, pregnancy, carbon monoxide, fever, obesity, trauma, ascites

Presentation

- Presentation varies with the underlying cause
- Tachypnea
- Tachycardia
- Accessory muscle use
- Abnormal or decreased breath sounds, wheezing, or crackles
- Inability to speak in full sentences
- Skin may appear pale or cyanotic
- Stridor (upper airway obstruction)
- Chest pain if PE, MI, trauma, or pneumothorax are present
- Fever may indicate infection
- Mental status changes may indicate hypoxia
- Cardiac murmur, orthopnea, PND may indicate CHF

Diagnosis

- Thorough history and physical exam to limit the differential
- Pulse oximetry may reveal hypoxemia
- Peak expiratory flow rate to measure airway obstruction
- Arterial blood gas may reveal hypoxemia and respiratory alkalosis (decreased pCO_2)
  - Calculate A-a gradient: $(713 \times F_{IO_2}) - (PaCO_2 \times 1.25) - PaO_2$ (normal gradient should approach age/10 + 10 on room air)
  - Respiratory acidosis (increased pCO_2) in a tachypneic patient may indicate impending respiratory failure
- CXR may show evidence of causative disease (e.g., vascular congestion in CHF, consolidation in pneumonia)
- Chest CT will identify intrinsic lung disease and may rule out pulmonary embolus
- ECG and echocardiogram may be used to exclude cardiac etiologies
- CBC, electrolytes, BUN/creatinine, and LFTs are usually ordered

Treatment

- Goal of therapy is to provide adequate oxygenation and ventilation with PaO_2 >60 mmHg and appropriate pCO_2
- Administer supplemental O_2
- Airway interventions
  - Noninvasive positive pressure ventilation (CPAP or BiPAP) may prevent the need for intubation in some patients, especially those with COPD or CHF
  - Endotracheal intubation and mechanical ventilation may be necessary if other measures fail
- Treat the underlying cause
  - Bronchodilators and steroids for asthma or COPD
  - Antibiotics for pneumonia and other infections
  - Steroids, epinephrine, and H_1/H_2 blockers for anaphylaxis
  - Nitroglycerin and loop diuretics for CHF or pulmonary edema
  - Tube thoracostomy for pneumothorax
  - Aspirin, nitroglycerin, β-blockade, or cardioversion for cardiac disease
  - Anxiolytics for psychogenic causes

Disposition

- Disposition depends on underlying cause (admission may be required to treat co-morbid conditions)
- Admit patients who are hypoxemic, appear to be tiring, or require mechanical ventilation

24. Acute Respiratory Failure

Etiology & Pathophysiology

- Failure of either oxygenation (PaO_2 <60 mmHg despite supplemental O_2) or ventilation (acute elevation of $PaCO_2$ >50 mmHg)
- Failure of oxygenation
  - Due to poor gas exchange [e.g., ventilation-perfusion (V/Q) mismatch, impaired diffusion capacity, carbon monoxide]
  - Most commonly caused by cardiac disease, pulmonary embolus, or intrinsic lung pathology
- Failure of ventilation
  - Due to inadequate minute ventilation or severe V/Q mismatch
  - Causes include respiratory muscle fatigue/weakness, abnormal neurologic control of respiration, pleural space disease, or chest wall injury

Differential Dx

- CNS: CVA, bleed, spinal trauma, encephalopathy
- Neuromuscular: Guillain-Barré, myositis, myasthenia gravis
- Cardiovascular: CHF, PE, valve disease, cardiomyopathy
- Pulmonary: Asthma, COPD, ARDS, pneumonia, pleural effusion, pneumothorax, inhalation injury
- Toxins: Drug abuse, CNS depressants (e.g., opiate overdose), organophosphates
- Sepsis
- Trauma

Presentation

- Dyspnea
- Tachypnea, bradypnea, or apnea
- Abnormal breathing patterns (e.g., Cheyne-Stokes)
- Inability to speak in full sentences
- Cyanosis
- Accessory muscle use
- Thoracoabdominal paradox
- Diaphoresis
- Hypertension
- Altered mental status due to hypoxia or hypercarbia
- Abnormal lung findings may include wheezing, rhonchi, rales, decreased air movement, decreased breath sounds

Diagnosis

- Pulse oximetry may reveal hypoxemia—saturation <92% is associated with pO_2 of <60 mmHg
- Arterial blood gas
  - Will show hypoxemia
  - May show either low pCO_2 due to tachypnea or elevated pCO_2 due to inadequate minute ventilation
  - Serial ABGs should be used to monitor respiratory status and response to therapy; however, changes may occur late and clinical judgment should guide management decisions
- CXR may reveal the underlying cause of the respiratory failure (e.g., pulmonary vascular congestion, pneumothorax, pleural effusion, or infiltrate)
- Chest CT or V/Q scan may be necessary to rule out pulmonary embolus
- EKG may show the presence of cardiac ischemia

Treatment

- Supplemental O_2 (a non-rebreather face mask will deliver the highest oxygen concentrations)
- Noninvasive positive pressure ventilation (CPAP or BiPAP) may prevent the need for intubation in some patients, especially those with COPD or CHF
- Endotracheal intubation and mechanical ventilation may be necessary if other measures fail
  - Rapid sequence intubation (RSI) is a safe procedure with high success rate and minimal complications
  - Orotracheal intubation is most common
  - Blind nasotracheal intubation may be useful when oral access is limited, but is associated with a higher complication rate and a lower success rate than orotracheal intubation
- Surgical airway (e.g., cricothyroidotomy, tracheostomy) may be necessary if other airway management attempts fail
- Once the airway is controlled, administer specific therapy to address the underlying cause of the respiratory failure

Disposition

- Admit all patients with acute respiratory failure to an ICU
- Outcomes depend on the underlying pathology and co-morbid conditions
- Rapid restoration of adequate oxygenation may prevent complications
- Labwork should not replace clinical judgment regarding management and need for intubation

25. Acute Pulmonary Edema

Etiology & Pathophysiology

- Leakage of fluid from the pulmonary capillaries into the pulmonary interstitium and alveolar air spaces
- Due to elevated hydrostatic pressure in pulmonary capillaries (cardiogenic pulmonary edema) or abnormal pulmonary capillary permeability (non-cardiogenic pulmonary edema)
    - Cardiogenic pulmonary edema may be caused by myocardial ischemia/infarction, valvular disease (e.g., aortic stenosis), cardiomyopathies, pericardial effusion, pericarditis, high output states (e.g., beriberi, thyrotoxicosis), volume overload, or hypertensive emergencies
    - Non-cardiogenic pulmonary edema may be caused by sepsis, inhalation injuries, drugs (e.g., opioids, salicylates, tocolytics), renal failure, high altitude, aspiration, seizure, trauma, CNS injury, airway obstructions (e.g., croup, foreign body), lung re-expansion

Differential Dx

- COPD
- Asthma
- Pneumonia
- ARDS
- Pulmonary embolism
- Myocardial ischemia/infarction
- Pericardial tamponade
- Restrictive lung disease

Presentation

- Dyspnea
- Weakness
- Anxiety
- Diaphoresis
- Cyanosis
- Tachypnea
- Tachycardia
- Accessory muscle use
- Crackles
- Wheezing
- Cardiogenic causes may result in cough (may be productive of frothy pink sputum), jugular venous distension, peripheral edema, and cardiac murmur or rub

Diagnosis

- Pulse oximetry may reveal hypoxemia
- CXR is generally the first test ordered
    - Mild congestion may result in cephalization of pulmonary vessels, pleural effusion, and azygous vein enlargement
    - As congestion worsens, interstitial edema, loss of distinct vascular margins, alveolar infiltrates, and Kerley B lines (short linear markings in lung periphery) will appear
    - Congestion is usually perihilar in cardiac-induced cases
    - Enlarged cardiac silhouette may be present in chronic CHF
- ABG may reveal hypoxemia and respiratory alkalosis (low pCO_2) due to tachypnea (respiratory acidosis is an ominous sign of tiring and impending respiratory failure)
- ECG may show signs of ventricular hypertrophy, atrial enlargement, conduction abnormalities, or ischemia/infarction
- Serum B-type natriuretic peptide (BNP) helps differentiate cardiac pulmonary edema from non-cardiac pulmonary edema

Treatment

- Administer supplemental O_2
- Positive pressure ventilation for patients who remain hypoxemic or hypercarbic despite supplemental oxygen
    - Non-invasive means include continuous positive airway pressure (CPAP) or bilevel positive airway pressure (BiPAP)—these may decrease the need for intubation
    - Endotracheal intubation for those with respiratory failure
- Cardiogenic edema requires medical therapy
    - Vasodilators (e.g., IV nitroglycerin or nesiritide) decrease hydrostatic pressure by venodilation
    - Loop diuretics (e.g., IV furosemide) decrease afterload by volume reduction and also cause venodilation
    - Morphine decreases the subjective sensation of dyspnea and causes venodilation
    - Inotropes decrease congestion by improving cardiac output (dopamine for hypotensive patients, dobutamine for normotensive patients)
- Non-cardiogenic edema generally requires only supportive care (diuretics are minimally helpful and steroids have no benefit)

Disposition

- Discharge is acceptable in patients with known CHF who have complete resolution of mild pulmonary edema, normal O_2 saturation levels without supplemental oxygen, and no new ECG changes
- Patients with first time episodes, new ECG changes, or symptoms resistant to treatment should be admitted
- Patients with severe disease and/or those who require mechanical ventilation should be admitted to an ICU

26. Asthma

Etiology & Pathophysiology

- Chronic airway inflammation, characterized by bronchial hyperreactivity and reversible airway obstruction
- Acute exacerbations may occur due to environmental triggers, exercise, infection, temperature, or medication noncompliance
- Status asthmaticus is a life-threatening attack that is unresponsive to initial therapy
- Immunologic reaction (allergic/extrinsic asthma) begins with mast cell activation and release of histamines, leukotrienes, prostaglandins, and thromboxane A_2 and progresses to bronchoconstriction, inflammation, and mucus production by eosinophils, neutrophils, and mononuclear cells
- Non-immunologic (intrinsic asthma) reactions result in bronchoconstriction without inducing the above immunologic cascade (e.g., exercise, cold, respiratory infections, air pollutants, and drugs)

Differential Dx

- Pneumonia
- Pulmonary embolism
- COPD exacerbation
- Bronchitis
- Bronchiolitis
- Pneumothorax
- Hypersensitivity pneumonitis
- CHF
- Allergic reaction/angioedema
- Vocal cord dyskinesia
- Carcinoid tumor
- Foreign body
- Anxiety attack

Presentation

- Classic triad of cough, dyspnea, and wheezing
- Chest tightness
- Diaphoresis
- Tachypnea, tachycardia
- Accessory muscle use, nasal flaring
- Wheezing may be absent in cases of severe obstruction (due to insufficient air movement)
- Severe acute exacerbations present with inability to speak in full sentences, decreased air movement, hyperinflation (increased AP diameter of thorax), altered mental status (due to hypoxia), and pulsus paradoxus (fall in systolic BP by 10 mmHg during inspiration)

Diagnosis

- Pulmonary function tests are the best measure of airway obstruction (peak flow meters are used in the ED)
    - Perform at baseline and before and after each treatment
    - In young adults, peak flow 400–600 is normal, 100–300 indicates a moderate exacerbation, <100 a severe exacerbation
- Continuous pO_2 monitoring via pulse oximetry
- Chest X-ray
    - Required in new onset asthma, febrile patients, patients unresponsive to treatment, or those with a suspicion of pneumonia or other lung pathology
    - May show hyperinflation and atelectasis from mucus plugging
- ABG is indicated in moderate to severe exacerbations
    - May show hypoxia and respiratory alkalosis (decreased pCO_2)
    - Normal or elevated pCO_2 levels indicate severe obstruction or respiratory fatigue with impending respiratory failure
- CBC should be evaluated if pneumonia is suspected (note that steroid use may increase the WBC count in absence of infection)

Treatment

- Administer supplemental O_2
- Airway interventions may include noninvasive positive pressure ventilation or endotracheal intubation
- Bronchodilator therapy via nebulizer or inhaler
    - Short-acting β-agonists (e.g., albuterol)
    - Inhaled anticholinergics (e.g., ipratropium)
- Steroids are a mainstay of treatment but effect is not seen for 2–6 hours
    - Mild exacerbations are usually managed with a short course of oral steroids
    - Moderate to severe exacerbations are generally treated with IV steroids; however, oral steroids are reportedly as effective as IV
- Magnesium sulfate is used in children with moderate to severe disease (shown to decrease need for intubation)
- Heliox (helium-oxygen mixture) is used in moderate to severe cases (may also decrease need for intubation)
- Epinephrine or terbutaline injections in the critically ill
- Leukotriene modifiers, cromolyn, and methylxanthines are not used in acute exacerbations due to slow onset

Disposition

- Disposition depends on history, response to therapy, and access to medical care
- Discharge patients who have a good response to treatment (peak flow ≥70% of predicted or personal best) and reliable follow-up (discharged patients require a 5–7 day course of oral steroids)
- Continue to monitor and reassess patients with peak flow greater than 40% but below 70%
- Admit patients with peak flow <40% at 4 hours (other considerations for admission include significant tachycardia, history of frequent admissions or prior intubations, and concurrent pneumonia)
- Admit patients with mental status changes, respiratory arrest, intubation, hypercapnia, or arrhythmias to an ICU

27. COPD Exacerbation

Etiology & Pathophysiology

- Progressive, irreversible airway destruction characterized by varying degrees of chronic bronchitis and emphysema
  - Emphysema involves destruction of alveolar walls with bronchial collapse, loss of elastic recoil, and hyperinflation
  - Chronic bronchitis involves endobronchial inflammation with secretion buildup (due to increased production and decreased mucociliary removal)
  - Airway edema and bronchospasm also contribute to obstruction
  - Patients may also have concurrent bronchiectasis and/or asthma
- Reduction of total minute volume and increased work of respiration (due to airway resistance and ventilation/perfusion mismatching) result in alveolar hypoventilation, hypoxemia, and hypercapnia
- Acute exacerbations may be idiopathic, infectious, or environmental in nature and often present with significant respiratory distress
- Cigarette smoking is the major cause of the disease

Differential Dx

- CHF
- Acute coronary syndrome
- Asthma
- Acute bronchitis
- Pneumonia
- Bronchiectasis
- Pulmonary embolism
- Pneumothorax
- Restrictive lung disease

Presentation

- Dyspnea (with exertion or at rest)
- Tachypnea
- Wheezing
- Pursed lip breathing
- Accessory muscle use
- Fever may be present with concurrent pneumonia or bronchitis
- Cyanosis
- Productive cough
- Poor air movement
- Hypoxia presents as tachypnea, tachycardia, cyanosis, and agitation
- Hypercapnia presents as confusion, tremor, and decreased respirations

Diagnosis

- Pulse oximetry reveals hypoxemia (COPD patients may be chronically hypoxic with baseline saturation below 90%)
- Arterial blood gas
  - Hypoxemia may be the only abnormality in early stages
  - Respiratory alkalosis (due to hyperventilation) or respiratory acidosis (insufficient ventilation to exhale CO_2) may occur
  - Even at baseline, pCO_2 may be elevated and pO_2 decreased
  - Progressive worsening of pCO_2 or pO_2 requires intubation
- CXR: Chronic changes include hyperinflation, hyperlucency of lung fields, bullae, increased AP diameter, flattened diaphragm, and small heart (may also show concurrent pneumonia)
- Serum BNP (elevated in CHF but normal in COPD), cardiac enzymes, electrolytes, and theophylline level
- ECG is used to rule out coronary ischemia; COPD patients may have low QRS voltage, RV strain, and RV hypertrophy

Treatment

- Supplemental O_2 is always indicated
  - Titrate to PaO_2 >60 mmHg (SaO_2 >90%)
  - Increasing FiO_2 may slightly increase $PaCO_2$ due to increased dead space (V/Q mismatch) and transient depression of respiratory drive
- Inhaled bronchodilators should be used immediately (anticholinergics are more effective than β-agonists, but the best bronchodilation is achieved by combining both agents)
- Systemic corticosteroids may be beneficial in some patients
- Antibiotics (e.g., azithromycin, doxycycline) should be administered, particularly in severe exacerbations
- Methylxanthines (e.g., theophylline) are not beneficial in acute attacks
- Ventilatory assistance may be necessary
  - Non-invasive mechanical ventilation via CPAP (continuous positive airway pressure) or BiPAP (bilevel positive airway pressure) may avoid the need for intubation
  - Orotracheal intubation for cases of respiratory failure

Disposition

- All patients should be strongly considered for admission, especially those with severe exacerbations, failed outpatient management, existing co-morbid disease, or inability to accomplish activities of daily living
- ICU admission is necessary for intubated patients or those with progressively worsening respiratory function, mental status changes, or poor response to initial ED therapy
- Discharge may be acceptable in patients with good response to ED therapy, access to home oxygen and bronchodilators, and close follow-up
- Smoking cessation is essential

28. Pneumonia

Etiology & Pathophysiology

- Infection of lung parenchyma, resulting in inflammation, alveolar exudates, and consolidation
- May be community-acquired, hospital-acquired (i.e., due to residence in any healthcare facility or nursing home in the preceding 10–14 days), or due to aspiration
- The most common community-acquired organisms are *Streptococcus pneumoniae, Haemophilus influenzae,* and *Mycoplasma pneumoniae;* other causative organisms include *Chlamydia pneumoniae, Moraxella catarrhalis, N gonorrhea, Klebsiella, Legionella, S aureus,* and viruses (e.g., influenza, parainfluenza)
- Gram negative rods and anaerobes are more common in hospital-acquired pneumonia
- Fungi and anaerobes are less common causes
- Altered level of consciousness (e.g., intoxication, stroke, seizure, anesthesia) predisposes to aspiration pneumonia

Differential Dx

- CHF
- Bronchitis
- COPD
- Asthma
- Lung cancer
- Pulmonary embolism
- Vasculitis
- Foreign body aspiration

Presentation

- Fever
- Dyspnea
- Tachypnea
- Cough (with or without sputum)
- Tachycardia
- Increased work of breathing
- Pleuritic chest pain in some
- Constitutional symptoms may include rigors, diaphoresis, fatigue, and malaise
- Pulmonary exam findings include decreased breath sounds, rhonchi, dullness to percussion, and egophony
- Mental status changes may be the only symptom in elderly patients

Diagnosis

- Pulse oximetry often reveals hypoxemia
- Chest X-ray may show opacities with air bronchograms
    - May see dense, lobar, fluffy, patchy, or diffuse infiltrates
    - There may be an associated pleural effusion
    - Findings are not specific for the specific causative organism
- CBC will often show leukocytosis
- Sputum cultures and sputum gram stain are rarely helpful in identifying the organism but are recommended in published guidelines
- Blood cultures are positive in only 10% of patients and the results rarely alter patient management; however, they are recommended in published guidelines for all hospitalized patients
- Legionella urinary antigen
- Serologies for *Legionella, Mycoplasma,* and *Chlamydia* have poor sensitivity and specificity

Treatment

- Administer supplemental O_2
- Isolation is necessary if there is a clinical suspicion for TB
- Community-acquired pneumonia
    - Outpatient meds: Macrolide, doxycycline, or a quinolone
    - Inpatients without complications: Either a 3rd generation cephalosporin plus a macrolide or single agent therapy with a 2nd generation quinolone (e.g., levofloxacin)
    - ICU patients: Macrolide or quinolone plus either a cephalosporin or β-lactam/β-lactamase inhibitor
    - Aspiration pneumonia: 2nd generation quinolone plus either clindamycin or a β-lactam/β-lactamase inhibitor
    - Patients with underlying structural lung disease should receive an anti-pseudomonal penicillin or cephalosporin plus an anti-pseudomonal quinolone
- Hospital-acquired pneumonia is generally treated with a 3rd generation cephalosporin plus clindamycin or with a β-lactam/β-lactamase inhibitor; severe cases require coverage for pseudomonas and MRSA
- Patients with known or suspected HIV infection should have antibiotic coverage for *Pneumocystis carinii*

Disposition

- Discharge patients who are not toxic-appearing, are well oxygenated, and are without co-morbid conditions
- Admission is necessary for patients who are hypoxemic, toxic-appearing, hemodynamically unstable, have co-morbid conditions, or fail outpatient therapy
- Pneumonia severity index (PSI) is a scoring system used to determine the risk of mortality and need for admission
    - Risk class I (age <50 and absence of co-morbidities): Discharge
    - Risk classes II–V use a point system based on age, sex, coexisting disease, and abnormal vitals, exam, or labs
    - Class II (mortality <1%): Discharge
    - Class III: Discharge or short admit
    - Class IV (mortality 9%): Hospitalize
    - Class V (mortality 30%): Hospitalize

29. Tuberculosis

Etiology & Pathophysiology

- Caused by *Mycobacterium tuberculosis,* an acid-fast, aerobic, non-spore forming rod that does not produce endo- or exotoxin
- Other rare causes include *M bovis* and *M Africanum*
- Transmission is via respiratory droplets containing the bacterium
- Bacilli can remain airborne for prolonged periods
- Replicates within alveolar macrophages following phagocytosis
- CD8 suppressor T-cells kill infected macrophages and destroy local tissue, resulting in formation of caseating necrotic granulomas
- 1° TB: Asymptomatic or self-limited illness causing latent disease
- Active TB: Clinical symptoms plus positive sputum or chest X-ray
- Latent TB: Positive PPD but no clinical, CXR, or culture proof of active infection; active disease may occur when immune system is weakened
- Disseminated TB: Systemic spread of bacilli due to inadequate host defense mechanisms (e.g., HIV or other immunocompromised states)

Differential Dx

- Bacterial pneumonia
- Fungal infection (e.g., *Histoplasma, Coccidioides*)
- Non-tuberculous mycobacteria (e.g., *M kansasii, M avium* complex)
- Lymphoma
- Sarcoidosis
- HIV
- Bronchogenic carcinoma
- Vasculitis (e.g., Wegener's granulomatosis)
- Silicosis

Presentation

- 1° TB is often asymptomatic but may be associated with mild fever and malaise
- 2° (active) TB presents with anorexia, weakness, fever/chills, night sweats, malaise, fatigue, weight loss, headache, and cough
- As the disease progresses, symptoms may include productive cough, pleuritic chest pain, dyspnea, and hemoptysis
- Complications of disease include pneumothorax, empyema, pericarditis, massive hemoptysis
- Extrapulmonary organ involvement may occur

Diagnosis

- PPD (purified protein derivative) skin test is a screening test that is read 48–72 hours after injection; thus, application is limited in ED
  - Exposure to TB will cause induration at injection site (erythema alone is not considered positive)
  - Previous BCG vaccine may cause a false positive PPD; however, the vaccine is considered unreliable, so BCG recipients should be treated as if the PPD is a true positive
  - Patients who are HIV-positive or immunocompromised may be anergic; therefore they require less induration for a positive result
- Sputum analysis may reveal acid-fast bacilli; cultures grow very slowly and have limited sensitivity
- CXR may show hilar or mediastinal adenopathy in 1° disease
  - 2° disease classically causes lesions (may be cavitary) in the upper lobes
  - Miliary disease causes small nodules throughout lungs

Treatment

- Four-drug regimen (at least) should be initiated in patients with active TB until drug susceptibility tests return
  - Begin therapy with isoniazid, rifampin, pyrazinamide, and either streptomycin or ethambutol
  - Treatment should continue for at least 6 months
  - Non-compliance with medication regimens is common and contributes to multi-drug resistant TB (MDRTB); directly observed therapy should be strongly considered in potentially unreliable patients
- Preventive therapy with isoniazid should be initiated in anyone in close contact to patients with active disease, recent PPD converters (i.e., patients with latent disease), and in anergic individuals with known TB contacts
  - 6 months for adults
  - 9 months for children
  - 12 months for immunocompromised
- Surgical resection has high cure rates for patients with multi-drug resistant TB and localized disease

Disposition

- 10–15% of latent disease eventually becomes active; treatment cures >95%
- Most patients are treated as outpatients
- Hospitalization should be considered for patients who are acutely ill, MDRTB, elderly, homeless, substance abusers, or patients with children at home
- Adequate follow-up and access to health resources, along with clear instructions on home isolation procedures and drug regimens must be ensured before discharge
- Patients are considered contagious for at least 2 weeks after starting therapy
- Close contacts should be screened for active disease, and, if negative, placed on preventative treatment
- All cases of active TB must be reported to the health department

30. Pneumothorax

Etiology & Pathophysiology

- Free air in the intrapleural space
- May occur spontaneously or following trauma or iatrogenic causes
- Primary spontaneous PTX is not associated with an underlying lung disease (usually caused by rupture of an apical pleural bleb); more common in young, thin, healthy men and smokers
- Secondary spontaneous PTX is associated with other pathology, such as COPD, infection, or neoplasm
- Traumatic PTX is caused by penetrating or blunt chest trauma
- May be classified as simple (closed), communicating (pleural space communicates with atmosphere), and tension (intrathoracic pressure increases, resulting in lung collapse, mediastinal shift, and impeded cardiac venous return)
- Risk factors include trauma, smoking, changes in atmospheric pressure, and genetic predispositions (e.g., Marfan's syndrome, α_1-antitrypsin deficiency)

Differential Dx

- Pneumonia
- Pulmonary embolus
- COPD exacerbation
- Asthma exacerbation
- Pleuritis
- Myocardial infarction
- Pericarditis
- Aortic dissection
- Rib fracture
- Muscle strain
- Diaphragmatic hernia
- Subphrenic abscess
- Acute abdomen (e.g., cholecystitis, perforated ulcer)

Presentation

- Chest pain (sudden, pleuritic pain localized to the affected side)
- Dyspnea and tachypnea
- Cough is present in some patients
- Tachycardia
- Decreased breath sounds, decreased tactile fremitus, hyperresonance to percussion on affected side
- Respiratory distress or failure may occur, especially in patients with underlying lung disease
- Tension PTX: Hypotension, absent breath sounds, JVD, tracheal deviation (towards the unaffected side), diaphoresis, cyanosis, cardiovascular collapse

Diagnosis

- PTX should be strongly suspected in trauma patients and in symptomatic patients with known lung disease
- Chest X-ray often suggests the diagnosis
  – Presence of a thin radiolucent pleural line
  – Absence of vascular lung marking peripheral to the radiolucent line
  – Upright position and expiration may help visualize the PTX
  – Lateral decubitus chest X-ray with affected side up may also aid in visualization
- Chest CT is very sensitive and may detect very small PTXs not seen on chest X-ray
- ABG may reveal hypoxemia due to V/Q mismatching
- Tension PTX is a clinical diagnosis and a true emergency—must be treated immediately; diagnosis is confirmed by hemodynamic improvement and a rush of air following needle decompression or chest tube insertion

Treatment

- Supplemental O_2 administration accelerates reabsorption of intrapleural air (natural reabsorption rate is ~1.25% of volume per day but this rate can be increased fourfold with the administration of 100% O_2)
- Treatment options include observation without therapy, catheter aspiration, and insertion of chest tube
- Primary spontaneous PTX
  – Observation with repeat CXR is acceptable for patients with <15% collapse and minimal symptoms
  – Catheter aspiration may be attempted in patients with 15–30% collapse or expanding PTX; chest tube should be inserted if unsuccessful
  – Chest tube is required for patients with >30% collapse
- Secondary spontaneous PTX is more dangerous than primary PTX due to the decreased pulmonary reserve in patients with lung disease; most patients require a chest tube
- Traumatic PTX should be treated with a chest tube in most cases; small PTXs may be observed
- Tension PTX requires immediate needle decompression and insertion of chest tube

Disposition

- Healthy, asymptomatic patients with small, stable PTX and no co-morbidities may be discharged if a follow-up CXR (6 hours after presentation) shows no progression of PTX
- Patients with chest tubes, large PTX, or progressive PTX should be admitted for further management and additional X-rays
- Patients with poor respiratory reserve or co-morbid conditions require admission
- Half of spontaneous PTXs may recur
- Definitive therapy (e.g., pleurodesis, thoracoscopy, or surgery) may be required to prevent recurrence

31. Pleural Effusion

Etiology & Pathophysiology

- Excess fluid in the pleural space (normally <15 ml of fluid)
- Pleural fluid is formed by systemic capillaries at the parietal pleural surface and absorbed by pulmonary capillaries of the visceral pleural
- The underlying causative pathologic process must be identified—most common causes are CHF, pneumonia, cancer, and PE
- Transudative effusions occur in the setting of a normal pleural surface; an underlying process (see DDx section) results in either increased capillary hydrostatic pressure (in the systemic or pulmonary circulation) or decreased colloid oncotic pressure
- Exudative effusions occur as a result of pleural inflammation with an increase in capillary wall permeability (due to inflammation or neoplasm) or disruption of lymphatic drainage (i.e., as occurs when a neoplasm invades mediastinal lymph nodes)
- Empyema: A grossly purulent pleural effusion
- Hemothorax: Blood in the pleural space

Differential Dx

- Transudative effusions
  - –CHF
  - –PE
  - –Cirrhosis
  - –Nephrotic syndrome
  - –Hypothyroidism
- Exudative effusion
  - –Pulmonary: Pneumonia, TB, neoplasm, PE
  - –Cardiac: Pericarditis, CABG
  - –GI: Pancreatitis, esophageal rupture
  - –Other: Trauma, subphrenic abscess, uremia, RA/SLE, drugs (e.g., amiodarone)

Presentation

- Small effusions are generally asymptomatic; symptoms of the causative condition may be present
- Large effusions may cause compromised pulmonary function, resulting in dyspnea on exertion or at rest
- Chest pain (pleuritic or dull/achy)
- Nonproductive cough in some
- Large effusions may cause mediastinal shift (deviated trachea, displaced PMI, hypotension)
- Lung exam may reveal decreased breath sounds at the bases, egophony, dullness to percussion, and diminished tactile fremitus

Diagnosis

- Pulse oximetry may reveal hypoxemia
- CXR will show blunting of costophrenic angles
  - –Posterior costophrenic angle is initially affected (obliterated by as little as 200 ml of fluid)
  - –Lateral decubitus films can detect very small amounts of fluid and will show shifting of the effusion if it is not loculated
- Chest CT is more sensitive for effusion and will show loculations
- Diagnostic thoracocentesis should be considered for unexplained effusions or if patient has not responded as expected to therapy
  - –Fluid analysis for LDH and protein identifies exudate versus transudate—criteria for exudates include LDH >200 U, fluid:serum LDH ratio >0.6, or fluid:serum protein ratio >0.5
  - –Other tests on fluid are helpful in identifying the cause of exudates and may include amylase, glucose, cell count with differential, triglycerides, gram stain, cytology, RF, and ANA
  - –Ultrasound may help locate the best insertion site
  - –Post-procedure CXR to rule out iatrogenic pneumothorax

Treatment

- Treatment must address the underlying cause of the effusion
- Transudative effusions need only be drained if they cause significant symptoms
- Exudative effusions may require therapeutic thoracentesis
  - –Large symptomatic effusions require thoracentesis
  - –Large parapneumonic effusions (>10 cm) require thoracentesis and possibly a chest tube to prevent development of more complex, loculated effusions, which may require surgical intervention
  - –Chest tube insertion is required for hemothorax, empyema, and complicated parapneumonic effusions (positive gram stain/culture, loculations, glucose <40, pH <7.0–7.2, or LDH >1000)
- Recurrent effusions (e.g., in malignancy) may require repeated throacentesis and may benefit from pleurodesis or surgery
- Hemothorax usually requires a chest tube for drainage
- Rapid draining of large effusions may cause re-expansion pulmonary edema

Disposition

- Discharge should be considered for small effusions with known cause, minimal symptoms, and without evidence of respiratory compromise
- Admission is required for unknown etiologies, underlying etiologies or co-morbidities that require hospitalization, presence of hypoxia or impaired respiratory function, or empyema
- Severe hemodynamic or respiratory compromise requires ICU admission

32. Pulmonary Embolus

Etiology & Pathophysiology

- Thrombus of the deep venous system embolizes to the lungs, causing infarction of lung parenchyma and ventilation/perfusion mismatch
- 90% of emboli originate in the iliofemoral veins (may also come from pelvic or upper extremity veins)
- Virchow's triad describes the predisposing factors to venous thrombosis (risk factors are present in >90% of cases)
  - Venous stasis: Immobility, pedal edema, CHF, paraplegia
  - Hypercoagulability: Obesity, malignancy, hypercoagulable states, pregnancy, estrogen replacement therapy or OCPs
  - Endothelial damage: Recent trauma or surgery, burns, indwelling catheters, IV drug abuse
- 600,000 cases per year; up to 50% of cases are undiagnosed

Differential Dx

- Acute coronary syndrome
- CHF
- Aortic dissection
- Pericarditis/pericardial tamponade
- Pneumonia
- Asthma
- Pleurisy
- COPD exacerbation
- Pneumothorax
- Musculoskeletal pain
- Anxiety attack
- GERD/esophagitis

Presentation

- Most common symptom is dyspnea (present in up to 90% of patients)
- Other common symptoms include chest pain (usually pleuritic), apprehension, cough, hemoptysis, and syncope
- Most common sign is tachypnea (present in >90% of patients)
- Other common presenting signs include localized wheezing, tachycardia, low-grade fever, diaphoresis, leg swelling, and JVD
- 10% of patients present in shock

Diagnosis

- Pulmonary angiogram is the gold standard but only used if diagnosis is uncertain (invasive, may miss small distal emboli)
- Ventilation-perfusion scan (V/Q): Interpretation of results depends on clinical pretest probability; in general, a normal scan rules out PE and a high probability scan is diagnostic for PE (many patients will require further testing)
- Helical (spiral) CT is very sensitive for proximal PE but sensitivity and specificity for peripheral PE is unclear
- D-dimer is non-specific; only the ELISA assay has sufficient sensitivity to rule out PE and only in low-risk patients
- Lower extremity venous duplex scanning is used if initial test (V/Q scan or CT) is unclear: Diagnostic if positive but a negative study does not rule out PE
- ABG: Increased A-a gradient (may be normal in up to 15%)
- CXR is usually normal; may show pleural effusion, wedge-shaped infiltrate (Hampton's hump), area of decreased vascularity (Westermark sign), atelectasis, or cardiomegaly
- ECG may show tachycardia, RV strain, or a $S_1Q_3T_3$ pattern

Treatment

- Anticoagulation is used in all patients unless contraindicated; prevents clot propagation but does not reverse existing clot
  - Initiate anticoagulation with unfractionated heparin or low molecular weight heparin
  - Attain therapeutic levels within 24 hrs to reduce mortality
  - Warfarin therapy should be instituted concomitantly with heparin and continued for at least 6 months
- Inferior vena cava filter is indicated if anticoagulation is contraindicated, recurrent embolus occurs while on adequate anticoagulation, massive PE has occurred, or patient has poor baseline cardiac/respiratory status
- Hypotensive patients require IV fluids and vasopressors (e.g., norepinephrine); consider thrombolysis or surgery if hypotension is refractory
- Systemic thrombolysis (tPA or streptokinase) is only indicated for cases of refractory hemodynamic compromise if the potential benefits outweigh the risks of bleeding
- Pulmonary embolectomy is occasionally used in capable institutions in patients with refractory shock

Disposition

- Mortality is 2–10% in treated patients; 20–30% in untreated patients
- Clinical symptoms depend on the size of the embolus and the cardiopulmonary reserve of the patient
- All patients must be admitted
- Stable patients should be admitted to a general floor bed for monitoring of anticoagulation
- Patients who present in shock should be admitted to an ICU
- Normotensive patients with right ventricular dysfunction may need a higher level of care than is available on a general medical floor
- Surgical consultation for possible embolectomy may be necessary for unstable patients who have contraindications to thrombolytics

33. Hemoptysis

Etiology & Pathophysiology

- Expectoration of blood from below the vocal cords
- Degree of hemoptysis determines management and disposition
- Massive hemoptysis is variously defined as greater than 100–500 cc of hemoptysis in 24 hours (patients are often inaccurate in estimating blood volumes)
- The majority of cases are due to malignancy or non-tuberculous infections
- Bleeding from the high-pressure bronchial vessels accounts for 90% of cases; bleeding from the low-pressure pulmonary vessels is much less common
- Blood accumulates in the alveolar spaces and impedes oxygen exchange
- Up to 30% of cases have no identifiable etiology

Differential Dx

- Infection: Bronchitis (50% of cases), TB (5%), pneumonia, fungi, parasites, abscess
- Lung cancer (10–20% of cases)
- Vascular: PE, ruptured thoracic aneurysm, lung AVM, SLE, Wegener's or Goodpasture's
- Coagulopathy/anticoagulant use
- Trauma/instrumentation
- Foreign body
- CHF
- Mitral stenosis
- Bronchiectasis
- Pseudohemoptysis (e.g., GI or nasopharyngeal bleed)

Presentation

- May present as streaking of sputum or frank blood
- Crackles
- Associated symptoms are related to the underlying cause
  - Pneumonia and acute bronchitis: Cough, fever, purulent sputum
  - Chronic bronchitis and bronchiectasis: Chronic cough
  - TB and carcinoma: Fevers, weight loss, night sweats
  - Tracheolaryngeal mass or foreign body: Stridor
  - Vasculitis: Associated with renal disease and hematuria
- Massive hemoptysis may result in hypotension and shock

Diagnosis

- CBC, electrolytes, urinalysis, and coagulation studies are only required for cases of massive hemoptysis
- CXR may reveal parenchymal pathology (e.g., mass, cavitary lesion, infiltrate) and will localize areas of massive bleeding
- CT scan provides better information on focal areas of bleeding (shows alveolar filling) but is only performed on stable patients
- Sputum examination (gram stain, acid-fast stain for TB, cultures, and cytology) may be helpful but has limited sensitivity and often does not affect ED management
- Bronchoscopy can be both diagnostic and therapeutic (via balloon tamponade or vasoconstrictor injection) but is only performed emergently in cases of massive hemoptysis
- Algorithm for patients with massive hemoptysis
  - Active bleeding requires emergent bronchoscopy
  - Stable patients may undergo chest CT if there is no active bleed, followed by bronchoscopy

Treatment

- Massive hemoptysis requires emergent treatment
  - Secure airway and provide supplemental O_2
  - Insert 2 large bore IVs and type/cross-match blood
  - Position patient with the bleeding side in a dependent position to prevent blood from draining into opposite lung
  - Intubation if necessary to protect the airway; the tube may be placed into the main bronchus of the non-bleeding lung to protect it from blood
  - Transfuse blood and platelets as necessary and correct coagulopathies with fresh frozen plasma
  - Emergent bronchoscopy (rigid or flexible) is used to localize and control bleeding via epinephrine-induced vasoconstriction or balloon tamponade
  - Definitive therapy for persistent bleeding may require arteriography with embolization or emergent thoracic surgery
- Minor hemoptysis only requires treatment of the underlying etiology; outpatient elective bronchoscopy may be indicated

Disposition

- Stable patients with minor hemoptysis and normal CXR can be discharged with close follow-up
- Patients with risk factors (age >40, tobacco use, recent weight loss, anemia, persistent symptoms) require follow-up with elective bronchoscopy to rule out neoplasm
- Patients with massive hemoptysis must be admitted to the ICU (even if bleeding has subsided) because they remain at high risk for re-bleeding
- Massive hemoptysis is a medical emergency (30% mortality); death usually results from asphyxiation due to alveolar flooding and hypoxemia
- Patients with minor hemoptysis from TB, mycetomas, and bronchiectasis should be admitted due to risk of sudden massive hemoptysis

Gastrointestinal Emergencies

MATTHEW STUPPLE, MD
MEHUL M. PATEL, MD

34. Abdominal Pain

Etiology & Pathophysiology

- Extremely common (5–10% of all ED visits)
- Visceral pain: Distension of a hollow organ (e.g., intestine, stomach) results in autonomic nerve stimulation causing poorly characterized, diffuse, intermittent pain
- Parietal (somatic) pain: Direct irritation of the parietal peritoneum results in localized, intense, constant pain
- Referred pain: Overlap of innervation results in pain at a distance from the true source of pathology (e.g., diaphragmatic irritation from cholecystitis may result in right shoulder pain)
- Distinguish serious etiologies and those requiring acute surgical intervention from non-emergent causes
  - Life-threatening causes include ruptured AAA, perforated viscus, intestinal obstruction, ectopic pregnancy, mesenteric ischemia, appendicitis, and myocardial ischemia

Differential Dx

- Gastrointestinal
- Gynecologic
- Genitourinary
- Cardiac
- Vascular
- Infectious
- Abdominal wall
- Metabolic
- Trauma

Presentation

- Note location, onset, duration, quality, and intensity of pain; similarity to past episodes; and aggravating and alleviating factors
- Note bowel sounds, abdominal tenderness, rebound, guarding, distension, blood on rectal exam, and cervical/adnexal tenderness
- Associated symptoms may include nausea/vomiting, dysuria, vaginal discharge, diarrhea, constipation
- Atypical presentations are common in the elderly, alcoholics, and the immunocompromised
- Hypotension may be due to sepsis, vomiting, diarrhea, blood loss, or 3rd spacing

Diagnosis

- Pregnancy test in all females of reproductive age
- Urinalysis may show signs of UTI, pyelonephritis, or urolithiasis, but is nonspecific (e.g., appendicitis may cause pyuria)
- Leukocytosis is generally present in cases of inflammation (e.g., appendicitis, diverticulitis); however, a normal WBC count does not rule out inflammatory or infectious disease
- Liver function tests, amylase, and lipase may indicate liver, biliary, or pancreatic disease
- Imaging
  - Abdominal CT will often establish a diagnosis (e.g., nephrolithiasis, AAA, diverticulitis, appendicitis, mesenteric ischemia, obstruction)
  - Ultrasound is the initial test-of-choice for biliary tract disease, AAA, ectopic pregnancy, or free peritoneal fluid
  - Plain films are used only to rule out perforation or obstruction

Treatment

- Hemodynamically unstable patients should receive rehydration with normal saline; consider transfusion for GI bleeding or vasopressors for shock
- Place NG tube in cases of obstruction or persistent vomiting
- Symptomatic treatment of emesis (e.g., promethazine, metoclopramide, odansetron) and pain
  - Colicky pain responds well to NSAIDs (especially IV ketorolac)
  - H2 blockers/antacids for burning epigastric pain
  - Add narcotics as necessary—there is no evidence to show that pain control with narcotics will hinder exam findings or "mask" an acute abdomen
  - Intestinal cramping often responds to anticholinergics (e.g., donnatol) or antispasmodics (e.g., dicyclomine)
- Administer broad-spectrum empiric antibiotics for suspected intra-abdominal infections (cover gram-negatives and anaerobes)

Disposition

- Prompt surgical or obstetric consultation as necessary
- In most cases in the ED, specific diagnoses are not obtained
- Patients with surgical abdomens (e.g., peritoneal signs, perforation) should be admitted for surgical evaluation
- Non-surgical medical causes may be admitted for medical management or discharged home with close follow-up
- Any discharged patient should be instructed to return to the ED if symptoms change or worsen
- Consider cardiac causes of abdominal pain in all patients with cardiac risk factors
- Serious and life-threatening etiologies must be ruled out prior to discharge

35. GI Bleeding

Etiology & Pathophysiology

- Ranges from occult, microscopic bleeding to profuse hemorrhage
- May originate from anywhere in the upper (from the esophagus to the ligament of Treitz) or lower GI tract (distal to the ligament of Treitz)
- Sources of life-threatening upper GI bleeding
    - Peptic ulcer disease (most common cause of upper GI bleeding)
    - Esophageal varices, secondary to portal hypertension and cirrhosis
    - Mallory-Weiss tears, due to forceful vomiting
- Sources of life-threatening lower GI bleeding
    - Diverticular bleeding, due to erosion of a diverticula into a vessel
    - Angiodysplasia (arteriovenous malformation) is common in elderly
    - Aortoenteric fistula (GI bleeding in a patient with past aortic surgery should be assumed to be an aortoenteric fistula secondary to an infected aortic stent until proven otherwise—they often have a small herald bleed that precedes massive hemorrhaging)

Differential Dx

- Upper GI bleed
    - Peptic ulcer
    - Esophageal varices
    - Gastric erosions/gastritis
    - Mallory-Weiss tear
    - Esophagitis
- Lower GI bleed
    - Diverticulosis
    - Angiodysplasia (AVM)
    - Cancer/polyps
    - Anorectal disorders
    - Inflammatory bowel disease
    - Aortoenteric fistula
    - Infectious diarrhea

Presentation

- Symptoms may range from occult, microscopic bleeding or minor blood on toilet paper to frank bloody vomitus or bloody stools
- Signs of upper GI bleeding include hematemesis and melena (dark, tarry stools)
- Hematochezia (bright red blood per rectum) indicates a lower GI bleed or brisk upper GI bleeding
- Hypovolemia due to hemorrhage (e.g., pallor, dizziness, weakness, syncope) and signs of shock (e.g., hypotension) may be present
- Nonspecific complaints may include dyspnea, abdominal pain, chest pain, and fatigue

Diagnosis

- Tachycardia or orthostasis may occur with >15% blood loss; hypotension occurs with >40% blood loss
- History may reveal causative factors, such as medications (e.g., aspirin, NSAIDs, steroids, anticoagulants), alcohol use, liver disease, or bleeding diathesis
- Blood type and cross/screen should be immediately ordered
- PT/PTT may be prolonged due to a coagulation disorder
- BUN may be elevated in upper GI bleed
- ECG should be evaluated in the elderly, patients with a history of cardiac disease, and those who present with chest pain or shortness of breath
- NG tube may be inserted to aspirate and test gastric contents in order to identify if upper GI bleeding has occurred
- Endoscopy (done by gastroenterology) is the diagnostic and often therapeutic procedure of choice for upper GI bleeding
- Colonoscopy, angiography, and red cell bleeding scans are used to identify sources of lower GI bleeding

Treatment

- Establish 2 large bore IVs and bolus with normal saline
- Blood transfusion may be added if hypotension persists despite IV fluid administration (replenish platelets and fresh frozen plasma for every 6 units of blood given)
- NG tube placement is controversial; often used in cases of severe active bleeding or severe nausea/vomiting
- Medication is often used but lacks evidence for efficacy in most settings
    - Anti-acid therapy (proton pump inhibitors or H2 blockers)
    - Octreotide infusion (causes splanchnic vasoconstriction) may be of benefit for bleeding varices and ulcers
    - Vasopressin (causes splanchnic and systemic vasoconstriction) (may result in myocardial ischemia)
- Emergent endoscopy (i.e., with ligation or sclerotherapy) is the preferred treatment for severe upper GI bleeds
- Balloon tamponade with Sengstaken-Blakemore tube may also be used for uncontrolled variceal bleeding
- Severe lower GI bleeding may be controlled by arteriographic embolization
- Surgery may be required for any persistent uncontrolled bleeding

Disposition

- Gastroenterology and surgery consult in patients with moderate to severe bleeding
- Most patients with GI bleeding should be admitted
- Very low risk patients may be discharged (e.g., patients with hemorrhoids, fissures, or proctitis)
- Patients with normal vital signs, no comorbid conditions, negative gastric aspirate and normal stool guaiac, good medical access, and understanding of their condition can be discharged
- All patients with systolic BP <100, tachycardia, >4 units transfused, or active bleeding should be admitted to an ICU

36. Foreign Body Ingestion

Etiology & Pathophysiology

- Ingested foreign bodies may lodge in the GI tract (potentially resulting in obstruction or perforation) or pass spontaneously
- Populations at risk include children (80% of all cases), alcoholics, psychiatric patients, patients with altered mental status, and inmates
- Coins are ingested in >50% of cases
- Objects often lodge at levels of physiologic esophageal narrowing
  - Cricopharyngeal level is most common in children—may cause airway obstruction and respiratory failure
  - Aortic arch and carina (T4 level) is most common in adults
  - Proximal to the gastroesophageal junction
- Foreign bodies that pass to the intestine are rarely problematic and can be managed expectantly
- Button batteries deserve special consideration as they may cause alkaline burns and/or rupture of the esophagus within 4–6 hours

Differential Dx

- Coins
- Food
- Pins
- Batteries
- Button batteries
- Drug packing (cocaine, heroin)
- Dislodged esophageal stent
- Bezoars (especially trichobezoars in hair chewers)

Presentation

- Discomfort and anxiety
- Retching and vomiting
- Coughing and gagging
- Drooling
- Retrosternal pain
- Look for signs and symptoms of esophageal or GI perforation
- Children may have acute airway obstruction if the object lodges at the cricopharyngeous muscle
- Young children may present only with poor feeding, choking, stridor

Diagnosis

- Examine oro/nasopharynx, neck, and soft tissue for subcutaneous air (indicating esophageal perforation) and examine the abdomen for peritoneal signs (indicating GI perforation)
- Direct or indirect laryngoscopy is used if the patient feels the foreign body is in the throat/pharynx or has airway symptoms
- Chest X-ray and lateral neck X-ray will identify radio-opaque objects (e.g., coins)
  - On an AP view, coins often align in the coronal plane if in the esophagus or sagittal plane if in the trachea
- Endoscopy by a gastroenterologist may be both diagnostic and therapeutic
- Gastrograffin swallowing study may be used if plain films are negative and endoscopy is unavailable
- CT scan is very effective at locating objects and damage to the surrounding tissue (may soon replace endoscopy)
- Handheld metal detectors are effective at localizing metal objects

Treatment

- Endoscopic removal is required in unstable patients or those who have ingested a sharp object
- Objects in the esophagus
  - Button battery requires emergent removal
  - Smooth, blunt objects (e.g., coins) may be managed expectantly if <24 hrs have passed or by endoscopic removal if beyond 24 hrs
  - Food bolus requires endoscopic removal, pharmacologic treatment with IV glucagon to cause reflex contraction of esophageal muscle to expel the bolus, or sphincter relaxing agents (e.g., nitroglycerin, nifedipine) to allow passage of the bolus
  - Avoid meat tenderizers (may cause perforation)
- Objects that have passed to stomach can often be managed with observation alone
  - Endoscopic removal is indicated if object is wider than 2 cm, longer than 6 cm, or sharp (e.g., razors, safety pins)
  - Remove button battery if lodged in stomach for >48 hrs
- Foreign objects in the intestines may be observed without surgical intervention unless perforation is suspected

Disposition

- 80–90% of objects pass spontaneously
- 10–20% require intervention
- 1% require surgical intervention
- Esophageal objects may be managed in the ED or admitted
- Patients with objects distal to the esophagus that do not require removal may be discharged
  - Monitor stool and obtain outpatient serial radiographs to ensure passage
  - Objects that fail to progress after 1–2 weeks may require removal
- Immediate surgery is required if signs of perforation or obstruction are present
- Body packers/stuffers of illicit drugs should be admitted for close observation; manage either expectantly or with surgical removal (avoid endoscopy as bags may break)

37. Dysphagia

Etiology & Pathophysiology

- Difficulty swallowing due to oropharyngeal or esophageal etiologies
- Oropharyngeal (transfer) dysphagia results from abnormal transfer of a food bolus from the pharynx to the esophagus
  - Due to lesions of the neurological reflex arc involving the afferent nerves (cranial nerves V, IX, X, XI), CNS swallowing center, efferent nerves (V, VII, IX, XI, XII), or responding muscles
- Esophageal (transport) dysphagia results from disordered propulsion of the food bolus from the upper esophagus to the stomach
  - Motility disorders lead to abnormal peristalsis or esophageal muscle tone (resulting in difficulty with solids and liquids)
  - Obstructions physically impede transport (difficulty with solids)
  - Achalasia: Dysphagia due to a spastic lower esophageal sphincter
  - Diffuse esophageal spasm: Multiple areas of esophageal spasm due to GERD, stress, alcohol, connective tissue disease, DM, or idiopathic

Differential Dx

- Oropharyngeal dysphagia
  - CVA
  - Sjogren's syndrome
  - Parkinson's disease
  - Multiple sclerosis or ALS
  - Diabetic neuropathy
  - Dermato/polymyositis
  - Myasthenia gravis
- Esophageal dysphagia
  - Achalasia
  - Diffuse esophageal spasm
  - LES hypertension
  - Obstructions (e.g., food bolus, tumor, stricture)
  - Severe esophagitis

Presentation

- Oropharyngeal
  - Gagging, drooling
  - Multiple swallowing attempts
  - Head and neck turning to facilitate swallowing
  - Liquids more difficult than solids
  - Exacerbated by temperature extremes
- Esophageal
  - Chest pain
  - Sensation of food sticking
  - Odynophagia (painful swallow)
  - Retrosternal fullness
  - Worse during stress or rapid eating
  - Solids worse or equal to liquids

Diagnosis

- History and physical examination will narrow the differential
- Rule out cardiac causes if chest pain is present
- Plain imaging
  - Neck X-rays to rule out foreign bodies
  - CXR may show mediastinal mass, aortic aneurysm, or foreign body in cases of obstructions
  - CXR may show absent gastric air in cases of achalasia
- Further GI testing may be necessary to determine etiology (not generally done in ED)
  - Videofluoroscopy is the gold standard to diagnose most cases of dysphagia, especially oropharyngeal causes
  - Barium swallow will show a "bird beak" sign in achalasia and a "corkscrew" sign in diffuse esophageal spasm
  - Endoscopy is used to diagnose esophageal dysphagia
  - Manometry will help evaluate achalasia and esophageal spasm

Treatment

- Protect airway if there is any risk of aspiration
- Administer IV fluids if the patient is dehydrated
- Oropharyngeal (transfer) dysphagia require a swallowing evaluation to determine risk of aspiration
- Acute obstructions (e.g., foreign body)
  - Glucagon may cause forceful expulsion of a food bolus
  - Alternatively, Ca^+-channel blockers and other muscle relaxants may be used to relax smooth muscle
- Motility disorders/spasm
  - Nitrates or Ca^+-channel blockers are used to relax smooth muscle and prevent spasms
  - Anticholinergics are only minimally helpful
- Achalasia
  - Medical therapy with Ca^+-channel blockers
  - Esophageal dilation or lower esophageal sphincter myotomy provides definitive treatment
- Esophageal strictures/masses require dilation and possible esophageal stent placement

Disposition

- Admit patients who are at risk for aspiration or unable to safely swallow oral fluids
- Most patients can be discharged home with referral to a gastroenterologist
- Complications may include malnutrition, dehydration, weight loss, and aspiration pneumonia

38. Esophageal Perforation

Etiology & Pathophysiology

- Results in leakage of acid and non-sterile secretions into the mediastinum, a life-threatening emergency that can rapidly lead to infection and overwhelming sepsis
- Perforations are iatrogenic in over 80% of cases
  - Especially common in patients undergoing endoscopy who have underlying pathologies that weaken the esophageal or gastric wall (e.g., carcinoma, esophagitis, strictures)
  - Esophageal wall thinning and perforation may also occur with sclerotherapy (e.g., for varices), pill esophagitis, and radiation
- Spontaneous perforation (Boerhaave's syndrome) may occur secondary to forceful vomiting or other maneuvers that increase intra-esophageal pressure (e.g., straining, weightlifting, childbirth, severe coughing)
- Further causes include trauma, caustic ingestions, tumors, foreign bodies, and aortic aneurysms

Differential Dx

- Myocardial infarction
- Dissecting aortic aneurysm
- Pancreatitis
- Pneumothorax
- Perforated peptic ulcer
- Pericarditis
- Pneumonia
- Pulmonary embolism
- Lung abscess
- Esophageal hematoma
- Esophageal bleeding (e.g., Mallory-Weiss tear, varices)

Presentation

- Classic triad of pain, fever, and subcutaneous air
- Other symptoms may include dysphagia, respiratory distress, nausea/vomiting, hoarseness, and hematemesis
- 25% of patients present in shock
- Pain is the most common symptom
  - Severe, persistent pain
  - Cervical rupture results in neck pain and tenderness
  - Thoracic rupture results in back, substernal, or abdominal pain
- Hamman's crunch: Crunching sound due to mediastinal air during auscultation of the heart

Diagnosis

- High level of clinical suspicion is essential—suspect perforation in any patient with pain following esophageal instrumentation (e.g., endoscopy), prolonged vomiting, or coughing
- Chest X-ray should be ordered initially: Signs of perforation include subcutaneous emphysema, mediastinal widening, mediastinal air-fluid levels, pneumomediastinum, and pleural effusion
- Esophagography (a swallowing study that is initially performed with water-soluble contrast) will confirm the diagnosis and delineate the location of the lesion, but is falsely negative in up to 20% of cases
- Chest CT may show abscess, mediastinal air, air-fluid collections
- Endoscopy is reserved for patients with high clinical suspicion but negative CT and esophagography
- Thoracentesis of associated pleural effusions will reveal a high amylase level if the effusion is due to a perforation
- Leukocytosis and acidosis may signal evolving sepsis

Treatment

- Avoid oral intake
- Nasogastric tube is generally placed to decompress the stomach
- Treat shock with IV fluids (normal saline) and vasopressors
- Administer broad-spectrum IV antibiotics to cover gram positives, gram negatives, and anaerobes in cases of proven or suspected perforation
- All patients with perforation require immediate surgical consultation—controversy exists regarding operative versus non-surgical treatment
  - Non-surgical approach should be considered in patients with minimal symptoms, absence of shock and sepsis, and with well-contained or cervical tears
  - Surgery is the treatment of choice in patients with large, non-contained perforations or clinical signs of shock or sepsis

Disposition

- Esophageal rupture results in a full-thickness tear of the esophagus (in contrast to Mallory-Weiss syndrome, which results in a partial thickness tear)
- All patients should be admitted
- ICU admission for severe cases and following surgery
- Consider admission and empiric IV antibiotics in patients with high clinical suspicion, but negative chest X-ray and esophagography since these tests are not definitive—further evaluation by ENT or GI may be indicated
- High morbidity and mortality

39. GERD/Esophagitis

Etiology & Pathophysiology

- GERD: Symptomatic reflux of gastric contents into the esophagus
  - Lower esophageal sphincter (LES) dysfunction is the #1 cause—exacerbated by alcohol, caffeine, tobacco, fatty foods, pregnancy, chocolate, hiatal hernia, meds (e.g., anticholinergics, Ca^+-channel blockers), prolonged gastric emptying (e.g., DM), scleroderma
- Esophagitis: Esophageal inflammation
  - Most commonly secondary to GERD
  - Pill esophagitis is also common (e.g., NSAIDs, antibiotics, iron)
  - Barrett's esophagus may result from chronic inflammation of the esophageal mucosa, resulting in replacement of columnar epithelium with precancerous squamous epithelium
  - Infectious esophagitis (often *Candida*) generally occurs in immunocompromised patients (e.g., HIV, diabetes)
  - Chemical esophagitis occurs with ingestion of mucosal irritants (e.g., alcohol, tobacco, hot fluids), alkali, acids, medications

Differential Dx

- Acute coronary syndrome
- Esophageal motility disorder
- Foreign body ingestion
- Esophageal tear/perforation
- Esophageal cancer
- Peptic ulcer disease
- Gallbladder disease
- Dissecting aortic aneurysm
- Pulmonary embolus
- Less common causes of infectious esophagitis include cryptosporidium, HSV, CMV, or pneumocystis carinii

Presentation

- Burning, subxyphoid pain ("heartburn")
  - May radiate to back
  - Usually occurs 10–30 minutes after ingesting specific foods
  - Often relieved with antacids or resolves spontaneously
- GERD is one of the most common causes of chronic cough
- Regurgitation, hypersalivation, belching, and acid taste in mouth
- Odynophagia/dysphagia
- Pain and associated symptoms may mimic a cardiac syndrome
- Atypical presentations include asthma, sinusitis, dental erosions, hoarseness, and chronic cough

Diagnosis

- Initial examination should be aimed at ruling out cardiac ischemia by history, physical exam, and appropriate diagnostic tests (e.g., ECG and enzymes in patients at risk)
- After cardiac causes are ruled out, diagnosis is usually made clinically and the patient is discharged
- Diagnostic testing may be done on an outpatient basis
  - Omeprazole challenge test: 1 week of proton pump inhibitor therapy—if pain resolves, GERD is the diagnosis
  - Endoscopy allows direct visualization and biopsy of esophageal and gastric mucosa to diagnose Barrett's esophagus or esophagitis
  - Barium esophagram will demonstrate high-grade esophagitis, ulceration, or stricture formation but is insensitive for reflux
  - 24-hour pH monitoring correlates esophageal pH to symptom onset to diagnose reflux

Treatment

- Lifestyle modification is the 1st line therapy
  - Eliminate/minimize alcohol, tobacco, caffeine, onions, peppermint, chocolate, and other inciting foods
  - Avoid postprandial recumbancy
  - Elevate head of bed 30°
  - Do not eat within 2–4 hours of bedtime
  - Lose weight if obese
  - Eliminate medications that may decrease LES tone (e.g., Ca^{++}-channel blockers)
- Proton-pump inhibitors (most effective) and H2-receptor blockers (may be better for nighttime symptoms) will block acid production to improve symptoms
- Promotility agents (e.g., metoclopramide) have not been proven to be effective and have many side effects
- Severe GERD may require surgical fundoplication
- Infectious esophagitis requires appropriate antifungal agents (oral ketoconazole or fluconazole) or antibiotics
- Pill esophagitis: Avoid pills, use small, non-gelatin coated pills, and take pills with fluids while in upright position

Disposition

- Severity of symptoms does not necessarily correlate with degree of esophageal injury
- Start most patients on a PPI for 2–4 weeks with GI follow-up
- Patients require long-term follow-up to manage the condition and obtain recommended screening endoscopies if chronic symptoms occur
- Refer patients with persistent symptoms to GI for endoscopy
- Infectious esophagitis may require admission for IV antibiotics and/or antifungals, pain control, IV fluids, and hyperalimentation if unable to swallow

40. Peptic Ulcer Disease

Etiology & Pathophysiology

- Erosion and ulceration of the gastric or duodenal mucosa
- Occurs secondary to a disrupted balance between parietal cell acid formation and production of mucus (to coat and protect the mucosa) and bicarbonate (to buffer the acid)
- *H. pylori* infection is the most common cause of PUD
  - A urease producing gram-negative rod
  - Disrupts the mucosal protective barrier
  - Responsible for 95% of duodenal ulcers and 85% of gastric ulcers
- Other causes include NSAIDs (inhibit prostaglandin formation, disrupting bicarbonate and mucus production), gastrin-secreting tumors (e.g., Zollinger-Ellison syndrome, gastrinoma), Crohn's disease of the stomach or duodenum, tobacco, stress, family history, renal failure, COPD

Differential Dx

- Acute gastritis (due to shock, trauma, steroids, burns, alcohol, NSAIDs)
- Gastric cancer
- Pancreatitis
- Esophagitis/GERD
- Esophageal motility disorder
- Non-ulcer dyspepsia
- Biliary colic/cholecystitis
- Hepatitis
- Aortic dissection/AAA
- Acute coronary syndromes
- Pneumonia
- Mesenteric ischemia
- Small bowel obstruction

Presentation

- Dyspepsia (burning/gnawing epigastric pain without radiation)
  - Relieved by food, milk, antacids
  - Often worse at night
- Epigastric tenderness
- Gastric ulcer pain often occurs immediately after eating
- Duodenal ulcer pain often occurs 1½–3 hours after eating or at night
- Vomiting, chest or back pain, and bloating may be present (nausea and belching are notably absent)
- GI bleeding may occur (guaiac positive stool, melena, hemoptysis, hematochezia, and/or hypotension)
- Perforation with peritoneal signs may occur

Diagnosis

- Unstable patients with GI bleeding may require emergent surgery prior to the completion of a full diagnostic workup
- ED workup is aimed at ruling out other potential causes of pain
  - Amylase/lipase (pancreatitis)
  - LFTs and abdominal ultrasound (hepatic and biliary disease)
  - ECG and serial enzymes (cardiac ischemia)
  - Urine HCG (pregnancy)
- CBC may reveal anemia due to chronic blood loss
- Ulcer visualization by endoscopy or barium swallow (upper GI series) is diagnostic; however, these are not usually done in ED
- *H. pylori* testing
  - IgG serology should be ordered in patients not previously treated for *H. pylori;* since IgG remains positive even after appropriate therapy, it is not useful in previously treated pts
  - Previously treated patients require outpatient urease breath test or endoscopic biopsy to determine if active *H. pylori* is present

Treatment

- Lifestyle changes include bland diet (e.g., low-fat, non-acidic foods) with frequent small meals and avoidance of alcohol and tobacco
- Avoid aspirin, NSAIDs, and steroids (COX-2 inhibitors may be less ulcerogenic)
- Begin antacid therapy with high-dose proton pump inhibitors or H2 blockers
- Sucralfate (a mucosal protective agent that binds to ulcer and forms a protective barrier against acid) may also be used
- Treat *H. pylori* if present with triple antibiotic therapy for 10–14 days, multiple regimens are available
  - Bismuth subsalicylate, metronidazole, and tetracycline
  - Ranitidine, tetracycline, and either clarithromycin or metronidazole
  - Omeprazole, clarithromycin, and either metronidazole or amoxicillin
- Indications for surgery include intractable bleeding, gastric outlet obstruction, perforation, Zollinger-Ellison syndrome

Disposition

- Eradication of *H. pylori* decreases ulcer recurrence from 50–80% to <10%
- Admit patients with severe symptoms indicating possible or imminent perforation/hemorrhage (e.g., recent weight loss, persistent vomiting, GI bleeding)
- Majority of patients are discharged with close follow-up for definitive diagnosis and ongoing management
- Patients who continue to have symptoms for greater than a month despite PPI therapy require referral for endoscopy
- Complications may include pancreatitis, perforation, gastric outlet obstruction, GI bleed, and gastric cancer (secondary to chronic inflammation)

41. Infectious Diarrhea

Etiology & Pathophysiology

- Acute diarrhea lasts less than 4 weeks; chronic lasts more than 4 weeks
- Due to increased secretion, decreased absorption, osmotic diarrhea, or abnormal intestinal motility
- Gastroenteritis: Intestinal inflammation that results in diarrhea and vomiting
- Dysentery: Invasive diarrhea (due to *Campylobacter, Salmonella, Shigella,* enterohemorrhagic *E coli* (O157:H7), *Yersinia, C difficile,* or *Vibrio parahemolyticus*) that results in bloody, mucous stools
- Invasive diarrhea may occur with severe systemic effects
- Non-inflammatory/non-invasive diarrhea: Due to superficial mucosal invasion by viruses (e.g., Norwalk, rotavirus) and or toxin release by bacteria ("traveler's diarrhea" due to enterotoxigenic *E coli* or food poisoning due to *B cereus, S aureus, E coli, Clostridium perfringens, Vibrio cholerae*)
- Giardia infection

Differential Dx

- HIV
- Malabsorption syndromes
- Ischemic bowel
- Adrenal insufficiency
- Hyperthyroidism
- Vasculitis
- Inflammatory bowel disease
- Neoplasia
- Irritable bowel syndrome
- Appendicitis
- Medications (e.g., laxatives, antibiotics, anticholinergics, chemotherapy)

Presentation

- Frequent watery stools
- Vomiting, nausea, and crampy pain
- Viral disease is often epidemic, resulting in non-invasive, secretory diarrhea with nausea and vomiting
- Non-invasive (toxin-mediated) disease causes diarrhea and cramps with minimal other symptoms
- Invasive disease is associated with fever, dysentery, seizures (*Shigella*), abdominal tenderness
- Giardiasis is chronic and associated with foul-smelling stools and flatulence
- Patients may present with signs of dehydration, such as orthostasis, tachycardia, or hypotension

Diagnosis

- Both invasive and non-invasive diarrhea may be food related
- Proper history should include travel history, woodland exposure (Giardia), immune status, and other sick contacts
- Fecal leukocytes indicates invasive/bacterial diarrhea or inflammation of the mucosa (e.g., inflammatory bowel disease)
- Acute non-invasive diarrhea generally does not require further work-up, except in toxic or immunocompromised patients, children, and diarrhea lasting beyond 3 days
- Stool evaluation for ova and parasites (for *Giardia* and *Cryptosporidium*) should be considered in at-risk patients with persistent diarrhea
- Stool cultures may identify *Salmonella, Shigella,* or *Campylobacter*
- Test stool for *C difficile* toxin, if suspected (e.g., recent antibiotic)
- Stool osmolar gap is elevated in osmotic and malabsorptive diarrhea and decreased in infectious/secretory diarrhea

Treatment

- Treatment is generally supportive
- Fluid resuscitation—oral if possible or IV with isotonic crystalloid (e.g., normal saline or lactated Ringer's)
- Antimotility agents include opiates (e.g., loperamide) and parasympathetic inhibitors (e.g., diphenoxylate plus atropine); concerns that these agents may slow the clearance of pathogens have been disproven in recent studies
- Antibiotic therapy is generally reserved for severe or invasive disease
  - Most authorities recommend empiric treatment with a fluoroquinolone or TMP-SMX in patients with severe or bloody diarrhea, fever, or fecal leukocytes (will shorten the duration of illness)
  - If *Giardia* or *C difficile* is suspected, treat empirically with metronidazole
  - Antibiotic therapy does increase the risk of hemolytic-uremic syndrome in children with *E coli* O157 infection
  - There is no good evidence that antibiotics prolong the carrier state in *Salmonella* infections

Disposition

- Admit patients with hemodynamic instability, systemic toxicity, or inability to tolerate sufficient fluids to keep up with GI losses
- Patients who are hemodynamically stable and can tolerate sufficient oral fluids can be treated and discharged
- Advise patient to hydrate with glucose-containing, caffeine free beverages and to avoid lactose, sorbitol-containing gum, and raw fruit until symptoms subside
- Complications include hemolytic-uremic syndrome (in children with *E coli* O157) and mesenteric adenitis (*Yersinia*)
- Consider *E coli* O157 in any patient with bloody diarrhea but without fever

42. Bowel Obstruction

Etiology & Pathophysiology

- Obstruction may be mechanical or paralytic (i.e., ileus)
  - Mechanical small bowel obstructions include adhesions (most common cause), hernia, tumor, stricture, intussusception, foreign bodies, SMA syndrome, lymphoma, and gallstones
  - Mechanical large bowel obstructions include colon cancer, volvulus, diverticulitis, fecal impaction, intussusception, and ulcerative colitis
  - Adynamic (paralytic) ileus may be caused by peritonitis, uremia, electrolytes, surgery, MI, renal colic, trauma, meds (e.g., opiates)
- Increased intraluminal pressure causes wall dilatation, decreased absorption, and 3rd spacing of fluid into the bowel lumen and wall—this results in volume depletion, hypotension, and possibly translocation of bacteria into the systemic circulation with sepsis
- Strangulation may occur if the blood supply is compromised, resulting in bowel ischemia and necrosis

Differential Dx

- Acute gastroenteritis
- Pseudo-obstruction (a chronic disorder of intestinal motility due to collagen vascular diseases, diabetes, drugs)
- Appendicitis
- Mesenteric ischemia
- Perforation with peritonitis and secondary obstruction
- Pancreatitis
- Cholecystitis
- Perforated peptic ulcer
- Pelvic inflammatory disease

Presentation

- Mechanical obstructions
  - Colicky, intermittent pain
  - Increased bowel sounds with high-pitched rushes
- Paralytic ileus
  - Crampy, constant pain
  - Decreased or absent sounds
- Bilious vomiting in proximal obstructions
- Feculent vomiting may be present in obstructions of ileum or colon
- Abdominal distension
- Constipation or decreased flatus
- Tenderness is minimal to severe
- Peritoneal signs in perforation
- May have signs of shock

Diagnosis

- Flat and upright abdominal films are often diagnostic
  - Dilated loops of bowel (small bowel has plicae circulares extending completely across the lumen; large bowel has haustra that only partially cross the lumen)
  - May have air-fluid levels (stepladder pattern in small bowel)
  - "String of pearls" sign due to gas trapping in small bowel
  - Complete obstructions may have absence of gas in the rectum
  - May also show masses and help localize the site of obstruction
- Chest X-ray is the best view to evaluate for perforation (free air)
- Abdominal CT may be used if plain films are unclear—may demonstrate the obstruction, show intramural gas or wall thickening in ischemia, or identify other pathology
- Labs should include CBC, electrolytes, and renal function
  - Significant leukocytosis suggests bowel ischemia or infection
  - Consider lactate level to rule out mesenteric ischemia
- Gastrograffin enema may be used to diagnose colonic obstruction

Treatment

- NG tube decompression to decrease intraluminal pressure and stop vomiting
- Isotonic IV fluids should be administered aggressively to replace fluid lost by vomiting and 3rd spacing into bowel lumen and wall
- Correct electrolyte abnormalities as necessary
- Broad-spectrum IV antibiotics are indicated in complete mechanical obstructions or if perforation has occurred
  - Penicillin/anti-penicillinase
  - 3rd generation cephalosporin plus either clindamycin or metronidazole
- Partial mechanical obstructions may be closely observed without specific treatment
- Complete mechanical obstructions, strangulation, or sepsis require immediate surgery
- Adynamic ileus may be observed for resolution following nasogastric decompression

Disposition

- All patients with complete or partial obstructions should be admitted
- Mortality increases dramatically (from 10% to 50%) if bowel ischemia is present
- Adynamic ileus has a good prognosis
- Complications may include perforation and peritonitis, sepsis, hypovolemia, and intestinal ischemia/infarction

43. Hernia

Etiology & Pathophysiology

- Herniation of abdominal viscera occurs in areas of weakness or disruption in the fibromuscular tissue of the abdominal wall
- Reducible hernia: Hernia can be replaced to its proper location
- Irreducible (incarcerated) hernia: Hernia cannot be reduced
- Strangulated hernia: Blood supply to the herniated bowel becomes compromised, resulting in ischemia and gangrene
- Inguinal hernia: Herniation through Hasselbach's triangle and the external inguinal ring (direct inguinal hernia) or internal inguinal ring (indirect); more common in males; low risk of incarceration
- Femoral hernia: Herniation into the femoral canal, below the inguinal ligament; more common in females; high risk of incarceration
- Umbilical and epigastric hernias: Herniation through midline fascia; high risk of incarceration
- Spigelian hernia: Herniation below arcuate line, lateral to the rectus
- Incisional hernia: Herniation through a wound closure site

Differential Dx

- Genital pathology (e.g., testicular torsion, epididymitis, hydrocele, varicocele, cryptorchidism, testicular tumor, undescended testes)
- Lymphadenitis
- Femoral artery aneurysm
- Small bowel obstruction
- Large bowel obstruction

Presentation

- Inguinal hernia is usually asymptomatic
  - May have inguinal pain
  - Bulge in scrotum/labia (increased by straining, lifting)
  - Incarcerated hernias may cause pain, tenderness, nausea, vomiting, obstructive symptoms
- Femoral: Femoral bulging/pain
- Spigelian: Anterior abdominal wall pain with a mass below the arcuate line
- Strangulated hernias may result in pain, tenderness, fever, tachycardia, and hypotension
- Children with hernia may present only with irritability

Diagnosis

- Detailed history and physical exam is often diagnostic
  - Palpate the affected area (e.g., groin, incisional area) for tenderness, discomfort, and masses while the patient is supine and upright (while straining)
  - For inguinal hernia, place finger through external inguinal ring and palpate for hernia while asking patient to cough
  - Outright pain with a simple hernia is unusual—consider incarceration or strangulation in patients with pain
- Vomiting or dehydration may result in electrolyte abnormalities
- Strangulated hernias may cause leukocytosis with left shift
- Urinalysis may be ordered if suspect GU infection
- Abdominal CT may show herniation of bowel
- Abdominal X-ray may be ordered if suspect bowel obstruction
- Testicular ultrasound if suspect testicular torsion or tumor
- Inpatient studies may include herniography, ultrasound, or MRI if the diagnosis is unclear

Treatment

- Reducible hernias may be treated in the ED
  - Provide analgesia and sedation (opiates and benzodiazepines) if required
  - Place the patient in a supine position (hernia may spontaneously reduce in this position)
  - Place constant gentle pressure at the site of herniation until it is reduced
- Attempt reduction of newly incarcerated hernias; however, old incarcerated hernias should not be reduced because the gut may already be ischemic
- Surgical consultation is warranted if reduction is unsuccessful or strangulation is suspected
- Surgical repair is the definitive treatment for all hernias
  - Emergent repair for strangulated hernias—insert NG tube, begin IV fluids and keep patient NPO, begin IV antibiotics (usually a 3rd generation cephalosporin), and consult surgery for immediate intervention
  - Elective repair for reducible hernias
  - Some hernias (e.g., in patients who are not good candidates for surgery) are managed expectantly

Disposition

- Criteria for admission
  - Any strangulated or incarcerated hernia
  - Bowel obstruction
  - Peritonitis
  - Fever
  - Vomiting
  - Intractable pain
- Discharge if successful reduction is accomplished in the ED
- Discharged patients require close follow-up, re-examination in 24–48 hours, and surgical referral for elective repair
- Strangulated bowel can become necrotic and gangrenous in as little as 6 hours—rapid and accurate diagnosis is essential

44. Appendicitis

Etiology & Pathophysiology

- Appendicitis is the most common abdominal surgical emergency
- Affects 10–15% of the population over their lifetime
- Most common between ages 10–30
- Obstruction of lumen (due to fecalith, neoplasm, foreign object) leads to distention, increased intraluminal pressure, venous engorgement and impaired arterial blood supply
- Bacterial invasion of appendix wall ensues, with eventual necrosis, rupture, and peritonitis (usually within 36 hours)
- Multiple possible presentations are possible due to varied locations of the appendix (e.g., retrocecal, retroileal, or pelvic)—fewer than 50% of patients present with the "classic" history and physical findings

Differential Dx

- Gastroenteritis
- Pelvic inflammatory disease
- Nephrolithiasis
- Terminal ileitis (Yersinia infection or Crohn's disease)
- Intestinal obstruction
- Pancreatitis
- Cholecystitis
- Irritable bowel syndrome
- Tubo-ovarian abscess
- Ovarian cyst/torsion
- Pregnancy/ectopic pregnancy
- Testicular torsion
- UTI/pyelonephritis

Presentation

- Classic presentation: Vague, periumbilical or epigastric pain that migrates to right lower quadrant (i.e., McBurney's point)
- Low-grade fever, anorexia, N/V
- Retrocecal appendix may present with poorly localized or right flank pain; positive psoas sign
- Retroileal appendix: Scrotal pain
- Pelvic appendix: LLQ pain, urge to urinate/defecate, rectal tenderness, obturator sign
- In pregnancy, appendicitis pain may be anywhere in abdomen
- Perforation: High fevers and rigors, peritoneal signs on exam

Diagnosis

- History and physical exam generally suggest the diagnosis
  - Rovsing's sign: RLQ pain upon LLQ palpation
  - Psoas sign: RLQ pain with right hip extension
  - Obturator sign: RLQ pain with hip flexion, internal rotation
- CT with oral contrast is >90% sensitive and specific; may show periappendiceal inflammation ("fat-streaking"), appendiceal dilatation/thickening, abscess; may also show other pathology
- Ultrasound is diagnostic if positive but does not rule out appendicitis if negative
- Abdominal X-ray may show fecalith, appendiceal gas, blurred psoas line, or ileus; however, it has very poor sensitivity and is therefore not indicated
- Leukocytosis and/or neutrophilia (90%) are usually present; however, a normal CBC does not rule out appendicitis
- Urinalysis may show microscopic hematuria and pyuria
- Urine hCG in all females of reproductive age to rule out pregnancy; however, pregnancy does not rule out appendicitis

Treatment

- Administer IV fluids and avoid oral intake
- Narcotics for pain control (studies show that narcotics will *not* mask appendiceal pain and obscure the diagnosis)
- Evaluation and treatment pathway
  - If history and physical exam clearly suggest appendicitis, consult surgery for immediate appendectomy
  - If the diagnosis is uncertain after history and exam, obtain imaging (CT or ultrasound) to prove the diagnosis
  - If diagnosis is still uncertain following imaging, continue with serial abdominal exams and consider short hospital stay for observation
- Appendectomy is treatment-of-choice
  - Surgery before perforation occurs (may occur within 24 hours of symptom onset) will limit morbidity and mortality
- Antibiotics against enteric organisms (gram negatives, anaerobes, and enterococcus) should be given in all patients
  - Administer a 3rd generation cephalosporin
  - In cases of perforation, add metronidazole, clindamycin, gentamycin, or ampicillin

Disposition

- Most patients are admitted for immediate surgery or observation and further workup
- Patients may be discharged if there are no signs of appendicitis on imaging, symptoms do not worsen on serial abdominal exams, and they are able to tolerate oral intake
- Follow-up within 24 hours; return earlier if symptoms worsen
- Complications of perforation include longer recovery times and increased risk of ileus, abscess formation, and sepsis
- Pediatric appendicitis is difficult to diagnose (the only symptoms may be lethargy or decreased activity); most cases result in perforation
- The elderly may also have atypical, unimpressive presentations

45. Inflammatory Bowel Disease

Etiology & Pathophysiology

- Chronic GI inflammation of unknown etiology, possibly autoimmune
- Chronic, relapsing-remitting conditions with flare-ups occurring due to stress, infections, NSAIDs, or medication noncompliance
- Ulcerative colitis (UC): Inflammation of the colon and rectum (called *ulcerative proctitis* if rectum alone is involved)
  - Continuous mucosal inflammation (no skip areas)
  - Involves only the mucosa and submucosa—*not* full-thickness
  - No small bowel involvement
  - Crypt abscesses are formed but there is no granuloma formation
- Crohn's disease: Inflammation may occur anywhere in the GI tract
  - Usually involves the terminal ileum and colon and spares rectum
  - Noncontinuous inflammation (skip lesions)
  - Cobblestoning and fissuring of mucosa
  - Transmural (full-thickness) involvement is characteristic, increasing the risk of perforation, stricture, and fistula formation

Differential Dx

- Bacterial diarrhea (*Shigella, Salmonella, Campylobacter, Yersinia, E. coli*)
- Parasitic or viral GI disease
- *C. difficile* colitis
- Appendicitis
- Diverticulitis
- Mesenteric ischemia
- Colon cancer
- Irritable bowel syndrome
- Pelvic inflammatory disease
- Endometriosis
- Radiation colitis
- Collagen vascular disease

Presentation

- Age peaks of diagnosis occur at ages 15–30 and >55
- Abdominal pain, fever, weight loss, and diarrhea are common to both
- Symptoms of obstruction, megacolon, peritonitis, shock, and/or sepsis may be present
- Ulcerative colitis: Intermittent bouts of bloody, mucous diarrhea with periods of constipation and tenesmus
- Crohn's disease: RLQ mass (may mimic appendicitis) and steatorrhea may be present if there is extensive ileum involvement

Diagnosis

- Electrolyte abnormalities may include hyponatremia, hypokalemia, and decreased bicarbonate due to diarrhea
- CBC may show leukocytosis and anemia of chronic disease
- Fecal leukocytes will be present in these conditions as well as in infectious diarrhea
- Stool cultures for bacteria and ova/parasites if diagnosis unclear
- Abdominal X-rays if suspect perforation or obstruction
- Abdominal CT may show free air, abscesses, thickened bowel loops or mesentery (Crohn's), fistula formation (Crohn's), or toxic megacolon (UC)
- Definitive diagnosis of UC is made by colonoscopy with biopsy, revealing continuous inflammation with friability, exudates, and polyps
- Definitive diagnosis of Crohn's is made by colonoscopy, upper GI series with small bowel follow-through, and barium enema, showing nodularity, rigidity, cobblestoning, fistulas, and strictures

Treatment

- IV fluids as necessary to correct dehydration and electrolytes
- Antidiarrheal therapy (loperamide, diphenoxylate/atropine)
- Therapy is usually undertaken in consultation with GI
- Acute ulcerative colitis
  - Mild disease: Aminosalicylates such as mesalamine (fewer side effects) or sulfasalazine
  - Moderate-severe disease: Aminosalicylates plus an immunosuppressant (e.g., systemic glucocorticoids, azathioprine, or 6-mercaptopurine)
  - Fulminant disease: IV glucocorticoids plus cyclosporine
- Acute Crohn's disease
  - Aminosalicylates, antibiotics (metronidazole or ciprofloxacin), and an immunosuppresant
  - Infliximab (anti-TNF-α) may be useful in acute flares and possibly also as a maintenance therapy
  - IV cyclosporine in severe cases
- Azathioprine and 6-MP may be used to decrease the necessary dosage and duration of steroid therapy
- Colectomy is curative in UC; however, surgery is avoided in Crohn's disease as it will often recur in other areas

Disposition

- Admit patients with severe dehydration, persistent nausea/vomiting, failed outpatient management, or those who require surgery (e.g., for perforation, toxic megacolon, abscess, or fistula)
- Complications of UC include megacolon, perforation, cancer
- Complications of Crohn's include perforation, abscess, obstruction, fistula (to bowel, bladder, or vagina), perianal fissures/abscesses, malabsorption syndromes, and cancer
- Involvement of other organ symptoms occurs in 10% of patients: Arthritis, skin (erythema nodosum), eye (uveitis, iritis), liver (cholelithiasis, sclerosing cholangitis, pancreatitis), pulmonary embolus, anemia, bone (osteoporosis), or malnutrition

46. Diverticular Disease

Etiology & Pathophysiology

- Diverticulosis: Asymptomatic outpouchings of the colonic mucosa through the muscularis layer; occurs at sites where intramural blood vessels penetrate (and thereby weaken) the muscular layer
- Diverticulitis: Infection and inflammation of a colonic diverticulum (occurs in 20% of patients with diverticulosis)
- Diverticular bleeding is the most common cause of lower GI bleeding in the elderly
- Diverticula are caused by increased intra-colonic pressures (e.g., in low-fiber diets, small stool mass requires increased intra-colonic pressures to propel stool)
- Diverticula may be present anywhere in the colon (most common in the sigmoid)
- Complications of diverticulitis include perforation, fistula (colon to bladder, vagina, or skin), abscess formation, and sepsis

Differential Dx

- Appendicitis
- Angiodysplasia
- Renal colic/UTI/pyelonephritis
- Ischemic colitis
- Mesenteric ischemia
- Abdominal aortic aneurysm
- Colon cancer
- Inflammatory bowel disease
- Gastroenteritis
- *C. difficile* colitis
- Intestinal obstruction
- Irritable bowel syndrome
- Pelvic inflammatory disease
- Pregnancy

Presentation

- Diverticulosis is usually asymptomatic; may present with alternating diarrhea/constipation or LLQ pain relieved by bowel movements
- Diverticular bleeding is generally painless, with signs of lower GI bleeding
- Diverticulitis presents with fever, LLQ tenderness, and pain
  - An inflammatory LLQ mass may be present
  - Perforation presents with peritoneal signs, high-grade fever

Diagnosis

- Triad of LLQ pain, fever, and leukocytosis is often present in acute diverticulitis
- Abdominal CT with contrast is usually diagnostic for diverticulitis (will show pericolic fat inflammation or streaking, bowel wall thickening, presence of diverticula, or abscesses) and may rule out other pathologies
- Plain abdominal X-rays will not effectively delineate diverticula but will show obstruction (dilated loops of bowel) or perforation (free air) if present
- Barium enema will show diverticula but is contraindicated in the acute setting
- Sigmoidoscopy or colonoscopy are contraindicated in acute diverticulitis as they may increase the risk of perforation
- Check urine hCG in females of childbearing age
- Urinalysis may show pyuria due to ureteral inflammation

Treatment

- Antibiotics for patients with diverticulitis should cover GI aerobes and anaerobes
  - Oral antibiotics may be used in those not systemically ill (10–14 day course of amoxicillin/clavulanic acid alone or ciprofloxacin plus metronidazole)
  - IV antibiotics are indicated in patients with systemic signs/symptoms, old age, or significant co-morbidities (penicillin/anti-penicillinase, cefoxitin, cefotetan, or a combination of ciprofloxacin plus metronidazole)
  - Life-threatening disease should be treated with IV imipenem or a combination of ampicillin plus gentamycin plus clindamycin
- Surgery may be necessary for abscesses, fistulas, or persistent diverticular bleeding
- Pain control with narcotics as needed
- In suspected cases of diverticular bleeding, stabilize the patient, rule out upper GI bleed (insert NG tube), identify source of bleeding (via colonoscopy, angiography, or Tc-tagged RBC scan), and treat appropriately

Disposition

- Discharge patients who are non-toxic, without severe complaints, able to tolerate fluids, have no significant co-morbid diseases, have good follow-up, and have no evidence of peritonitis
- Admit patients with signs of systemic illness, evidence of peritonitis, inability to tolerate oral fluids, or co-morbidities
- Consult surgery if perforation or abscess is suspected
- All patients require follow-up with enema or colonoscopy after symptoms resolve
- Diverticulitis often recurs—colectomy may be indicated after the second bout (colectomy is suggested after the initial bout in young patients)
- Increase dietary fiber and use stool bulking agents (e.g., psyllium) to help prevent diverticula formation

47. Anorectal Disorders

Etiology & Pathophysiology

- The dentate line defines the junction of the rectum (columnar epithelium) with the anus (squamous epithelium)
- Hemorrhoids: Engorgement, prolapse, or thrombosis of the venous plexuses that drain the anorectum—may be internal (proximal to the dentate line) or external (distal to the dentate line)
  - Internal hemorrhoids are usually painless; pain occurs if they strangulate or thrombose
- Anal cryptitis: Mucosal fold infection due to diarrhea or hard stool
- Anal fissure (most common cause of anal pain): Tear in the anal epithelium distal to the dentate line, due to hard stools or diarrhea
- Anal fistula: Abnormal communication between the anal canal and skin, often associated with anorectal abscess, UC, or Crohn's disease
- Pruritus ani: Anal pruritus caused by anorectal disease, infection, dermatitis (e.g., contact, atopic, psoriasis, lichen planus), neoplasm
- Anorectal abscess may occur proximal or distal to the dentate line

Differential Dx

- Hemorrhoids
- Anal cryptitis
- Anal fissure
- Anorectal abscess
- Anal fistula
- Cancer (anus, rectum, colon)
- STD proctitis (HSV, gonorrhea, chlamydia, syphilis, HIV)
- Rectal foreign body
- Rectal prolapse
- Pruritus ani
- Crohn's disease of the anus
- Ulcerative proctitis
- Pilonidal cyst/abscess

Presentation

- General symptoms include pain that increases with bowel movements or sitting, bright red blood per rectum, and itching
- Hemorrhoids: Pain and bleeding
- Anal fissure: Midline posterior pain
- Pruritus ani: Red, edematous, excoriated skin
- Anal fistula: Malodorous discharge
- Anorectal abscess: Constant pain, fever, and tenderness
- STDs: Itching, irritation, pain, tenesmus, minimal bleeding or discharge

Diagnosis

- Physical exam should include digital rectal exam and anoscopy
- Hemorrhoids: May see prolapsed internal or visible external hemorrhoid, which will be swollen and tender if strangulated
- Cryptitis: Tender, swollen crypts just proximal to dentate line
- Anal fissure: Midline tenderness, anal sphincter spasm, and a sentinel pile (nodular swelling at the distal end of the fissure)
- Anal fistula: Communication of skin with rectum, malodorous discharge
- Anorectal abscess: Fluctuant mass, type depends on location:
  - Perianal abscess: Superficial tender mass on the posterior midline at the anal verge (distal to dentate line), without rectal involvement
  - Ischiorectal abscess: Abscess in lateral rectum/medial buttocks
  - Deep abscess: Tender mass on rectal exam +/− fluctuance
- Signs of STDs may be present (e.g., warts, chancres, vesicles)
- Obtain X-rays if foreign body is suspected

Treatment

- General conservative therapy is sufficient in many cases
  - Stool bulking agents, laxatives and high-fiber diet
  - Sitz baths (3–4 times/day and after bowel movements)
  - Local anesthetics
  - Topical steroids
  - Good anal hygiene after each bowel movement
- Processes that originate proximal to the dentate line (i.e., in the rectum) usually require surgical management
- Hemorrhoids: Conservative therapy for most cases
  - Internal: Reduce prolapsed hemorrhoids; urgent surgery is required if incarcerated, strangulated, or thrombosed
  - Thrombosed external: Consider incision with excision of clot in the ED
- Cryptitis and anal fissure may be treated conservatively
- Anorectal abscesses require drainage either by the ED physician (if simple perianal and distal to the dentate line) or by surgery
- STDs require appropriate antibiotics
- Rectal foreign body must be removed, surgically if necessary

Disposition

- Most patients can be discharged
- Admit patients with signs of systemic infection and consider admission in patients who require surgical intervention
- Urgent surgery is required for strangulated hemorrhoids and anorectal abscesses
- Any patient with rectal bleeding and age >40 or other risk factor for cancer requires a complete GI evaluation

48. Ischemic Bowel Disease

Etiology & Pathophysiology

- Celiac trunk supplies the stomach and duodenum; superior mesenteric artery (SMA) supplies the jejunum, ileum, and right colon; inferior mesenteric artery (IMA) supplies the left colon and rectum
- Acute mesenteric ischemia most commonly occurs due to embolic occlusion (e.g., secondary to Afib, CAD, clotting disorders, aortic dissection, CHF, or post-MI mural thrombus)
- Acute ischemia may also occur due to proximal vessel thrombosis (i.e., secondary to CHF, hypercoagulable states, trauma, pancreatitis) or non-occlusive states with low blood flow to the intestine (e.g., shock, sepsis, GI bleed, dehydration, arrhythmia, MI, CHF)
- Chronic mesenteric ischemia (intestinal angina) occurs due to atherosclerotic narrowing of mesenteric arteries
- Ischemic colitis is a non-occlusive (never embolic) process involving the IMA that occurs secondary to low-flow states
- Mesenteric venous thrombosis may also occur

Differential Dx

- Perforated viscus (e.g., duodenal/gastric ulcer)
- Intestinal obstruction
- Abdominal aortic aneurysm
- Aortic dissection
- Pancreatitis
- Cholelithiasis
- Inflammatory bowel disease
- Hernia
- Volvulus
- Intussusception
- Diverticulitis
- Colon cancer
- Infectious colitis

Presentation

- Acute mesenteric ischemia: Sudden (embolic) or subacute (thrombotic) onset of severe abdominal pain, vomiting, diarrhea, and occult blood; exam may be benign (pain out of proportion to exam); mental status changes may occur; peritonitis (guarding, rigidity, rebound) and hypotension occur late
- Chronic mesenteric ischemia: Dull, crampy, *postprandial* abdominal pain and extensive weight loss (fear of eating due to pain); abdominal bruit may be present
- Ischemic colitis: Episodic crampy LLQ pain, hematochezia, diarrhea

Diagnosis

- Elevated lactate levels (nearly 100% sensitive, 40% specific), LDH, WBCs, alk phos, and CPK; 50% have metabolic acidosis
- Abdominal X-ray is used to exclude perforation (free air) and obstruction (dilated loops of bowel)
- Abdominal CT is often normal early in the course, otherwise may show bowel wall thickening, mesenteric edema or streaking, free air, pneumotosis intestinalis (air in the intestinal wall), or venous thrombosis and may rule out other pathologies
- Angiography is the gold standard for diagnosis and may also be therapeutic (via injection of papaverine)
- Duplex Doppler ultrasound and/or angiography to diagnose chronic mesenteric ischemia
- Colonoscopy or barium enema is diagnostic for ischemic colitis; abdominal X-ray may show "thumbprinting" (edematous haustral folds)

Treatment

- Acute mesenteric ischemia
  - Replace intravascular volume with normal saline
  - Correct predisposing causes (e.g., hypotension—but avoid vasopressors as they may exacerbate ischemia)
  - IV antibiotics to cover gram negatives and anaerobes
  - Angiography with papaverine (a vasodilator that is especially useful in non-occlusive ischemia to decrease vasospasm) may be attempted as the initial treatment
  - Exploratory laparotomy for resection of dead bowel is necessary if peritoneal signs are present or if angiography fails
  - Intra-arterial thrombolytics are investigational
- Chronic mesenteric ischemia: Surgical revascularization is the definitive therapy (via percutaneous transluminal angioplasty, endarterectomy, or bypass)
- Ischemic colitis: Supportive care with antibiotics, bowel rest, and hydration; surgery is rarely needed
- Mesenteric venous thrombosis: Thrombolysis and long-term anticoagulation

Disposition

- Most patients are admitted
- Patients who are definitively diagnosed with ischemia should proceed to angiography or directly to surgery
- Discharge if mesenteric ischemia is effectively ruled out and no other serious abdominal pathology exists
- Mortality 50–100%
- Outcomes depend on an aggressive diagnostic and therapeutic approach—early angiography or surgery is essential
- Patients are at increased risk of sepsis due to intestinal mucosal breakdown with bacterial invasion

49. Abdominal Aortic Aneurysm

Etiology & Pathophysiology

- Dilation of the aorta >3 cm secondary to a weakened aortic wall
- 90% of aneurysms originate below the renal arteries; however, AAA may involve renal, mesenteric, and spinal arteries, resulting in organ ischemia (e.g., mesenteric ischemia causing abdominal pain, spinal ischemia causing lower extremity paralysis)
- Once present, aneurysms typically grow 0.3–0.5 cm/year
- Untreated AAAs may rupture, resulting in high mortality
- Risk factors include atherosclerosis, hypertension, connective tissue diseases (e.g., Takayasu's arteritis), Marfan syndrome, age >60, male sex, family history, tobacco use, peripheral vascular disease, vasculitis, and trauma
- Bacterial invasion accounts for 5% of AAAs (e.g., *Staphylococcus, syphilis*, and *Salmonella*)

Differential Dx

- Iliac artery aneurysm
- Renal colic
- Pancreatitis
- GI bleed
- Peptic ulcer disease/GERD
- Acute MI/myocardial ischemia
- Diverticulitis
- Mesenteric ischemia
- Cholecystitis/biliary colic
- Sepsis
- Aortic dissection
- Musculoskeletal back pain
- Other causes of syncope
- Herpes zoster

Presentation

- Unruptured AAA causes few symptoms
  - Vague abdominal/back pain
  - Pulsatile abdominal mass
  - Abdominal bruit
  - SMA syndrome (N/V, weight loss due to duodenal compression) may be present
- Ruptured AAA
  - Severe back, abdominal, or flank pain that may radiate to the groin
  - Hypotension and tachycardia
  - Syncope
  - Abdominal mass on exam
  - Retroperitoneal hematoma (Grey-Turner/Cullen's signs)

Diagnosis

- Obtain CBC, chemistries, coagulation factors, and type/cross
- Bedside ultrasound is diagnostic for AAA; however, it is insensitive for rupture
- Patients diagnosed with a AAA on ultrasound who exhibit signs and symptoms consistent with rupture should proceed to surgery immediately without further imaging studies
- Abdominal CT is also diagnostic for AAA and will detect nearly all cases of rupture
  - Used only in stable patients
  - Provides anatomic details, surgical landmarks, and arterial involvement of aneurysm
  - May detect alternative diagnoses
- Plain films have poor sensitivity and specificity for AAA: May demonstrate a dilated, calcified aortic wall, loss of psoas shadow, or paravertebral soft tissue mass

Treatment

- Asymptomatic AAAs discovered incidentally require only outpatient vascular surgery follow-up
  - If <5 cm, follow with serial ultrasounds, avoid tobacco, and manage hypertension and hyperlipidemia
  - If >5 cm, elective surgery is indicated due to risk of rupture
- Unstable patients require bedside ultrasound
  - If positive, emergent surgery is indicated
  - In hypotensive patients, maintain BP with blood products and normal saline
  - In hypertensive patients, BP control with antihypertensive medications have not been shown to limit hemorrhage or improve outcome
- Stable patients may undergo ultrasound and CT to further delineate the pathology
  - If rupture is confirmed on CT scan, emergent surgical repair is indicated (patient can rapidly decompensate)
- Current surgical techniques include placement of an extravascular or endovascular graft

Disposition

- Admit all patients with symptoms for further surgical/medical management
- Discharge patients with asymptomatic, incidentally identified AAAs with close follow-up
- Educate patient about warning signs/symptoms of impending rupture (e.g., increased abdominal/back pain)
- Rupture is fatal without surgery
- 50% perioperative mortality following rupture
- 5% elective perioperative mortality
- Graft infection (*S. epidermidis* is most common) carries a 30% mortality and may result in systemic infection
- Aortoenteric fistula formation (often due to infected graft) may result in GI bleeding—GI bleeding in any patient with aortic repair is a fistula until proven otherwise

50. Hepatitis

Etiology & Pathophysiology

- Inflammation of the liver due to viral, autoimmune, toxic (e.g., alcohol, *Amanita* mushrooms), medications (e.g., isoniazid, methyldopa, ketoconazole, acetaminophen), or ischemic insults
- Alcoholic and viral hepatitis are the most common causes in the US
- Damage may be due to direct toxic effects, infiltration, or cholestasis
- Acute hepatitis lasts <6 months and results in either resolution of disease or aggressive deterioration to liver failure
- Chronic hepatitis is a sustained inflammation of the liver for >6 mo
- Viral hepatitis: Hepatitis A, B, C, D, E; EBV; HSV; CMV
  - HAV: Self-limited, rarely fatal, not chronic, fecal-oral spread
  - HBV: May result in cirrhosis or chronic carrier state; transmission by sexual, IV drug use, and blood
  - HCV: Mild acute disease, but 70% develop chronic disease and some have liver failure after 15–25 years; blood transmission
  - HDV: Rapid liver failure; occurs only concurrently with HBV

Differential Dx

- Cholecystitis
- Cholelithiasis
- Cholangitis
- Biliary cirrhosis
- Steatohepatitis
- Reye's disease
- Tetracycline toxicity
- Hemolytic anemia
- Dubin-Johnson syndrome
- Carcinoma (e.g., biliary, head of pancreas)
- Biliary atresia and strictures

Presentation

- Acute hepatitis: Jaundice, dark urine/light stools, hepatomegaly, fatigue, malaise, lethargy, RUQ pain/tenderness, N/V, fever
- Liver failure/cirrhosis may occur: Ascites, edema due to hypoalbuminemia, hepatic encephalopathy (e.g., confusion, stupor, coma, rigidity, asterixis), spider angiomas, palmar erythema, esophageal varices/bleeding
  - Patients with liver failure require a workup for complications (see the *Cirrhosis* entry)
- History may reveal alcohol use, IV drugs, transfusions, high-risk sex, family history, toxic medications

Diagnosis

- Laboratory abnormalities
  - Elevated AST and ALT in liver inflammation (AST/ALT ratio >2 suggests alcoholic liver disease)
  - Elevated total and direct bilirubin in cholestasis, liver disease
  - Elevated alkaline phosphatase in biliary tract obstructions, cholestasis, primary biliary cirrhosis, sclerosing cholangitis
  - Hypoalbuminemia and elevated PT due to impaired synthesis of albumin and coagulation factors (II, VII, IX, X)
  - Hyperammonemia due to impaired NH_3 metabolism
- Hepatitis virus serologies
  - HAV: Elevated IgM in acute infection, IgG in prior exposure
  - HBV: IgM anti-HBc (core antibody) in acute infection; HBs Ag (surface antigen) in chronic hepatitis; HBe antigen indicates high infectivity; anti-HBs (surface antibody) indicates immunity (prior infection or vaccination)
  - HCV: IgG may be elevated after 6–8 weeks of infection
  - HDV: Positive IgM or IgG

Treatment

- Symptomatic relief of nausea, vomiting, and diarrhea; however, avoid hepatotoxic agents and all medications that are metabolized by the liver
- Avoid offending substances (e.g., alcohol, drugs)
- Correct clinical and metabolic abnormalities
  - Gentle hydration, correct electrolytes and acid/base status
  - Normalize coagulation with fresh frozen plasma
  - Treat hypoglycemia
  - Lactulose and neomycin to decrease ammonia in cases of hepatic encephalopathy
- Definitive inpatient therapies may include
  - HBV: Interferon and lamivudine
  - HCV: Recombinant interferon and ribavirin
  - Autoimmune hepatitis: Glucocorticoids
- End-stage liver failure may require liver transplant
- Contact prophylaxis is available for Hepatitis A and B
  - HAV: Complete vaccine 2 weeks prior to travel; immune globulin for household, institutional, day-care contacts
  - HBV/HDV: Vaccine and immune globulin following exposure (within 7 days)

Disposition

- Admit patients with any clinical or metabolic derangements (e.g., persistent nausea/vomiting, encephalopathy, renal failure, electrolyte disturbances)
- ICU admission for fulminant hepatic failure
- All pregnant or immunocompromised patients are admitted
- Patients with minor symptoms that can be controlled in the ED may be discharged with close follow-up
- All patients with unexplained liver function test elevations must be evaluated by gastroenterology
- Chronic inflammation eventually scars the liver, producing cirrhosis with cellular dysfunction, portal HTN, and portosystemic shunting of blood (see the *Cirrhosis* entry)

51. Cirrhosis

Etiology & Pathophysiology

- Cirrhosis is the end result of a hepatocellular injury that leads to fibrosis and nodular regeneration of the liver
- Clinical features result from hepatic cell dysfunction (synthetic or metabolic), portal hypertension, and porto-systemic shunting
- Most cases are due to chronic alcohol abuse or viral hepatitis; however, any chronic liver disease (e.g., Wilson's disease, hemochromatosis, medication use, PSC, PBC) or massive acute injury (e.g., drug overdose) may result in cirrhosis
- Complications
  - Variceal hemorrhage (esophageal vein rupture due to portal HTN)
  - Ascites (due to portal HTN, 3rd spacing, and volume overload)
  - Spontaneous bacterial peritonitis (SBP) (infected ascitic fluid)
  - Hepatic encephalopathy (due to accumulation of nitrogenous wastes)
  - Hepatorenal syndrome (renal failure despite normal kidneys; due to decreased intravascular volume plus renal vasoconstriction)

Differential Dx

- 1° biliary cirrhosis
- 2° biliary cirrhosis
- Noncirrhotic hepatic fibrosis (CHF and constrictive pericarditis may lead to hepatic fibrosis with resulting ascites and may be mistaken for cirrhosis)

Presentation

- Weakness, fatigue, weight loss
- Anorexia, nausea/vomiting
- Firm, nodular liver
- S/S of portal hypertension: Ascites (abdominal distension, dyspnea), hepatosplenomegaly, caput medusae, esophageal varices (GI bleed, hypotension)
- S/S of liver failure: Jaundice, spider angiomata, palmar erythema, gynecomastia, testicular atrophy, impotence, bruising, and hypocoagulation
- Hepatic encephalopathy: Coma, lethargy, confusion, asterixis
- SBP: Fever, abdominal pain and tenderness, mental status changes

Diagnosis

- Liver enzymes are elevated early due to chronic liver disease but may be normal once significant cirrhosis ensues
- Hypoalbuminemia, hypocholesterolemia, and decreased coagulation factors (increased PT/PTT) due to poor hepatic hormone and protein synthesis
- Azotemia and electrolyte disturbances (decreased Na^+ and K^+)
- CBC may reveal anemia, thrombocytopenia
- Ammonia level is elevated in hepatic encephalopathy
- To aid diagnosis, obtain hepatitis profile, iron studies, autoantibodies (ANA, ASMA, AMA), ceruloplasmin, copper
- Ultrasound may show gallstones or ductal dilatation, and provides evidence of abnormal liver architecture
- Abdominal CT will detect masses, fatty liver, dilated ducts, and other abdominal pathology
- Paracentesis of ascitic fluid to diagnose SBP (>1000 WBC, >250 PMNs, or organisms present)—should be obtained in the presence of ascites with unexplained fever or abdominal pain

Treatment

- Variceal bleed
  - Protect airway and intubate as necessary
  - Correct coagulation abnormalities with FFP
  - IV somatostatin (octreotide) will decrease variceal pressure and bleeding
  - GI for emergent EGD with sclerotherapy or band ligation
  - Sengstaken-Blakemore tube while awaiting endoscopy
  - β-blockers and nitrates may be used for prophylaxis
- Hepatic encephalopathy
  - Narcan, thiamine, and dextrose to rule out other causes
  - Oral lactulose (traps NH_3 in gut), and oral neomycin (decreases NH_3 production by gut bacteria)
- Ascites: Administer diuretics, restrict sodium intake, and consider paracentesis (may be diagnostic and therapeutic) with appropriate fluid studies
- Spontaneous bacterial peritonitis: IV antibiotics (e.g., cefotaxime, ceftriaxone, or penicillin/anti-penicillinase)
- Hepatorenal: Correct hypovolemia and stabilize electrolytes
- Avoid liver toxins (e.g., alcohol, medications)

Disposition

- Hospitalize for acute deterioration and to manage complications (e.g., encephalopathy, hepatorenal syndrome, SBP)
- Admit to ICU for GI bleed or advanced hepatic encephalopathy
- Mortality of variceal bleed is 30–60%
- Mortality of hepatorenal syndrome: 80%
- Discharge if cirrhosis is well-compensated and close follow-up is possible
- Liver transplant is the only cure for advanced cirrhosis

52. Gallbladder Disease

Etiology & Pathophysiology

- Cholelithiasis: Asymptomatic gallstones
- Choledocholithiasis: Gallstones lodged in the common bile duct
- Biliary colic: Intermittent blockage of the cystic or common bile ducts by gallstones, resulting in transient, colicky pain
- Acute cholecystitis: Persistent (>6 hrs), painful obstruction of the cystic duct, resulting in gallbladder inflammation and infection
- Cholangitis: Obstruction of the common bile duct resulting in inflammation and infection; may progress to sepsis and shock
- Gallstone pancreatitis: Blockage of pancreatic duct by a gallstone resulting in pancreatitis (2nd most common cause after alcohol)
- Risk factors: Female, fat, forty, fertile (pregnancy), rapid weight loss, diabetes, inflammatory bowel disease, cirrhosis
- Gallbladder disease may also result from biliary dyskinesia (abnormal contraction), acalculous cholecystitis, and sphincter of Oddi dysfunction

Differential Dx

- Abdominal aortic aneurysm
- Renal colic
- Pyelonephritis/UTI
- Pancreatitis
- Peptic ulcer disease/gastritis
- Perforated duodenal ulcer
- Hepatitis
- Appendicitis
- Diverticulitis
- RLL pneumonia
- Renal colic
- Pelvic inflammatory disease
- Mesenteric ischemia
- Pregnancy (normal or ectopic)

Presentation

- Biliary colic: Dull, achy RUQ pain that lasts <6 hrs and occurs >1×/week; usually occurs after a large, fatty meal; Murphy's sign (RUQ tenderness with inspiration) is present during episodes; anorexia, N/V, afebrile
- Acute cholecystitis: Severe, steady RUQ or epigastric pain lasting >6 hrs; may radiate to right scapula; positive Murphy's sign; may have rebound/guarding, N/V, fever
- Cholangitis: Charcot's triad (RUQ pain, fever, and jaundice); peritoneal signs may be present; may have decreased mental status and shock due to sepsis

Diagnosis

- Initial labs should include CBC, LFTs, bilirubin, amylase/lipase, urinalysis, and pregnancy test
  - Normal labs in biliary colic/cholelithiasis
  - May see elevated WBCs and LFTs in cholecystitis
  - Elevated amylase/lipase in gallstone pancreatitis
- U/S is the gold standard for diagnosis of gallbladder pathology
  - May show gallstones or ductal dilatation
  - In acute cholecystitis, will show distended gallbladder, thickened walls, and pericholecystic fluid
- CT scan may also be used but it is somewhat less accurate than ultrasound for gallbladder disease; will rule out other pathology
- Plain films are not useful for gallbladder disease; abdominal X-ray will rule out other abdominal pathology (e.g., intestinal obstruction/perforation), CXR will identify pulmonary disease
- Hepatobiliary nuclear scan (HIDA scan) may be used after admission to diagnose acalculous cholecystitis

Treatment

- Biliary colic generally only requires IV fluids, no oral intake until symptoms resolve, and analgesia
  - NSAIDs (especially ketorolac) plus narcotics for pain (meperidine is generally preferred as morphine may theoretically cause sphincter of Oddi spasm)
  - Antispasmodics (e.g., dicyclomine) and antiemetics
- Acute cholecystitis will require cholecystectomy
  - IV fluids, NPO, antiemetics, and analgesia as above
  - Administer IV antibiotics to cover gram negatives, anaerobes, and enterococcus (e.g., penicillin/anti-penicillinase, ceftriaxone plus metronidazole, imipenem, or ampicillin plus gentamycin plus metronidazole)
  - Cholecystectomy is generally delayed for 3–5 days to allow gallbladder inflammation to decrease
  - Unstable patients may require urgent surgical intervention (cholecystectomy or percutaneous drainage)
- Cholangitis requires emergent, aggressive intervention
  - Aggressive IV fluids and pressors as needed for shock
  - Broad-spectrum antibiotics and analgesia as above
  - Emergent biliary drainage if no improvement within 24 hrs

Disposition

- Admit patients with acute cholecystitis, acute cholangitis, common bile duct obstruction, or gallstone pancreatitis
- Discharge if there is no clinical evidence of gallbladder disease other than simple biliary colic, if pain has resolved, and if patient is able to tolerate oral intake
- Though many people have symptomatic cholelithiasis, few cases will result in cholecystitis—however, once infection occurs, surgery to remove the gallbladder is indicated
- Patients with recurrent biliary colic may undergo elective lithotripsy or cholecystectomy
- Complications include pancreatitis, ascending cholangitis, gallbladder empyema, or gangrene

53. Pancreatitis

Etiology & Pathophysiology

- Pancreatic inflammation associated with edema, autodigestion, necrosis, and possibly hemorrhage
- Varies from mild, self-limited disease to severe pancreatitis with systemic multiorgan failure and death
- 80% of acute attacks are due to cholelithiasis or alcohol
- Risk factors include alcohol use, cholelithiasis, abdominal trauma or surgery, hypercalcemia, ampullary stenosis, penetrating ulcers, pregnancy, SLE, parasite infection, ischemia, hyperlipidemia, drugs (e.g., OCPs, steroids, diuretics, aspirin), viral infections, scorpion bite, recent ERCP, family history
- Chronic pancreatitis is a slowly progressive destruction of pancreatic tissue from inflammation, fibrosis, and distortion of the pancreatic ducts, most commonly due to alcohol abuse
    - Classic triad of pancreatic calcifications, steatorrhea, and diabetes
    - Amylase and lipase may not be elevated in chronic disease

Differential Dx

- Gastritis
- Perforated viscus (acutely perforated duodenal ulcer)
- Acute cholecystitis
- Acute intestinal obstruction
- Aortic aneurysm rupture
- Renal colic
- Mesenteric ischemia
- Mesenteric thrombosis
- Ectopic pregnancy
- Myocardial infarction
- Pneumonia

Presentation

- Steady, severe epigastric pain that radiates to the back
    - Begins 1–4 hours after large meal or alcohol intake
    - Relieved by leaning forward
- N/V, distension, dyspnea
- Exam may reveal fever, decreased bowel sounds, tachycardia, bluish discoloration of umbilicus (Cullen's sign) or flank (Grey-Turner sign)
- Severe disease may present with signs of volume depletion, hypotension, peritonitis, and shock
- Chronic pancreatitis: Abdominal pain, N/V, anorexia, steatorrhea, constipation, jaundice, weight loss

Diagnosis

- Lipase and amylase are generally elevated in acute disease (lipase has higher specificity and sensitivity; amylase is also found in the salivary glands, adipose tissue, and elsewhere)
- Labs should include CBC, electrolytes, BUN/Cr, LDH, LFTs
    - Electrolyte abnormalities (e.g., hypokalemia, hypocalcemia)
    - Elevated LFTs and LDH in biliary disease
    - Decreased hemoglobin in hemorrhagic pancreatitis
- Plain films are nonspecific and may show isolated left pleural effusion, atelectasis, dilated sentinel bowel loop and will rule out pneumonia and perforation
- Abdominal CT may show inflammation but is insensitive for pancreatitis; indicated for critically ill patients to rule out necrotizing pancreatitis and other abdominal pathology
- U/S has poor sensitivity for pancreatic pathology but will show associated biliary tract disease (e.g., ductal dilatation, stones)
- Inpatient ERCP may be used to evaluate for biliary obstruction

Treatment

- Supportive care is the mainstay of treatment
    - Aggressive IV fluid replacement (normal saline) is necessary due to 3rd spacing into the retroperitoneal space—titrate fluids to maintain BP and urine output
    - Clear liquids in mild disease
    - Bowel rest (NG tube, NPO) in severe disease, ileus, N/V
    - Meperidine for pain (morphine may theoretically cause sphincter of Oddi dysfunction)
    - Antiemetics as necessary
    - Monitor and correct electrolytes (especially calcium)
- Indications for surgery after admission: To confirm disease in severe pancreatitis unresponsive to treatment, to relieve biliary or pancreatic duct obstruction, to drain abscess or debride necrotic pancreatic tissue, or for necrosis or sepsis
- Complications of pancreatitis include persistent ductal obstruction (may require ERCP with sphincterotomy), pseudocyst formation, abscess/necrosis (develops 2–4 weeks after acute episode and requires drainage and broad-spectrum antibiotics), and ARDS (3–7 days after initial event, most require intubation)

Disposition

- Most patients are admitted
- Patients with hemorrhagic or necrotizing pancreatitis, respiratory distress, or shock should be admitted to the ICU
- Discharge is acceptable for patients with mild pancreatitis without anatomical abnormalities who are able to tolerate clear liquids
- Ranson's criteria are used to assess severity and mortality
    - Mortality <1% if <3 criteria are present; nearly 100% if >6
    - Criteria at presentation: Age >55, WBC >16,000, glucose >200, LDH >350, and AST >250
    - Criteria after 48 hours: HCT decrease of more than 10%, BUN increase of >5 mg/dL, calcium <8, PaO_2 <60, base deficit >4, fluid deficit >6 L

Hematologic-
Oncologic
Emergencies

MICHAEL C. BOND, MD

54. Anemia

Etiology & Pathophysiology

- Hemoglobin (Hb) <12 mg/dL
- Due to decreased production of hemoglobin, increased destruction of RBCs, or blood loss
    - Decreased production (marrow failure): Pernicious anemia, thalassemia, chronic liver or renal disease, malignancy, folic acid deficiency, vitamin B_{12} deficiency, or iron deficiency
    - Increased destruction: Infection, sickle cell disease, and immune mediated hemolysis
    - Loss of blood: Hemorrhage, trauma, chronic GI bleeding, and excessive blood donation or blood draws
- Chronic anemia is much better tolerated than acute anemia
- Anemia is classified based on RBC size (i.e., microcytic, macrocytic, or normocytic) and hemoglobin concentration (i.e., hypochromic or normochromic)

Differential Dx

- Microcytic: Iron deficiency, anemia of chronic disease, lead poisoning, thalassemia
- Macrocytic: Vitamin B_{12} or folate deficiency, liver disease, alcohol, hypothyroidism, HIV
- Normocytic: Aplastic anemia, hemorrhage, anemia of chronic disease, hemolysis (drug-induced, autoimmune, SLE), marrow disease, infection, hypothyroidism, renal insufficiency, sickle cell disease, microangiopathy, membrane defects, DIC, TTP

Presentation

- Decreased exercise tolerance
- Easy fatigability
- Dyspnea on exertion
- Altered mental status
- Chest pain
- Cold intolerance
- Headaches
- Pallor
- Postural hypotension/syncope
- Tachycardia and hypotension
- Heme-positive stools (in cases of GI bleed)
- Jaundice (in cases of hemolysis)
- Glossitis (B_{12} deficiency)

Diagnosis

- Detailed history and physical exam, including rectal and guaiac
- CBC: Note red cell indices—MCV, MCH, RDW
- Peripheral smear may show characteristic cell types (e.g., spherocytes, schistocytes, multinucleated cells)
- Reticulocyte count is increased if anemia is due to blood loss or RBC destruction; decreased if due to marrow failure
- Further studies may include iron panel (iron, ferritin, transferrin saturation, TIBC), haptoglobin, B_{12} and folate levels, bilirubin, LDH, LFTs, TSH, renal function, blood type and cross, hemoglobin electrophoresis, bone marrow aspirate, GI workup
- Classify the etiology based on laboratory results
    - Iron deficiency: ↓ ferritin, reticulocytes, MCV, MCH; ↑ TIBC
    - Chronic disease: ↓ reticulocytes, TIBC; normal MCV, MCH
    - B_{12}/folate deficiency: ↓ reticulocytes; ↑ MCV
    - Marrow failure: ↓ reticulocytes; may involve other cell lines
    - Hemolysis: ↑ reticulocytes, bilirubin, LDH; ↓ haptoglobin in cases of intravascular hemolysis

Treatment

- Supplemental O_2
- In cases of ongoing acute blood loss: Establish 2 large bore IVs, monitor, and send for blood type and cross (note that change in Hb levels may lag behind actual blood loss)
- IV fluids as necessary to maintain blood pressure
- Blood transfusion is generally indicated for hemoglobin <8
    - Young, healthy patients should only be transfused if they are symptomatic or have ongoing acute blood losses
    - Cardiac patients may require transfusion at Hb <10
    - Avoid transfusing beyond a Hb of 12 as this may result in increased blood viscosity, which may impair O_2 delivery
- Therapy of hemolytic anemia may include systemic steroids, avoidance of precipitating drugs, and transfusions; therapy should be instituted only in consultation with a hematologist
- Supplement vitamin B_{12}, folate, and iron as necessary
- Patients with primary marrow disorders require transfusions, further evaluation, and possibly a bone marrow transplant

Disposition

- Most patients can be discharged home, assuming adequate outpatient follow-up is available
- Criteria for admission
    - Active blood loss
    - Initial unexplained Hb <8 mg/dL
    - Cardiac symptoms (e.g., SOB, CP)
    - Patients requiring transfusion
    - Symptomatic patients
    - Unstable vital signs
    - Aplastic anemia
    - Significant co-morbid disease
- Patients with unexplained iron deficiency anemia should be referred for outpatient colon cancer screening

55. Sickle Cell Disease

Etiology & Pathophysiology

- An autosomal recessive disorder resulting in defective hemoglobin
- Defect is in position 6 of the β-globin gene, where valine substitutes for glutamic acid; this defective hemoglobin has diminished solubility in the deoxygenated form, resulting in sickling of RBCs that have difficulty traversing the microvasculature
- Hemolytic anemia results as the spleen removes these abnormal cells
- Acute sickling ("vaso-occlusive crisis") results in occlusions and infarcts of the spleen, brain, kidney, lung, and other organs
- Causes of crises include hypoxia, acidosis, dehydration, infection, temperature changes, stress, pregnancy, alcohol, and menstruation
- Patients with sickle cell disease are at increased risk of infection with encapsulated organisms (e.g., *S pneumoniae, H influenzae, Salmonella*)
- Homozygotes are affected; heterozygotes are carriers
- Very common in African-American populations

Differential Dx

- Acquired hemoglobinopathies (methemoglobin, sulfhemoglobin, carboxyhemoglobin)
- Thalassemias
- Iron-deficiency anemia
- Bone marrow disease (leukemia)
- Other inherited hemoglobinopathies

Presentation

- Anemia: Pallor, fatigue
- Hemolysis: Jaundice, cholelithiasis
- Microvascular occlusion: Finger swelling, bone pain, leg ulcers, priapism, CVA, blindness
- Vaso-occlusive crisis: Pain in back, chest, abdomen, or extremities
- Acute chest syndrome: Severe pleuritic chest pain, hypoxemia, dyspnea, and tachypnea
- Splenic/hepatic sequestration crisis: Fever, splenomegaly, pallor, and abdominal pain
- Acute aplastic anemia (often due to infection): Rapid onset of profound anemia and fever

Diagnosis

- Prior diagnosis has usually been established upon presentation
- Definitive diagnosis via hemoglobin electrophoresis
- CBC with peripheral smear (baseline Hb usually 6–10 mg/dL)
    - Microcytic, hypochromic anemia; sickled cells
    - RBCs are often profoundly decreased during hemolytic and hypoplastic crises; normal in painful crises
    - WBC may be elevated due to crisis or to concurrent infection
- Reticulocyte count is increased in most crises (to replace sickled, damaged RBCs); decreased during hypoplastic crises
- Elevated bilirubin due to hemolytic anemia
- Blood cultures, urinalysis and urine culture, sputum samples, and lumbar puncture may be necessary to rule out infection
- CXR may show evidence of pneumonia or acute chest crisis
- Bone X-ray and/or bone scan may show evidence of bone infarction, osteomyelitis, or joint osteonecrosis
- Head CT to rule out hemorrhage during acute CVA

Treatment

- Blood type and cross
- Aggressive IV hydration with D5½NS or D5W is preferred due to hyposthenuria (defective renal concentration)
- Supplemental O_2 (sat >92%) minimizes peripheral sickling
- Antibiotics if suspect or cannot rule out infection: 3rd generation cephalosporin plus source-specific antibiotics
- IV narcotics for pain control: Morphine sulfate is the preferred agent (less addictive than meperidine); consider PCA pump so patient can control the dosing
- Blood transfusion if Hb <5, symptomatic anemia, aplastic anemia, or splenic sequestration crisis occurs; do not transfuse beyond HCT >25 as this may worsen symptoms due to increased blood viscosity
- Exchange transfusions to replace patient's sickled blood with donor blood should be considered in acute chest syndrome, acute CVA, priapism, or hepatic sequestration crisis
- Hydroxyurea is an antisickling agent that will increase production of fetal hemoglobin to augment O_2 delivery

Disposition

- Disease follows a relapsing/remitting course with acute exacerbations/crises and potential chronic complications
- Symptoms may last up to 4–6 days
- Admit for infection, uncontrolled pain, acute chest syndrome, splenic or hepatic sequestration crisis, severe anemia, aplastic crisis, acute CVA, priapism, cholecystitis, severe renal disease, or ophthalmic symptoms
- Discharge is acceptable if pain is easily controlled and underlying causes of crisis are adequately treated (e.g., dehydration, infection)
- Instruct patient to avoid possible triggers, such as infection, fever, hypoxia, dehydration, and low O_2 tension (i.e., high altitudes)

56. Platelet Disorders

Etiology & Pathophysiology

- Thrombocytopenia is most commonly due to accelerated platelet destruction; may also occur due to decreased marrow production or increased splenic sequestration
- Thrombotic thrombocytopenic purpura (TTP): Diffuse vessel wall injury results in thrombocytopenia, microangiopathic hemolytic anemia, fever, renal dysfunction, and CNS symptoms; idiopathic or due to infection, pregnancy, medication, or autoimmune diseases
- Idiopathic thrombocytopenic purpura (ITP): Platelet destruction caused by anti-platelet antibodies; often associated with viral illness
- Disseminated intravascular coagulation (DIC): Life-threatening disorder in which coagulation factors are inappropriately activated, resulting in ischemia (due to thrombosis of small vessels) and bleeding (due to consumption of clotting factors); caused by diffuse endothelial injury or release of tissue factors (e.g., sepsis, pregnancy, trauma, burns, malignancy)

Differential Dx

- Increased platelet destruction: Drugs (e.g., digoxin, HCTZ, PCN, antibiotics, clopidogrel, amiodarone, heroin, cocaine), ITP, TTP, DIC, HUS, sepsis, transfusion reaction, prosthetic valve, viral infections, HELLP syndrome, hypothyroidism
- Decreased marrow production: Myelodysplasia, alcohol, marrow infiltration by cancer cells, cytotoxic drugs
- Sequestration: Leukemia, lymphoma, portal HTN

Presentation

- Superficial bleeding
  - Skin: Easy bruising, petechiae developing into purpura
  - Mucous membranes: Epistaxis, gingival bleeding, GI bleeding
  - Genitourinary: Menorrhagia
- Splenomegaly (in cases of splenic sequestration)
- TTP: Fever, jaundice, confusion, headache, coma
- DIC: Bleeding phenomena (e.g., skin/mucous membrane bleeding; hemorrhage from surgical scars, puncture sites, and IV sites) and thrombotic phenomena (e.g., gangrenous digits, genitalia, and nose; peripheral acrocyanosis)

Diagnosis

- CBC, electrolytes, BUN/creatinine, LDH
- Peripheral smear: Fragmented RBCs (schistocytes) in DIC, TTP
- Prolonged bleeding time in all cases
- PT and PTT are increased in DIC; normal in other etiologies
- TTP: Anemia, thrombocytopenia, increased bilirubin and LDH, increased BUN and creatinine, hematuria, and proteinuria
- ITP: Peripheral smear shows large platelets without hemolysis or schistocytes; history of viral illness/URI; normal LDH
- DIC: Increased fibrin split products and D-dimer; decreased fibrinogen
- Bone marrow exam as an inpatient may be required if etiology is uncertain
- Abdominal CT to rule out hypersplenism due to platelet sequestration
- Head CT to rule out intracerebral bleed if there are any mental status changes

Treatment

- Treat the underlying disorder (e.g., infection, placental abruption) or avoid causative medications
- Platelet transfusion is indicated if platelet count is <10,000 due to risk of major hemorrhage; if platelets >30,000, transfusion is indicated only if bleeding
- DIC: Bleeding can usually be controlled with fresh frozen plasma, platelets, and/or cryoprecipitate
  - Heparin therapy has no proven benefit in DIC treatment
- TTP: Plasma exchange is the treatment of choice; IVIG may be helpful; avoid platelet transfusions (may worsen disease) except in cases of severe bleeding
  - Steroids have not been proven to be effective
- ITP: Systemic steroids +/- IVIG; immunosuppressive agents may be required; danazol or splenectomy for persistent disease
  - It is unclear if asymptomatic patients need treatment
  - Self-limited in children—no therapy required

Disposition

- Consult hematology for significant thrombocytopenia
- Admission criteria
  - Significant bleeding
  - Need for IV medication/transfusion
  - Unclear future course of platelet levels
  - Poor outpatient follow-up
  - Platelets <30,000
  - Diagnosis of DIC or TTP
- ICU admission may be needed for close monitoring depending on the cause
- ITP: Acute course with self-limited remission in children; often chronic and persistent in adults
- DIC is often progressive and fatal; treatment is supportive until the underlying cause can be reversed
- Close follow-up for discharged patients

57. Hemophilia and von Willebrand's Disease

Etiology & Pathophysiology

- Hemophilia A and B are clinically indistinguishable, x-linked recessive disorders in which a decrease in clotting factors prevents stabilization of the platelet plug
  - Hemophilia A (85% of cases) is due to factor VIII deficiency
  - Hemophilia B is due to factor IX deficiency
- von Willebrand's disease is a deficiency of von Willebrand's factor
- von Willebrand's factor mediates platelet adhesion to sites of injury and stabilizes and carries clotting factor VIII
  - Type I (autosomal dominant): Deficiency of vWF
  - Type II (autosomal dominant): Defective vWF
  - Type III (autosomal recessive): Complete absence of vWF
  - Acquired defects (often iatrogenic or secondary to medical illness) occur rarely

Differential Dx

- Acquired coagulation disorders (e.g., DIC, liver disease, vitamin K deficiency)
- Factor XI deficiency
- Factor XII deficiency
- Thrombocytopenia (including ITP, TTP, or idiopathic)
- Platelet aggregation disorders (e.g., afibrinogenemia, drugs)
- Damage to endothelium (e.g., DIC, HUS, TTP, HSP)
- Granule release disorders (e.g., Chediak-Higashi syndrome, aspirin, NSAIDs, uremia)

Presentation

- Delayed bleeding
- Symptoms of von Willebrand's disease
  - Skin: Petechiae/purpura/bruising
  - Mucous membranes: Gingival bleeding, epistaxis, GI bleeds
  - GU bleeding: menorrhagia
  - Excessive bleeding after dental extraction, surgery, or trauma
- Symptoms specific to severe hemophilia
  - Hemarthrosis
  - Chronic joint disease
  - Large superficial ecchymoses
  - Muscle hematomas
  - CNS bleeds with minor trauma
  - Compartment syndrome

Diagnosis

- Hemophilia
  - Prolonged PTT (may be normal if factor levels are >30% of normal)
  - PT, platelet count, and bleeding time are usually normal
  - Decreased factor VIII or IX levels
- von Willebrand's disease
  - Prolonged bleeding time in moderate to severe cases
  - PT is normal
  - PTT is generally normal but may be increased
  - Specific von Willebrand factor assays (e.g., vWF Ristocetin cofactor assay) will identify the presence of von Willebrand's disease in equivocal cases
- Head CT should be obtained in any case of trauma (even minor trauma)

Treatment

- Prevent trauma
- Avoid aspirin and other antiplatelet drugs
- Hemophilia: Treat bleeding episodes by supplementing coagulation factors
  - Factor VIII or IX concentrates (monoclonal purified factors or recombinant factors greatly decrease risk of HIV and hepatitis C transmission)
  - Fresh frozen plasma or cryoprecipitate may be administered if factor concentrates are not available (carry a risk of viral transmission)
- von Willebrand's disease
  - Desmopressin (DDAVP) increases levels of vWF in vWD types I and II
  - Humate-P, a factor VIII concentrate, is the preferred therapy in vWD type III

Disposition

- Most patients with severe symptoms are admitted
- Admission criteria: Severe or life-threatening bleeding, unable to self-administer factor replacements, and unreliable follow-up
- Consider HIV/AIDS in patients transfused prior to 1985
- Type I and II vWD are often subclinical and revealed after trauma or surgery
- Type III vWD causes bleeding during menses or any minor trauma
- Complications of therapy are common, including transfusion-related infections and chronic liver disease; however, newer treatments, which include recombinant factors, prevent these devastating side effects

58. Oncologic Emergencies—Hematologic/Infectious

Etiology & Pathophysiology

- Oncologic emergencies may be hematologic, infectious, metabolic, or due to compression of adjacent structures
- Hematologic emergencies include severe anemia, neutropenia, thrombocytopenia, DIC, and leukocytosis
  - May be due to direct tumor effects on the marrow, chemotherapy effects on the marrow, or immune-mediated cell destruction
  - Malignancy is also an independent risk factor for hypercoagulability, spontaneous DVT, and PE
- Infectious emergencies secondary to immunosuppression caused by chemotherapy toxicity, direct tumor suppression of the marrow, or ineffective white blood cells (i.e., leukemia)
  - Patients are prone to opportunistic infections (e.g., bacteria, yeast)
  - Neutropenic fever is defined as a temperature >38°C with an absolute neutrophil count (PMNs plus bands) <500

Differential Dx

- Hematologic emergencies
  - Anemia
  - DVT, PE, arterial thrombus
  - Neutropenia
  - Thrombocytopenia
  - DIC
  - TTP/ITP
- Infectious emergencies
  - Bacterial infections (e.g., pneumonia, UTI, bacteremia, sepsis)
  - Fungal infections
  - Viral infections
  - Fever of malignancy

Presentation

- Anemia: Fatigue, lethargy, pallor
- Thrombocytopenia: Petechiae, purpura, spontaneous bleeding
- Neutropenic fever: May be asymptomatic or may have rigors, malaise, fatigue, nausea/vomiting, shortness of breath, myalgias, and mental status changes
- DVT: Extremity edema and erythema, calf tenderness
- Pulmonary embolus: Pleuritic chest pain, shortness of breath, tachypnea, tachycardia

Diagnosis

- Detailed history, including type of cancer, staging, and date and types of last chemotherapy or radiation treatment
- CBC, electrolytes, and PT/PTT
- Blood cultures × 2 (prior to antibiotic administration in cases of neutropenic fever)
- Urinalysis and urine culture
- Chest X-ray may show infiltrate
- Head CT is indicated for mental status changes or weakness to rule out metastases and cerebral edema
- Chest CT or ventilation/perfusion scan if pulmonary embolism is suspected
- Venous Doppler of extremities if DVT is suspected
- Lumbar puncture if suspect meningitis, encephalitis or subarachnoid hemorrhage (always check head CT before LP to rule out mass lesions and avoid possible cerebral herniation)

Treatment

- Treat underlying disorders as appropriate
- Neutropenic fever requires broad-spectrum IV antibiotics until cultures become negative
  - Piperacillin and gentamicin
  - Piperacillin and ciprofloxacin
  - 3rd-generation cephalosporin, gentamicin, +/− vancomycin
  - 4th-generation cephalosporin alone
  - Penicillin/anti-penicillinase
  - Imipenem +/− vancomycin
  - Add antifungal agents in persistently febrile patients
  - Further therapy may include G-CSF or GM-CSF to stimulate WBC production
- Anemia: Transfuse symptomatic patients with Hb ≤8
- Thrombocytopenia: Transfuse platelets if platelet count is <10,000 or if ≤50,000 with spontaneous bleeding
- DVT or PE requires IV heparin followed by warfarin therapy
  - Place IVC filter if anticoagulation is contraindicated

Disposition

- Most patients are admitted
- Criteria for admission
  - Neutropenia with fever
  - Severe anemia (Hb <8)
  - Pulmonary embolus or new thrombus
  - Mental status changes
  - Persistent vomiting
  - Major metabolic disturbances
- Discharge is acceptable if patient is hemodynamically stable, afebrile, tolerating oral intake, and DVT or pulmonary embolus is unlikely
- Many neutropenic fever patients will have negative cultures; however, all patients are empirically treated with antibiotics due to the rapid progression of infection and sepsis
- Place on neutropenic precautions if neutropenic

59. Oncologic Emergencies—Metabolic

Etiology & Pathophysiology

- Tumor lysis syndrome: Following large scale destruction of tumor cells (1–5 days after chemotherapy or therapeutic radiation), large quantities of uric acid (from DNA breakdown), potassium (from cytoplasmic stores), and phosphate (from protein breakdown) are released, resulting in renal failure and electrolyte imbalances
  - Associated with leukemia and lymphoma; rarely with solid tumors
- Hyperviscosity syndrome: Increased blood viscosity due to elevated levels of blood cells or protein (e.g., immunoglobulins), resulting in sludging, decreased blood flow, ischemia, and end-organ damage
  - Causes include Waldenström's macroglobulinemia, polycythemia vera, multiple myeloma, leukemias, connective tissue disorders
- SIADH: Inappropriate ADH secretion, most commonly due to ectopic ADH production in small cell lung tumors; results in excess free H_2O and hyponatremia with normal total body H_2O
- Hypercalcemia: Occurs with bony metastases or ectopic PTH peptide

Differential Dx

- Tumor lysis syndrome
  - Dehydration
  - Drug-induced nephrotoxicity
  - Tumor infiltration of kidney
  - Anemia
- Hyperviscosity syndrome
  - CVA
  - Platelet disorders
  - Thrombosis
  - DIC
  - Sickle cell disease
  - Polycythemia
- SIADH: Other causes of hyponatremia

Presentation

- Tumor lysis: Weakness, mental status changes, renal failure, arrhythmias (due to hyperkalemia), and symptoms of hypocalcemia (e.g., tetany, cramps, seizures)
- Hyperviscosity: Fatigue, headache, mucosal bleeding, renal failure, poor vision, neurologic symptoms (e.g., ataxia, headache, confusion, seizure, coma), cardiac symptoms (e.g., angina, MI, arrhythmia, CHF), and dermatologic symptoms (e.g., Raynaud's, palpable purpura)
- SIADH: Mental status changes, edema, weakness, N/V, seizures
- Hypercalcemia: Weakness, N/V, abdominal pain, delirium

Diagnosis

- Tumor lysis: History of recent chemotherapy or radiation in a patient with hyperkalemia, hyperphosphatemia, and hyperuricemia is essentially diagnostic
  - Check electrolytes and renal function (hyperkalemia, hyperuricemia, renal failure)
- Hyperviscosity: A clinical diagnosis in patients with risk factors
  - Symptoms occur with blood viscosity >4–5 (normal 1.4–1.8)
  - CBC: Elevated WBC and RBC and/or RBC rouleaux formation (symptoms occur with granulocytes >100,000 or lymphocytes >750,000)
  - Check electrolytes, PT/PTT, and renal function
- SIADH: Requires six criteria for diagnosis
  - Hyponatremia
  - Euvolemia
  - Urine not maximally diluted (osmoles >300)
  - Exclusion of other causes of hyponatremia (e.g., renal or thyroid disease)
  - Elevated urine Na^+ (>20)
  - Decreased serum osmoles

Treatment

- Tumor lysis
  - Aggressive hydration; correct electrolyte abnormalities
  - Allopurinol: Inhibits xanthine oxidase to prevent breakdown of nucleic acids into uric acid
  - Sodium bicarbonate: Alkalinizes urine to prevent uric acid from precipitating in the kidney
  - Consider dialysis if K^+ >6, uric acid >10, creatinine >10, phosphate >10, or symptomatic hypocalcemia
- Hyperviscosity
  - Aggressive hydration
  - Treat bleeding complications
  - Leukopheresis for leukocytosis
  - Plasmapheresis for elevated protein
  - Phlebotomy in severe cases to replace blood with NS
- SIADH: Free water restriction is the cornerstone of therapy
  - 3% saline or normal saline plus loop diuretics if severe
  - Demeclocycline affects renal tubules; used by nephrology
  - Slowly correct Na^+ to avoid central pontine myelinolysis
- Hypercalcemia: See "Hypercalcemia" entry

Disposition

- All tumor lysis patients are admitted
  - Most patients admitted to ICU
  - Monitored floor admission is sufficient in mild cases
  - Consult nephrology early, in case dialysis is needed
- Hyperviscosity syndrome
  - Consider transfer to tertiary care center if your facility does not have plasmapheresis or an oncologist readily available
- SIADH
  - Admission is necessary for severe hyponatremia, symptomatic hyponatremia, or if likely to worsen
  - Mild, asymptomatic cases may be discharged

60. Tumor Compression Syndromes

Etiology & Pathophysiology

- Be suspicious of a tumor compression syndrome in any cancer patient with a new onset of weakness, numbness, or mental status changes, or with unexplained swelling of the head or extremities
- May be the presenting symptom of a malignancy
- Prompt diagnosis and initiation of therapy are required to prevent permanent disability and/or death
- Lymphoma, lung, and breast cancer are common causes
- Upper airway obstruction may be due to tumor mass
- Superior vena cava syndrome occurs when compression results in increased venous pressure in arms, head, and neck
- Spinal cord compression and cauda equina syndromes occur when a tumor mass or collapsed vertebral body intrudes on the spinal cord
- Malignant pericardial effusion with tamponade may occur
- Cerebral herniation may occur due to tumor mass and cerebral edema

Differential Dx

- Airway obstruction: Foreign body, infection, cord paralysis
- SVC syndrome: Deep venous thrombosis due to central line, TB, syphilis, sarcoidosis, aortic aneurysm
- Spinal cord compression: Herniated disc, vertebral fracture, epidural abscess, neuropathy
- Pericardial tamponade: PE, MI, pneumothorax
- Cerebral edema/herniation: Meningitis, encephalopathy, metabolic disturbances

Presentation

- Airway obstruction: Voice changes, stridor, wheezing, neck mass
- SVC/IVC syndrome: Headache, upper extremity and facial edema, fatigue, syncope, vision changes, mental status changes, shortness of breath, supraclavicular mass, cough
- Cord compression: Back pain (worse when supine) or tenderness, weakness, paresthesias, bowel or bladder incontinence
- Tamponade: Hypotension, JVD, pulsus paradoxus, distant heart beat
- Cerebral edema: Mental status changes, weakness, paresthesias, seizures

Diagnosis

- Airway obstruction may be demonstrated on lateral neck X-rays; fiber optic laryngoscopy is diagnostic
- SVC syndrome: Chest CT or CXR reveals an apical lung mass
- Spinal cord compression requires emergent MRI or CT myelogram in all suspected cases as they are the gold standard tests to identify cord compression; plain films may show vertebral body disease
- Pericardial tamponade is diagnosed by transthoracic echocardiogram; chest X-ray may show a "water-bottle" heart and signs of CHF
- Cerebral edema is diagnosed by head CT (with or without contrast) or MRI; lumbar puncture may be required to exclude infection and to obtain cytology
- CBC, electrolytes, BUN/creatinine, and LFTs to exclude metabolic disorders

Treatment

- Supportive care with IV fluids and supplemental O_2
- IV steroids will temporarily decrease swelling in most cases
- Treat underlying metabolic disorders or infections, if present
- Prompt neurosurgical consult is required for spinal cord compression, cauda equina syndrome, or cerebral edema
- Seizure prophylaxis with phenytoin if cerebral mass present
- Airway obstruction
  - Ensure airway patency—surgical airway may be needed
  - Therapy may entail resection, chemotherapy, or radiation
- Pericardial tamponade
  - Pericardiocentesis for temporary relief of symptoms
  - Pericardial window or pericardiotomy may be definitive
- SVC syndrome
  - Radiation therapy is the definitive treatment
  - Loop diuretics and steroids if cerebral edema is present
- Spinal cord compression: High dose IV dexamethasone; may need emergency surgical decompression or radiation therapy
- Cerebral edema: IV mannitol, IV dexamethasone, and hyperventilation to ↓ ICP; urgent radiation or chemotherapy

Disposition

- All patients should be admitted to an ICU or a tertiary care center that has neurosurgery and oncology services available
- Prognosis is dependent on tumor type and length of symptoms
- Patients with history of a compression syndrome have a 10–30% likelihood of recurrence
- In patients with cord compression, paralysis for greater than 24 hours indicates that function is unlikely to return

Endocrine Emergencies

JACK PERKINS, MD

61. Hypoglycemia

Etiology & Pathophysiology

- Whipple's triad: Symptoms consistent with hypoglycemia, low blood glucose, symptoms resolve with normalization of serum glucose
- Hypoglycemia causes release of glucagon, growth hormone, and catecholamines, which rapidly mobilize liver glycogen to provide fuel (elevated epinephrine causes the symptoms of hypoglycemia)
- Hypoglycemia rapidly causes neurologic dysfunction (may be irreversible) as glucose is the brain's primary source of energy
- Causes of hypoglycemia include excessive insulin administration (#1 cause), sulfonylurea administration, ethanol, insulinoma, sepsis, renal failure, malnutrition/fasting, factitious insulin administration, decreased glucagon, sarcomas, pituitary or adrenal insufficiency, hypothyroidism, and congenital hormone/enzyme defects
- Reactive hypoglycemia occurs 2–4 hrs after meals, due to delayed and exaggerated insulin release (associated with a family history of type II diabetes)

Differential Dx

- Infection (e.g., UTI, meningitis, sepsis)
- Alcohol intoxication
- Medication overdose (e.g., sympathomimetics)
- CNS disorder (e.g., CVA/TIA, seizure, hemorrhage)
- Dehydration
- Adrenal insufficiency/crisis
- Hypothyroidism
- Renal failure
- Hepatic failure
- Psychosis
- Depression

Presentation

- Tachycardia
- Diaphoresis
- Tremor, anxiety
- Hyperventilation
- Hyperthermia
- CNS symptoms may include dizziness, headache, confusion, convulsions, mental status changes, abnormal behavior, and coma

Diagnosis

- Immediately measure serum glucose in any patient with altered mental status—missed diagnosis may result in irreversible neurologic damage or unnecessary procedures (e.g., intubation)
- Clinical symptoms of hypoglycemia usually begin to occur when the blood glucose level reaches 50 mg/dL; however, in diabetics, symptoms may begin at higher blood glucose levels or not at all
- Measure glucose, C-peptide, and insulin prior to glucose infusion
  - Serum insulin is elevated by insulinomas (insulin:glucose ratio >0.3) and sulfonylurea or exogenous insulin administration
  - C-peptide is produced during endogenous insulin production; thus, it will be decreased following exogenous insulin use and increased in insulinoma and sulfonylureas
  - Urine testing for sulfonylurea levels
- CBC, electrolytes, and BUN/creatinine
- Consider LFTs, urinalysis, CXR, TSH, cortisol, alcohol level, drug screen, head CT, and lumbar puncture if etiology is unclear
- CT/MRI may be necessary to evaluate for insulinoma

Treatment

- Glucose therapy (goal of therapy is glucose >100 mg/dL)
  - Alert patients may be repleted with oral glucose (e.g., juice, tablets) or IV D_{50}
  - Patients with altered consciousness require IV D_{50} solution
  - In children, use 1 g/kg bolus of 25% dextrose
  - Frequently recheck blood glucose after instituting therapy
- Glucagon may be used to increase glucose release from the liver if unable to obtain IV access and the patient cannot tolerate oral glucose; less effective in alcoholic and malnourished patients
- Octreotide may be used to inhibit insulin release in cases of sulfonylurea-induced hypoglycemia
- Thiamine must be given with glucose in any suspected case of alcohol abuse or nutritional deficiency to avoid Wernicke's encephalopathy
- Hydrocortisone should be administered to rule out adrenal insufficiency if blood glucose remains persistently low

Disposition

- Patients must be observed and repeated normal plasma glucose levels must be confirmed before disposition
- Admission criteria include sulfonylurea or long-acting insulin ingestion, co-morbidities, repeated requirement for glucose, some specific causes (e.g., sepsis), suicidal ingestions, and lack of outpatient support or follow-up
- Many patients are suitable for discharge once their blood glucose has normalized and they are able to tolerate oral intake; ensure follow-up with PCP for further workup and adjust medications as necessary
- Elderly have a blunted catecholamine response to low blood glucose and are especially susceptible to hypoglycemia
- Sulfonylurea action is especially long lasting

62. Diabetic Ketoacidosis

Etiology & Pathophysiology

- Hyperglycemia, acidosis, ketosis, and dehydration due to insulin deficiency in patients with type I diabetes mellitus
- Pathogenesis: Insulin deficiency causes hyperglycemia and an increase in counter-regulatory hormones (glucagons, catecholamines, and cortisol); this leads to the release of free fatty acids with subsequent hepatic oxidation to ketone bodies and anion gap acidosis
- Osmotic diuresis due to hyperglycemia and glycosuria results in dehydration and total body electrolyte depletion
- Causes include stress, infection, MI, insulin non-compliance, trauma, surgery, new onset of diabetes, pancreatitis, hyperthyroidism, drugs (e.g., steroids), CVA
- May be the initial presentation of diabetes in up to 20% of cases

Differential Dx

- Causes of anion gap metabolic acidosis (MUDPILES)
    - Methanol intoxication
    - Uremia
    - DKA
    - Paraldehyde ingestion
    - Isoniazid/Iron
    - Lactic acidosis
    - Ethanol/ethylene glycol
    - Starvation acidosis
    - Salicylate overdose
- Nonketotic hyperosmolar coma
- Hypoglycemia

Presentation

- Polyuria
- Polydipsia
- Dehydration
- Generalized weakness
- Lethargy
- Nausea/vomiting
- Abdominal pain
- Blurred vision
- Tachycardia
- Hypotension
- Hypothermia
- Mental status changes and/or coma
- Decreased bowel sounds
- Fruity (acetone) breath
- Kussmaul respirations (rapid, shallow breathing)

Diagnosis

- Hyperglycemia (glucose >200)
- Electrolyte abnormalities should be repeatedly monitored
    - Anion gap ($Na^+ - HCO_3 - Cl^- >12$) metabolic acidosis
    - Hyponatremia (secondary to hyperglycemia)
    - Total body potassium is invariably depleted; however, hyperkalemia is often present secondary to acidosis and lack of insulin; hypokalemia may occur in cases of severe total body potassium depletion
    - Increased BUN/creatinine ratio (due to dehydration)
    - Magnesium and phosphate levels may be decreased
- CBC may reveal leukocytosis due to ketosis and/or infection
- Serum ketones (acetone or β-hydroxybutyrate) are elevated
- Urinalysis reveals glucosuria and ketonuria
- ABG reveals metabolic acidosis (pH usually <7.3)
- Consider U/A, blood culture, and CXR to rule out infection
- ECG may show signs of hyper- or hypokalemia

Treatment

- Rehydration with NSS to correct fluid deficit (typically 5–10 L); give an initial bolus of 1–2 L and replete the remaining deficit over the next 6–12 hours
- IV insulin administration once hypokalemia is ruled out (as insulin will further decrease potassium level)
    - Administered as a bolus followed by an IV infusion
    - Do not administer insulin bolus in children (due to risk of cerebral edema from rapid shift of serum osmoles)
    - Continue insulin infusion until the acidosis clears, even if serum glucose is normal (add dextrose to IV fluids once serum glucose is <250 mg/dL to prevent hypoglycemia)
- Aggressive potassium repletion is essential—begin replacement as soon as hyperkalemia resolves, even if serum K+ is in the normal range (levels will further drop due to insulin therapy and correction of acidosis)
- Phosphorus administration as necessary
- Bicarbonate infusion is controversial; may increase intracellular acidosis and further diminish serum potassium; consider administering in older patients or if acidosis is causing cardiovascular collapse

Disposition

- Goal of therapy is to resolve acidosis— continue insulin therapy until acidosis resolves (even if glucose normalizes)
- Mortality is 10%, with increased rates among the elderly and patients with co-morbid conditions
- Search for the precipitating event
- Admission is required in all patients; strongly consider telemetry or intensive care setting for frequent glucose and electrolyte monitoring
- Complications of therapy may include hypoglycemia, hypokalemia, non-cardiogenic pulmonary edema, and cerebral edema (brain swelling due to osmotic fluid shifts)
- Children are the most likely to suffer from cerebral edema, which results in significant mortality; replace fluid slowly and do not give an insulin bolus

63. Hyperglycemic Hyperosmolar Nonketotic Coma

Etiology & Pathophysiology

- Systemic stress in type II diabetics results in hyperglycemia over days to weeks, leading to osmotic diuresis with severe dehydration, hyperosmolarity, and mental status changes
- Differentiate from DKA
  - Presence of some (but insufficient) insulin in HHNKC prevents the ketosis and acidosis seen in DKA
  - More severe dehydration and hyperosmolarity in HHNKC
  - Glucose is typically higher in HHNKC (>600 mg/dL)
  - Mental status changes may be more severe in HHNKC
- Most common in the elderly, who have impaired thirst mechanisms and/or difficulty obtaining fluids
- Precipitating stressors include infection (e.g., pneumonia, UTI), MI, CVA, GI hemorrhage, uremia, medications (e.g., diuretics, cimetidine, propanolol, corticosteroids), dialysis, burns, alcohol ingestion, pancreatitis, and hypothermia

Differential Dx

- Diabetic ketoacidosis
- CVA
- Infection
- Sepsis
- Dehydration
- Medication overdose
- Drug ingestion
- Organic brain syndrome
- Meningitis
- Uremia
- Liver failure

Presentation

- Polyphagia, polydipsia, polyuria
- Neurologic findings may include focal deficits, tremor, seizures, mental status changes, obtundation, and coma (degree of obtundation directly correlates with increased serum osmolality)
- Dehydration (e.g., dry membranes, tenting of skin, flat jugular veins, sunken eyes)
- Hypotension and tachycardia due to dehydration and/or sepsis
- Fever

Diagnosis

- CBC, electrolytes, renal function, urinalysis, serum osmolality
- Consider ABG, CPK, cardiac enzymes, blood cultures, CXR
- Serum glucose is generally >600 mg/dL
- Serum osmolality is generally >320 mOsm/kgH$_2$O
- Sodium is usually decreased due to extreme hyperglycemia (decrease of 1.6 meq/L for every 100 mg/dL of glucose elevation beyond 100 mg/dL); presence of hypernatremia indicates severe dehydration; however, regardless of serum sodium level, the patient is in a hypertonic state due to severe water loss
- Potassium may be normal, decreased, or increased; however, the patient will invariably be total body depleted (see DKA entry)
- Acid base status is normal (i.e., not acidotic as in DKA)
- Urinalysis shows few or absent ketones
- Leukocytosis may be present due to underlying infection
- Further workup for infection is generally indicated
- ECG may reveal MI or electrolyte-induced arrhythmias
- Neurologic findings may require head CT and LP

Treatment

- Immediate fluid replacement to correct severe dehydration
  - Total fluid deficit is often greater than 10 L
  - 1 L normal saline is administered in the first hour with an additional bolus if the patient is in hypovolemic shock
  - Replace half of fluid deficit over the first 12 hours and the remainder over next 24 hours
  - Administer normal saline if the patient is hyponatremic or half-normal saline if Na$^+$ is normal or elevated
  - Goal of therapy is to decrease serum osmoles by no more than 3 mOsm/kgH$_2$O/hr
- Aggressively replace potassium even if in normal range, as patients are total body depleted and insulin administration will further decrease serum potassium
- Judicious IV insulin administration to decrease serum glucose by 50–80 mg/dL per hour; overaggressive insulin administration puts patients at risk for hypokalemia, cerebral edema, and acute tubular necrosis
- Continuous ECG monitoring and serial glucose, electrolyte, and serum osmolality monitoring are indicated

Disposition

- Mortality is approximately 15%
- Admission is required in all patients; most will require ICU admission for intensive monitoring and therapy
- Complications of therapy include hypoglycemia, hypokalemia, volume overload, and cerebral edema
- Continue therapy until serum osmoles are <315 mOsm/kgH$_2$O, patient has normal mental status, and patient can tolerate subcutaneous insulin
- Precipitating cause should be identified prior to discharge

64. Hyperthyroidism/Thyroid Storm

Etiology & Pathophysiology

- Pituitary TSH controls thyroid hormone release—the primary synthesized form of thyroid hormone is T_4, which undergoes peripheral conversion to the more active T_3; both are bound to carrier proteins, though only the unbound form is biochemically active
- Thyroid hormone affects all organ systems and is responsible for increasing metabolic rate, heart rate and contractility, and muscle and CNS excitability
- Thyroid storm is a severe, life-threatening, acute state of thyrotoxicosis that may be caused by adrenergic hyperactivity or altered peripheral response to thyroid hormone
- Precipitating factors of thyroid storm include infection (#1 cause), thyroid surgery for hyperthyroidism, DKA, hypoglycemia, hyperosmolar coma, radioactive iodide treatment, PE, thyroid hormone overdose, withdrawal of anti-thyroid meds, iodinated contrast medium, vascular accidents, stress, toxemia of pregnancy

Differential Dx

- Infection
- Sepsis
- Cocaine use
- Psychosis
- Pheochromocytoma
- Neuroleptic malignant syndrome
- Hyperthermia
- Hyperthyroid states include Graves' disease, toxic multi-nodular goiter, toxic adenoma, subacute thyroiditis, acute Hashimoto's thyroiditis, factitious T_4 ingestion, thyroid cancer, pituitary neoplasm

Presentation

- General: Diaphoresis, weight loss, heat intolerance, fever
- CV: Palpitations, tachycardia, wide pulse pressure, PVCs, Afib, heart block, CHF, circulatory collapse
- CNS: Restlessness, anxiety, poor concentration, fatigue, agitation, tremor, mania, psychosis, coma
- GI: Diarrhea, N/V, abdominal pain
- Pulmonary: Dyspnea
- Muscle weakness
- Exophthalmos (in Graves' disease)
- Goiter may be present
- Thyroid storm: Exaggerated symptoms of above plus delirium, seizures, hypertension, lethargy

Diagnosis

- Thyroid storm is a clinical diagnosis in patients with pre-existing hyperthyroidism
- Thyroid studies, TSH, CBC, electrolytes, and LFTs
    - TSH is increased in primary pituitary disorders
    - Serum T_4 and T_3 (bound and unbound) are increased
    - Free T_4 level (measures unbound active T_4) will correct for falsely elevated T_4 level caused by changes in binding proteins
    - T_3 resin uptake estimates free T_4 levels by measuring unoccupied thyroxine binding sites and is also used to account for changes in binding protein concentration
    - Thyroid stimulating antibodies (Graves' disease), anti-microsomal antibodies (Hashimoto's disease), and serum thyroglobulin are increased in some primary thyroid diseases and normal in overdoses of T_4
- Consider cultures, urinalysis, and CXR to rule out infection
- ECG to rule out MI or arrhythmia
- Radioactive iodine uptake scan may be done as inpatient

Treatment

- Vigorous IV hydration and non-aspirin antipyretics
- Thioamides inhibit thyroid hormone production
    - Propylthiouracil (PTU) is the drug of choice—inhibits thyroid hormone synthesis and peripheral conversion of T_4 to T_3
    - Methimazole inhibits hormone synthesis but not peripheral conversion
- Iodide inhibits release of stored thyroid hormone if given 1 hour after PTU administration (otherwise it increases hormone release); used in severe cases
- β-blockers are used to treat symptoms (e.g., tachycardia, tremor); propranolol is preferred as it also decreases peripheral T_4 conversion
- IV steroids (dexamethasone or hydrocortisone) inhibit hormone release and peripheral conversion
- Dialysis and plasmapheresis are last resorts for patients that do not respond to the above treatments
- Radioactive iodine ablation therapy or surgery may be necessary for definitive cure

Disposition

- Without treatment, thyroid storm is fatal in nearly all patients; even with treatment, mortality is about 10%
- All patients diagnosed with thyroid storm require admission to the ICU
- Complete recovery can take up to one week based on how long it takes to deplete the circulating levels of thyroid hormones
- Admit patients with hyperthyroidism if they have serious complaints (e.g., chest pain) or risk factors (e.g., history of coronary artery disease)
- Hyperthyroid patients with minimal symptoms can be discharged

65. Hypothyroidism/Myxedema Coma

Etiology & Pathophysiology

- Insufficient thyroid hormone production, causing slowed metabolism
- Causes include Hashimoto's thyroiditis, thyroid ablation (surgery or radioiodine), postpartum, viral infection, drugs (e.g., amiodarone, lithium), amyloidosis, sarcoidosis, thyroid neoplasm, hypopituitarism, congenital, and idiopathic
- Myxedema refers to swelling of the skin and soft tissues that may occur in hypothyroid patients
- Myxedema coma is a severe, life-threatening decompensation of a hypothyroid patient heralded by mental status changes, hypotension, and hypothermia; most common (almost 90% of cases) in elderly women during the winter
- Precipitants of myxedema coma include sepsis/infection, MI, CVA, hypothermia, surgery, trauma, burns, hypoglycemia, hyponatremia, hemorrhage, medications (e.g., β-blockers, sedatives, narcotics, phenothiazine, amiodarone), thyroid medication non-compliance

Differential Dx

- Sepsis
- Depression
- Adrenal crisis/insufficiency
- CHF
- Hypoglycemia
- CVA
- Hypothermia
- Drug overdose/effect
- Meningitis

Presentation

- Fatigue, lethargy, weakness, weight gain, cold intolerance, hoarseness
- Neurologic: Depression, poor memory, confusion, delayed relaxation of DTRs, ataxia
- Cardiac: Bradycardia, distant heart sounds, pericardial effusion
- GI: Constipation, ileus
- Dermatologic: Dry skin, facial swelling, ptosis, macroglossia, periorbital edema, hair loss
- Non-pitting lower extremity edema
- Myxedema coma: Bradycardia, hypotension, hypothermia (usually <35.5°C), hypoventilation, and severely altered mental status, possibly resulting in coma

Diagnosis

- Hypothyroidism: Elevated TSH (may be decreased in hypopituitary states), decreased free and total T_4, variable T_3, increased T_3 resin uptake
- Myxedema coma
  - Thyroid panel: Significantly elevated TSH, decreased free and total T_4 and T_3, and increased T_3 resin uptake (consider hypothalamic or pituitary dysfunction if TSH, T_4, and T_3 are all low)
  - CBC: Anemia with increased MCV, leukopenia
  - Electrolytes: Hyponatremia, hypoglycemia, elevated CPK, elevated creatinine, elevated LFTs
  - Serum cortisol is often decreased due to hypothyroid-induced adrenal suppression
  - ABG reveals respiratory acidosis (due to muscle weakness)
  - Investigate precipitating causes: Cultures (rule out infection), head CT and LP (rule out hemorrhage, CVA, and infection), cardiac enzymes, renal and hepatic function

Treatment

- Hypothyroidism should be treated with oral T_4 (start with lower dose in the elderly and patients with CAD); may take weeks for the medication to take effect
- Myxedema coma
  - IV thyroid hormone must be administered immediately (Levothyroxine (T_4) has better cardiac safety than T_3, which may cause arrhythmias or an MI in large doses)
  - Intubation may be required due to mental status changes
  - Supplemental O_2 and cardiac monitoring (arrhythmias may develop due to IV T_4 administration)
  - Treat hypothermia by passive rewarming (active rewarming may cause hypotension due to reversal of cold-induced vasospasm)
  - Administer IV fluids (usually D_5 normal saline) to correct blood pressure and hypoglycemia
  - Administer IV hydrocortisone due to possible concurrent adrenal insufficiency
  - Consider empiric antibiotics as infection is a common precipitating cause (lack of fever does not rule out infection due to blunted fever response in these patients)

Disposition

- Myxedema coma carries a high mortality, ranging from 30–60% depending on co-morbid diseases; factors such as advanced age, bradycardia, and persistent hypotension suggest an unfavorable prognosis
- All patients with myxedema coma require ICU admission
- Milder hypothyroidism may be discharged and followed by a PCP

66. Adrenal Insufficiency/Adrenal Crisis

Etiology & Pathophysiology

- The adrenal gland synthesizes glucocorticoids (e.g., cortisol), mineralocorticoids (e.g., aldosterone), and androgens
  - Glucocorticoids (regulated by ACTH) maintain metabolism, potentiate catecholamine action, and control H_2O distribution
  - Mineralocorticoids (regulated by renin/angiotensin and serum K^+) control sodium and volume balance
- Primary adrenal insufficiency (Addison's disease): Intrinsic adrenal gland failure, resulting in decreased cortisol and aldosterone (due to infection (e.g., TB), drugs, adrenal hemorrhage (use of warfarin, sepsis, trauma), sarcoid, autoimmune, metastases, CAH)
- 2° adrenal insufficiency: Failure of pituitary stimulation of the adrenals, resulting in cortisol deficiency only (due to withdrawal of steroid therapy, pituitary disease, trauma, Sheehan syndrome)
- Adrenal crisis is a life-threatening exacerbation of adrenal insufficiency due to increased physiologic demand (e.g., infection) or decreased supply (e.g., discontinuation of steroid therapy) of cortisol

Differential Dx

- Shock
- Sepsis
- Dehydration
- Medication overdose
- Uremia
- Hypothyroidism/myxedema coma
- Gastrointestinal disease (e.g., appendicitis, peptic ulcer disease, pancreatitis, liver disease, gallbladder disease)
- Myocardial infarction
- Pulmonary embolus
- CHF

Presentation

- Cortisol deficiency: Weight loss, lethargy, weakness, mental status changes, abdominal pain, N/V
- Aldosterone deficiency: Dehydration, orthostasis, syncope
- 1° insufficiency: Symptoms of diminished cortisol and aldosterone and increased ACTH (skin hyperpigmentation)
- 2° insufficiency: Symptoms of diminished cortisol only; may have symptoms of pituitary lesions (e.g., HA, visual changes, galactorrhea)
- Adrenal crisis: Severe hypotension (refractory to vasopressors), dehydration, weakness, circulatory collapse, delirium, abdominal pain

Diagnosis

- CBC, electrolytes, serum cortisol, serum ACTH, ECG, U/A, and CXR are generally indicated; obtain cultures if suspect infection
- Serum cortisol >20 rules out adrenal insufficiency
- Hypoglycemia is often present due to cortisol deficiency
- Primary adrenal insufficiency: Hyponatremia, hyperkalemia, and elevated BUN (due to aldosterone deficiency)
- Secondary adrenal insufficiency: Hypernatremia, hypokalemia
- Adrenal crisis: Hypoglycemia is generally present but other labs are variable (may see $\downarrow Na^+$, $\uparrow K^+$, and elevated BUN)
- ECG changes are generally related to potassium imbalances (e.g., prolonged QT, peaked T waves, heart block in hyperkalemia)
- CT scan may be used to evaluate for adrenal hemorrhage/infarct
- Cosyntropin (synthetic ACTH) stimulation test is an inpatient study to evaluate adrenal response to ACTH and distinguish primary from secondary disease

Treatment

- Begin therapy immediately in any suspected case of adrenal crisis (prognosis is related to the rapidity of treatment onset)
- Hydrocortisone is the drug of choice for cases of adrenal crisis or insufficiency (provides both glucocorticoid and mineralocorticoid effects)
- Dexamethasone may also be used in adrenal crisis (this is the only steroid that will not confound the results of the cosyntropin stimulation test)
- Administer IV fluids
- Vasopressors should be administered following steroid therapy in patients unresponsive to fluid resuscitation (norepinephrine, dopamine, and neosynephrine are preferred)
- Patients may require lifelong glucocorticoids +/− mineralocorticoid supplementation
- Increased maintenance doses of chronic steroids are required during periods of stress (e.g., illness, surgery, trauma, GI upset) to satisfy the increased physiologic need for cortisol

Disposition

- Admit all patients with adrenal crisis to an ICU
- Patients with adrenal insufficiency generally require admission for IV steroid administration, confirmation of diagnosis, and identification of etiology
- Discharge is warranted for mild cases with previously identified etiologies
- Iatrogenic adrenal insufficiency is caused by withdrawal of chronic steroid use and may persist for up to one year after the steroids have been discontinued
- These patients are often unable to mount a sufficient fever response; therefore, infection should not be ruled out by lack of fever alone

Neurologic
Emergencies

GEORGE SMALL, MD
SALIMA KASSAB, MD

67. Altered Mental Status

Etiology & Pathophysiology

- Delirium: An acute, transient alteration in cognitive ability secondary to a physiologic event
  - Inciting event often does not directly involve the CNS (e.g., urinary tract infection, electrolyte abnormality, medications)
  - Presence of delirium mandates a thorough search for its cause
- Dementia: A chronic, irreversible change in memory and cognitive function caused by destruction of brain tissue
  - Most commonly due to Alzheimer's disease
  - Other causes include multiple vascular infarcts, Huntington's or Parkinson's disease, multiple sclerosis, hydrocephalus, metabolic disease (uremia, vitamin B_{12} or folate deficiency, thyroid disease), chronic infection (e.g., neurosyphilis, HIV), vasculitis, neoplasms
- Coma: A state of depressed level of consciousness with inappropriate or absent responses to environmental stimuli caused by global brain dysfunction involving the brainstem or bilateral hemispheres

Differential Dx

- Infection (meningitis, UTI, pneumonia, sepsis)
- Electrolyte abnormalities
- Endocrine disorders (abnormal glucose, adrenal, or thyroid)
- Hepatic encephalopathy
- Uremia
- Drugs (e.g., narcotics, steroids, cardiac drugs, anticholinergics)
- Hypoxemia/hypercarbia
- Hypotension or severe HTN
- CNS causes (CVA, trauma, hemorrhage, seizure)
- Depression or psychosis
- Toxin or poison ingestion

Presentation

- Delirium: Acute, recent onset
  - Altered short-term memory
  - Perceptual disturbances
  - Disturbed sleep/wake cycle
  - Psychomotor changes
  - Disorientation, agitation
  - Decreased consciousness
- Dementia: Insidious onset
  - Altered short-term memory
  - Disorientation, mood swings, behavioral changes, delusions
  - Impaired attention and language
- Coma: Involuntary or absent movement, decorticate or decerebrate posturing, progressive hemiparesis, sluggish or absent pupillary reflex

Diagnosis

- Signs and symptoms may provide clues to the inciting event
- Detailed history from family/caretakers
- Calculate Glasgow coma score (motor, verbal, eye opening)
- Lab studies depend on symptoms and patient characteristics
  - Rule out infection with CBC, urinalysis, CXR, blood/urine cultures, RPR, HIV serologies, and/or lumbar puncture
  - Rule out metabolic causes with glucose, electrolytes, renal function, LFTs, ammonia level, vitamin B_{12} and folate levels
  - Urine drug screen
  - ABG for suspected hypoxemia, hypercarbia, carbon monoxide, or acid-base disturbances
- ECG to rule out cardiac ischemia or arrhythmia
- Head CT without contrast is indicated in all unexplained mental status changes to identify hemorrhage, mass lesions, or abscess
- MRI of the brain with and without contrast may further delineate intracerebral processes (usually not performed in ED)

Treatment

- The key to proper treatment is identifying and treating underlying pathology
- Delirium
  - Minimize external stimulation
  - IV or IM haloperidol and/or benzodiazepines
  - Restrain as necessary for patient and caregiver safety
  - Treat underlying disorders (e.g., antibiotics for infection, removal of offending drug, antidotes for specific toxins)
- Dementia
  - Agitated patients may be sedated as above
  - Ensure that reversible causes are properly identified and treated (e.g., vasculitis, vitamin deficiencies, EtOH abuse)
  - Alzheimer's type: Long-term use of tacrine improves cognitive function
- Coma
  - Ensure airway, breathing, and circulation are maintained
  - Intubate for GCS <9
  - Administer empiric thiamine, glucose, and naloxone
  - Emergent therapy for increased intracranial pressure

Disposition

- Delirium
  - Admission is usually necessary
  - Admit any patient whose symptoms have not resolved in the ED or those with serious or unclear etiologies
- Dementia
  - Admission may be necessary
  - Discharge patients who are at their baseline mental status
  - Reversible causes include drugs, electrolyte/metabolic disturbances, emotional causes, trauma, nutritional deficiencies, infection, alcohol abuse
  - Irreversible causes include Alzheimer's, vascular infarcts, MS, Huntington's, and Parkinson's
- Coma
  - Stabilize patient in ED
  - Admit to appropriate ICU (e.g., neurosurgery, neurology, MICU)

68. Migraine Headache

Etiology & Pathophysiology

- An episodic headache associated with neurologic, GI, or autonomic changes—note that associated migraine symptoms may present *without* headache
- Classified as migraine with aura, migraine without aura, or migraine variant (retinal migraine, ophthalmoplegic migraine, or familial hemiplegic migraine)
- Etiology is unclear; thought to be due to an imbalance between brainstem nuclei that regulate vascular control; the prodrome is likely due to vasoconstriction followed by vasodilatation
- Occurs in 10–20% of the population; more common in women
- Precipitating factors include stress, menstruation, OCPs, fatigue, decreased sleep, hunger, head trauma, foods (e.g., nitrites, glutamate, aspartate, tyramine), medications (e.g., vitamin A, nitroglycerin, histamine, estrogens, hydralazine, steroid withdrawal), perfumes, smoke, and certain pungent odors

Differential Dx

- Other headaches (e.g., cluster, tension, hypertensive)
- Subarachnoid hemorrhage
- Subdural or epidural hematoma
- CVA
- Meningitis
- Brain tumor
- Pseudotumor cerebri
- Sinusitis
- Acute angle closure glaucoma
- Temporal arteritis
- Carbon monoxide exposure
- Hypoxia
- TMJ syndrome
- Cervical spondylosis

Presentation

- Headache (unilateral in 70%, bifrontal or global in 30%)
- Pain is exacerbated by rapid head motion, straining, and exertion
- May be dull, deep, and steady or throbbing and pulsatile
- Aura symptoms may be present, including visual scotomas, aphasia, and parasthesias
- Autonomic features may include nasal stuffiness, rhinorrhea, tearing, color and temperature change, and change in pupil size
- Complicated migraines may result in ophthalmoplegia, hemiplegia (persistent unilateral motor or sensory symptoms), or posterior circulation symptoms (e.g., ataxia)

Diagnosis

- International Headache Society diagnostic criteria
  - Migraine without aura (common migraine): Severe, unilateral, pulsating pain exacerbated by activity; last 4–72 hrs; no apparent underlying cause; presence of nausea/vomiting, photophobia, or phonophobia; and presence of at least 5 attacks fulfilling the above criteria
  - Migraine with aura (classic migraine): Typical aura symptoms followed by headache within 1 hour
- Head CT is indicated for patients with abnormal neurologic exam or atypical headache features in order to rule out serious etiologies
- MRI/MRA is indicated if a posterior fossa or vascular lesion is suspected
- Consider ESR (to rule out temporal arteritis), ABG (to rule out hypoxia and carbon monoxide exposure), CBC (to rule out anemia), and lumbar puncture (to rule out meningitis)

Treatment

- Treatment is more effective if administered early; a larger single dose is more effective than multiple small doses
- Analgesics (NSAIDs, acetaminophen, +/− caffeine)
- Antiemetics (e.g., prochlorperazine, metoclopramide) are generally very effective to relieve headaches; however, they may cause dystonic reactions or extrapyramidal side effects
- Triptans (e.g., Sumatriptan) are serotonin agonists that cause vasoconstriction; avoid in patients with CAD or HTN
- Ergotamine also causes vasoconstriction; contraindicated in CAD and HTN; side effects include vascular occlusion and rebound headaches
- Prophylactic treatments may decrease headache frequency by 30–40% (e.g., β-blockers, calcium-channel blockers, tricyclic antidepressants, and valproic acid)
- Ergots, triptans, and NSAIDs are contraindicated in pregnancy; acetaminophen and opioids should be used
- Children should be treated with NSAIDs and/or metoclopramide

Disposition

- Majority of patients are discharged
- Patients who are discharged with residual headache are twice as likely to have continued pain at 24 hrs
- Possible indications for admission include persistent vomiting or dehydration, inability to tolerate oral intake, suspected organic cause of headache, failed outpatient treatment, or headache accompanied by a significant medical or surgical problem

69. CVA/Stroke

Etiology & Pathophysiology

- Caused by an abrupt, focal interruption of cerebral blood flow
- Presentation depends on the specific arteries and brain areas involved (anterior, middle, or posterior cerebral artery; cerebellum; brainstem)
- Ischemic strokes constitute >80% of cases
    - Embolisms (most common sources are the heart, aorta, carotids, and vertebral arteries) account for up to 30% of cases
    - Thrombosis of an atherosclerotic artery
    - Small vessel lacunar infarction, usually due to long-standing systemic disease (e.g., HTN, diabetes)
    - Other causes include arterial stenosis with poor collateral flow, vasculitis, arterial dissection, venous occlusion, and polycythemia
- Hemorrhagic strokes (intracerebral or subarachnoid) account for 15%
- Transient ischemic attacks are episodes of transient, focal ischemia that resolve in less than 24 hours and are associated with increased risk of stroke in the future

Differential Dx

- Hypoglycemia
- Seizure
- Meningitis/encephalitis
- Intracerebral bleed
- DKA or hyperosmotic coma
- Complicated migraine
- Cerebral mass (tumor, abscess)
- Hypertensive encephalopathy
- Wernicke's encephalopathy
- Labyrinthitis
- Meniere's disease
- Demyelinating diseases
- Drugs (e.g., lithium, phenytoin, carbamazepine)

Presentation

- Anterior cerebral artery: Contralateral weakness (leg > arm) with facial sparing
- Middle cerebral: Contralateral hemiparesis and sensory loss (arm > leg), hemianopsia, dysarthria
- Posterior cerebral: Impaired vision and thought, visual agnosia, contralateral hemisensory loss
- Dominant hemisphere stroke: Aphasia (receptive, expressive, or global), apraxia, acalcula
- Nondominant hemisphere stroke: Contralateral hemineglect, spatial disorientation
- Cerebellar: N/V, nystagmus, ataxia
- TIA: Resolution of symptoms

Diagnosis

- Assess the patient using the NIH stroke scale
- Emergent head CT (without contrast) to rule out hemorrhage
    - Infarcts are hypodense (dark); blood is hyperdense (white)
    - Will be normal following TIA and early after ischemic CVA
- MRI is more sensitive than CT for ischemic CVA (usually done as an inpatient)
- Rule out other causes of altered mental status via CBC, glucose, electrolytes, ESR, uric acid, liver and thyroid function tests, and PT/PTT
- Urine toxicology screen (young patient with CVA suggests cocaine/amphetamine abuse)
- Full inpatient workup to determine etiology of stroke and identify possible sources of emboli
    - Cardiac workup with ECG and echocardiogram
    - Carotid ultrasound or MRA to evaluate the intra- and extracranial vasculature
    - EEG may be done if suspect seizure disorder

Treatment

- Airway, breathing, and circulatory support as necessary
- Thrombolytic therapy (rTPA)
    - Only used in strokes of moderate severity, within 3 hours of symptom onset, and in patients who meet entry criteria
    - One study (NINDS) demonstrated a benefit in neurologic recovery (but the increased risk of cerebral hemorrhage negated any decrease in mortality)
    - Another study found that use of rTPA in community EDs *increased* mortality due to violations in entry criteria
- Aspirin slightly decreases risk of recurrent stroke or death
- Heparin is often used but there is no evidence that it improves outcomes (decreased rate of stroke recurrence is offset by an increased rate of cerebral hemorrhage)
- Treat elevated blood pressure only when it exceeds 220/115 since HTN may be necessary to maintain cerebral perfusion (do not lower systolic BP below 180 mmHg)
- Treat hyperglycemia with insulin
- Ancrod (converts fibrinogen into fibrin) is investigational
- There is no evidence that other neuroprotective drugs (e.g., gangliosides, anti-free radical drugs) are effective

Disposition

- Dedicated stroke teams may improve speed of diagnosis and therapy, thereby improving outcomes
- 95% of new focal neurologic deficits are vascular in origin
- Admit all patients with CVA for close supervision of mental status and changes in focal deficits
- 50–70% of patients regain independence
- Up to 80% regain ability to walk
- New onset TIA requires inpatient or outpatient evaluation for cardiac and carotid sources of embolism formation; patients are admitted or may be discharged on antiplatelet therapy (e.g., aspirin, clopidogrel) with very close follow-up

70. Subarachnoid and Intracerebral Hemorrhage

Etiology & Pathophysiology

- SAH: Bleeding into the subarachnoid space
  - Most commonly due to rupture of a saccular aneurysm, trauma, or bleeding from an arteriovenous malformation
  - Other causes include ruptured mycotic aneurysm, and intracerebral hemorrhage with rupture into the subarachnoid space
  - Aneurysmal and traumatic SAH have different pathophysiology, treatments, and outcomes
- ICH: Bleeding into the brain parenchyma
  - Associated with chronic HTN; usually occurs in the elderly
  - Causes the majority of hemorrhagic strokes; occurs in small, deep intracerebral arterioles that have been damaged by chronic HTN
  - Other causes include amyloidosis, anticoagulation/thrombolytic use, arteriovenous malformations, cocaine, amphetamines, moyamoya disease, CNS vasculitis, leukemia, sickle cell disease, acquired thrombocytopenia and DIC

Differential Dx

- CVA
- Subdural or epidural hematoma
- Migraine
- Meningitis or encephalitis
- Intracerebral mass lesion
- Systemic infections (e.g., influenza)
- Carotid or vertebral artery dissection
- Hypertensive encephalopathy
- Cervical arthritis
- Temporal arteritis
- Labyrinthitis
- Acute angle closure glaucoma

Presentation

- SAH
  - Sudden, severe headache ("worst headache of life")
  - Cervical and occipital radiation
  - Physical exam is often normal
  - May have nuchal rigidity, photophobia, lethargy, N/V, altered mental status, or coma
  - Syncope or seizures may occur
- ICH symptoms and neuro findings depend on location of the bleed
  - Acute onset of headache; may progress to stupor, then coma
  - HTN, bradycardia, vomiting
  - Contralateral hemiplegia, hemianesthesia, hemianopsia, aphasia
  - Abnormal pupils

Diagnosis

- SAH
  - Head CT without contrast is the first test ordered and usually shows blood in the basilar cisterns (aneurysmal SAH) or in the hemispheric sulci and fissures (traumatic SAH)
  - Lumbar puncture should be performed in any patient with a negative CT but continued suspicion for SAH—reveals increased opening pressure, elevated RBC count, and xanthochromia (may not develop until 12 hrs after the bleed)
  - Cerebral angiogram is the gold standard but is generally only used if the diagnosis is in doubt
- ICH: Head CT without contrast will show hyperdensity (blood) in the brain parenchyma
- Lab studies may be needed to rule out other causes of symptoms: CBC, glucose, chemistries, PT/PTT, ECG, cardiac enzymes, chest X-ray, blood type/screen, and urine drug screen

Treatment

- ABCs, cardiac monitoring, pulse oximetry, and frequent neurologic checks
- Seizure prophylaxis with IV phenytoin
- Control elevated intracranial pressure with head elevation, moderate hyperventilation (pCO_2 30–35 mmHg), mannitol administration, and/or surgical drainage
- Reverse previous anticoagulation with fresh frozen plasma
- Aneurysmal SAH: Maintain blood pressure in the normal range (hypertension may cause the aneurysm to rebleed, hypotension may cause cerebral ischemia), and administer nimodipine within 48 hrs to prevent cerebral vasospasm
- Traumatic SAH generally requires only supportive care
- ICH
  - Maintain blood pressure at pre-hemorrhage levels (which is elevated in many patients) to prevent cerebral ischemia
  - Severe new hypertension may be treated judiciously with labetalol or nitroprusside—remember that hypertension may be a physiologic response to maintain cerebral perfusion pressure in patients with increased ICP

Disposition

- Admit all patients to neurosurgical ICU
- Mortality of SAH and ICH approaches 50%
- Aneurysmal SAH
  - Complications include rebleeding, cerebral vasospasm, intracerebral hematoma, hydrocephalus, cardiac arrhythmias, transient cardiomyopathy, SIADH, seizures, and persistent neurologic deficits
  - Definitive therapy may include angiography (with embolization or clipping) or surgery
- ICH
  - Complications include seizures, increased ICP, hydrocephalus, SIADH, and focal neurologic deficits
  - Acute surgical intervention is controversial

71. Subdural and Epidural Hematoma

Etiology & Pathophysiology

- Epidural hematoma
  - Usually due to a temporal-parietal skull fracture with laceration of the middle meningeal artery or vein
  - Rapid accumulation of blood in the epidural space results in a rapid rise in ICP, uncal herniation, and brainstem compression
  - Usually occurs in children, teenagers, and young adults
- Acute subdural hematoma
  - Most commonly due to severe head injury with tearing of the bridging veins that traverse the subdural space
  - Associated with damage to the underlying brain due to contusion, hematoma formation, diffuse axonal injury, and cerebral edema
- Subacute or chronic subdural: Slow accumulation of subdural blood
  - Occurs over 1–10 days following head trauma
  - Most common in elderly, alcoholic, and anticoagulated patients

Differential Dx

- Stroke
- Traumatic subarachnoid hemorrhage
- Coma
- Traumatic brain injury
- Complicated migraine
- Carotid or vertebral artery dissection
- Concussion
- Cerebral contusion

Presentation

- Headache, ipsilateral dilated pupil, posturing, vomiting, hemiparesis, and confusion
- Epidural
  - Initial head injury with LOC
  - 50% then have a lucid interval followed by gradual loss of consciousness as ICP increases
  - Sudden death may occur
- Acute subdural: Severe head injury with rapid LOC within 72 hrs, followed by progressive deterioration and deepening coma
- Subacute subdural: Slowly developing headache, drowsiness, mental status changes, and gradual neurologic deterioration

Diagnosis

- Detailed history by the patient or witnesses
- Glasgow coma scale (motor, verbal, and eye opening)
- Head CT without contrast
  - Epidural: Convex hyperdensity, shift of midline structures, compression of ipsilateral ventricular system, and dilation of contralateral ventricle
  - Subdural: Crescent-shaped concave hyperdensity (chronic subdural may be hypodense); cerebral edema may be present
- Cervical spine X-rays
- Further imaging may include skull films to look for fracture of temporal-parietal bones (in cases of epidural hemorrhage) or MRI (in cases of subdural hemorrhage)

Treatment

- Airway, breathing, and circulation
- Intubate if hypoxemic or unable to protect airway
- Frequent neurologic checks
- Treat hypotension with isotonic IV fluids (NSS or LR) to maintain cerebral perfusion
- Seizure prophylaxis (phenytoin or fosphenytoin)
- Treat increased intracranial pressure and/or impending herniation by elevation of head, intubation and moderate hyperventilation (pCO_2 30–35 mmHg), mannitol infusion, and possible neurosurgical drainage
- Epidural hematoma
  - Requires surgical decompression in most cases
  - Trephination with burr holes may be done in the ED if herniation is imminent and neurosurgical care is not immediately available
- Subdural hematoma
  - Acute subdural requires surgical drainage
  - Subacute or chronic subdural may be drained or may be managed conservatively with monitoring of neurologic status and serial CT scans

Disposition

- Admit all patients with intracranial hemorrhage
- Epidural hematoma has a 20% mortality rate
- Acute subdural has 50–80% mortality

72. Vertigo

Etiology & Pathophysiology

- A sense of impulsion (spinning), either of patient or environment
- Caused by conflicting inputs to the visual, vestibular (inner ear), or proprioceptive (position sense) mechanisms
- Dizziness is a nonspecific complaint, whose definition varies by patient (may refer to vertigo, pre-syncope, weakness, or confusion)
- Peripheral vertigo: Due to lesions of CN 8 or the vestibular apparatus
  - Benign positional vertigo: Due to crystals in semicircular canals
  - Vestibular neuronitis/labyrinthitis: Usually due to viral infection
  - Meniere's disease: Due to chronic, degenerative loss of hair cells
  - Cerebellopontine angle tumor (e.g., acoustic neuroma, meningioma)
  - Post-traumatic perilymphatic fistula
  - Drug ototoxicity
- Central vertigo: Caused by brainstem or cerebellar pathology including cerebellar infarct/hemorrhage, vertebrobasilar disease, CNS tumor, migraine, TIA/CVA, multiple sclerosis

Differential Dx

- Syncope or near-syncope
- Cardiac disease (ischemia, arrhythmia, valvular disease)
- Volume depletion/dehydration
- Delirium due to metabolic or infectious causes
- Brainstem CVA
- Seizure
- Migraine
- Panic attack or hyperventilation
- Sedative/hypnotic intoxication
- Ectopic pregnancy
- Hypoxia
- Age-related dysequilibrium

Presentation

- Peripheral vertigo
  - Acute, severe, intermittent vertigo
  - Increased with head movement
  - Nausea and vomiting
  - May have tinnitus (Meniere's disease) or hearing loss
  - Fatigable nystagmus (horizontal or rotatory)
- Central vertigo
  - Slow-onset, mild, constant vertigo
  - No change with head movement
  - Intact hearing
  - Non-fatigable nystagmus (vertical)
  - CNS signs/symptoms (e.g., vision changes, cerebellar signs, severe gait disturbance, oscillopsia)

Diagnosis

- Differentiate central from peripheral vertigo by a complete history and neurologic examination
- Dix-Hallpike maneuver is a test for peripheral vestibular disease
  - Move patient from sitting to supine with head hanging down
  - Positive test elicits findings when head is turned to either side
  - Findings in BPV or vestibulitis include nystagmus, transient worsening of symptoms, and fatigability of response
- Pneumatic otoscopy replicates symptoms in perilymphatic fistula or Meniere's disease
- ECG may be obtained to rule out arrhythmia in high-risk patients
- Head CT is required in patients with central vertigo, headache, focal neurologic findings, trauma, or risk factors for CVA
- MRI/MRA (usually not obtained in ED) should be considered for symptoms of cerebellar disease or cerebellopontine angle tumor, focal neurologic findings, CVA risk factors, or vertebrobasilar disease

Treatment

- Emergency room treatment of vertigo is generally supportive
- Be sure to exclude ominous central causes
- Vestibular suppressants are used to decrease symptoms
  - Antihistamines (e.g., meclizine or diphenhydramine)
  - Scopolamine patch
  - Benzodiazepines have *not* been proven to be effective
- Antiemetics for nausea and vomiting (e.g., promethazine)
- BPV
  - Epley maneuver (canolith repositioning) is a series of head and neck movements whose goal is to move canoliths (particle debris) into the utricle where they will not cause symptoms (50–80% success rate)
  - Vestibular exercises (repetition of the Hallpike maneuver) may fatigue the vertigo response and reduce symptoms
- Meniere's disease
  - Vestibular suppressants
  - Salt restriction and diuretic administration are controversial

Disposition

- Differentiate from near-syncope
- Admit for severe symptoms, unsafe ambulation, persistent vomiting, central vertigo, or unclear diagnoses
- Discharge patients with peripheral vertigo and adequate symptom control
- Consult neurology for vertigo associated with focal neurologic findings, headache, or unclear source
- ENT referral to exclude vestibular pathologies in cases of severe disease, persistent disease, or trauma
- BPV and vestibulitis are benign, self-limited diseases
- Meniere's disease follows a chronic, progressive course, eventually resulting in hearing loss

73. Seizures

Etiology & Pathophysiology

- Abnormal neuronal discharge leading to altered cerebral function
- Primary (idiopathic) seizure occurs without an evident cause
- Secondary seizure may be due to mass lesions, CVA, intracranial bleed, head trauma, alcohol or benzodiazepine withdrawal, infection, metabolic disturbances (e.g., hypoglycemia, hyponatremia, uremia), drugs (e.g., cocaine, anticholinergics), vasculitis, or eclampsia
- Generalized seizures involve loss of consciousness: Tonic-clonic (grand mal), absence (brief loss of consciousness without loss of postural tone), myoclonic, tonic, clonic, or atonic
- Partial seizures involve localized areas of the brain: Simple partial (no loss of consciousness, intact mentation), complex partial (impaired consciousness), or partial with generalization
- Epilepsy: A syndrome of recurrent, unprovoked seizures
- Status epilepticus: Seizure >30 minutes or recurrent seizures without return to baseline; commonly due to anti-epileptic non-compliance

Differential Dx

- Syncope
- Hypoglycemia
- Arrhythmia
- Pseudoseizure
- Hyperventilation syndrome
- Migraines
- Movement disorders
- Narcolepsy
- Cataplexy
- Decerebrate posturing
- Non-convulsive status epilepticus

Presentation

- May be preceded by aura or light-headedness
- Visual, olfactory, gustatory changes
- May have loss of sphincter tone
- Post-ictal state may consist of confusion, agitation, or prolonged alteration of consciousness
- Generalized tonic-clonic
  - LOC without warning/aura
  - Patient becomes rigid with extremities extended; falls; becomes apneic and cyanotic; may vomit, urinate, bite tongue
  - Rigidity progresses to symmetric, rhythmic (clonic) jerking of trunk and extremities
  - Generally lasts 1–3 minutes

Diagnosis

- Labs to evaluate for potential causes of seizure
  - Patients with new seizures or change in pattern of previously diagnosed seizure require electrolytes, glucose, pregnancy test
  - Consider CBC, BUN/Cr, ESR, LFTs, CK, RPR, urinalysis
  - Antiepileptic drug levels in patients taking anticonvulsants
  - Prolactin is often elevated in true seizure, not in pseudoseizure
  - Toxicology screen if drug overdose or withdrawal is suspected
- Lumbar puncture if meningitis or encephalitis is suspected
- Head CT without contrast is indicated in most first-time seizures, change in pattern of established seizures, fever, trauma, persistently altered mental status, cancer, history of anticoagulation, or severe headache
- EEG is used in the ED to rule out persistent status epilepticus
- MRI is the best imaging modality to detect underlying cerebral pathology in unexplained seizures but is seldom used in the ED

Treatment

- Airway, breathing, and circulation
- Intubation may be necessary
- Supplemental O_2, pulse oximetry, and cardiac monitoring
- Treat underlying systemic causes, if possible
- Administer thiamine in alcoholics, dextrose if hypoglycemic, and naloxone in suspected opiate overdose
- Anticonvulsants
  - Benzodiazepines (e.g., lorazepam or diazepam) are first line agents in the ED—IV, IM, or rectal
  - IV phenytoin or fosphenytoin are added if benzodiazepines are not quickly effective
  - IV phenobarbital is used if above medications ineffective
- Status epilepticus
  - Goal is control of seizure activity within 30 minutes
  - If initial anticonvulsants fail at maximal dosages, options include IV valproic acid, pentobarbital coma, propofol infusion, or benzodiazepine infusion
- Patients with known seizure disorder and subtherapeutic medication levels should be loaded to appropriate level

Disposition

- Admit patients with seizures due to hypoxia or hypoglycemia, persistent mental status changes, arrhythmias, alcohol withdrawal, acute head trauma, status epilepticus, or eclampsia
- Consult neurology for new onset seizures, persistent mental status changes, new focal neurological deficits, new intracranial lesions, and pregnant patients
- Discharge may be acceptable following loading dose of anticonvulsant if vital signs are stable and mental status is at baseline; ensure follow-up in 1 week
- Patients with uncontrolled seizure disorders must be reported to state DMV and instructed not to drive or operate hazardous machinery
- Less than half of first-time seizures will have a recurrence

74. Bacterial Meningitis

Etiology & Pathophysiology

- Causative organisms depend on patient characteristics
  - The majority of bacterial cases are due to *S. pneumoniae, N. meningitidis,* or *H. influenzae*
  - Post-surgical and trauma patients: *S. aureus,* gram-negatives
  - Neonates: Group B streptococcus, *Listeria, E. coli*
  - Alcoholic patients: *S. pneumoniae*
  - Additional organisms in immunocompromised include *M. tuberculosis, Cryptococcus neoformans,* HIV
- Nasopharyngeal source of infection is most common followed by hematogenous spread through the choroid plexus into the CSF
- Increased risk of infection in elderly and neonatal patients, adolescents *(N. meningitidis),* HIV patients, post-splenectomy, uremia, alcoholics, steroid or immunosuppressant therapy, simultaneous systemic infection with bacteremia, and recent neurosurgical procedures

Differential Dx

- Non-bacterial meningitis (e.g., viral, spirochetal, chemical, autoimmune, carcinomatous)
- Encephalitis
- Brain abscess
- Stroke
- Migraine
- CNS vasculitis
- Mass lesions
- Subarachnoid hemorrhage
- Intracerebral hemorrhage

Presentation

- Triad of headache, fever, and nuchal rigidity
- Emesis
- Photophobia
- Change in mental status
- Focal neurologic findings in 5%
- Severe dermal petechial eruption in *N. meningitidis* infection
- Kernig sign: With patient in supine position with hip and knee flexed to 90°, further extension of knee will cause neck and hamstring pain
- Brudzinski sign: Flexing the neck of a supine patient results in reflexive hip and knee flexion
- Elderly patients infrequently present with classic symptoms

Diagnosis

- Diagnosis is based on presentation and CSF findings
- Head CT is required prior to lumbar puncture in any patient who may have increased intracranial pressure
- Lumbar puncture
  - Bacterial: Increased opening pressure, cloudy appearance, elevated cell count, increased protein (>150), decreased glucose (<40), WBC >1000 PMNs, decreased CSF:serum glucose ratio (<0.4); gram stain may reveal organism
  - Viral: WBC <100 lymphocytes, protein ~200, normal glucose
  - TB, fungal, autoimmune, and chemical meningitis generally present with similar CSF findings as viral meningitis (low glucose in TB and fungal disease)
  - Consider fungal and acid-fast stains, TB culture, and cryptococcal antigen
- Blood cultures

Treatment

- Bacterial: Due to the severity of disease, rapid treatment based on the presumptive diagnosis is essential
  - Empiric treatment: 3rd generation cephalosporin (e.g., ceftriaxone) plus vancomycin (20% prevalence of cephalosporin-resistant *S. pneumoniae*)
  - Meropenim plus vancomycin in penicillin allergy
  - Ampicillin may be added to cover Listeria in elderly, immunocompromised, or newborn patients
  - Tuberculous meningitis requires isoniazid, pyrazinamide, and steroids to reduce inflammatory damage (further medications are necessary in HIV patients)
- Viral: Supportive care; begin empiric antibiotic therapy until cultures prove negative
- Fungal: IV fluconazole or amphotericin
- Chemical, allergic: Remove possible sources (i.e., NSAIDs, sulfa drugs, IVIG)
- Add steroids in childhood cases to avoid chronic hearing loss
- Treat dehydration aggressively
- Anticonvulsants may be required to treat seizures

Disposition

- Bacterial: Admit for IV antibiotics, culture of organism, treatment of seizures, and frequent neurological exams (look for signs of ↑ ICP)
- Viral: Admit and begin empiric antibiotics; discharge after 24 hrs if no organism is found and CSF is consistent with viral disease
- TB, fungal: Admit as for bacterial disease; complications and mortality are high if recognized late
- Overall mortality is now as low as 10%; however, untreated mortality is $>90\%$
- Course may be complicated by DIC or concurrent infections
- CNS sequelae may include blindness, deafness, hydrocephalus, seizures, and cranial nerve palsies (rare if treated)
- Prophylaxis with rifampin for contacts of patients with *N. meningitidis*

75. Encephalitis

Etiology & Pathophysiology

- Infection of brain parenchyma, resulting in gray matter inflammation
- DNA viruses
  - Herpes type 1 is the most common sporadic viral encephalitis
  - Herpes type 2 is more common in infants
  - Varicella-zoster may cause encephalitis with stroke-like onset
- RNA viruses include arboviruses (St. Louis encephalitis, eastern equine encephalitis, western equine encephalitis, California encephalitis, West Nile virus), HIV, measles, rabies, and others
- Non-viral causes: Tuberculosis, mycoplasma, fungal, and protozoa
- Post-infectious encephalitis may occur after a "viral syndrome," resulting in a single episode of mild or severe demyelination (acute disseminated encephalomyelitis)

Differential Dx

- Stroke
- Cerebral abscess
- Meningitis
- Cerebral vasculitis
- Dementia
- Sepsis
- Drug intoxication
- Seizure
- Lyme disease
- Acute subarachnoid hemorrhage
- Electrolyte disturbance
- Acute psychosis
- Non-cerebral infection

Presentation

- Triad of headache, fever, and altered mental status
- Seizures are common
- Meningeal signs may be present
- Confusion, impaired cognition
- Intact sensory and motor function
- Ataxia may be prominent in varicella-zoster encephalitis
- Herpes-1 has a predilection for frontal and temporal lobes, resulting in memory and personality changes and olfactory hallucinations
- Rabies: Retrograde viral transport from the area bitten results in paresthesias and muscle spasms, followed by CNS symptoms

Diagnosis

- Altered mental status with or without fever and headache should prompt an expeditious spinal fluid analysis—the decision to do a lumbar puncture is the most important consideration in a patient with suspected encephalitis
- CT is usually performed before lumbar puncture to rule out increased intracranial pressure and avoid cerebral herniation
- Lumbar puncture reveals lymphocytic pleocytosis with a mildly elevated protein and a relatively normal glucose level
- MRI may show characteristic changes in cases of herpes-1 encephalitis or other pathology (e.g., temporal lobe edema)
- EEG is always abnormal in encephalitis
- Identification of the causative organism may be possible via viral antibodies or culture, recognition of viral predilection for specific brain areas, and CSF PCR for HSV-1
- The presence of altered mental status or seizures in a patient with suspected "benign" viral meningitis changes the diagnosis to meningoencephalitis

Treatment

- Rapid diagnosis and supportive care are paramount
- Increased intracranial pressure may require intubation with moderate hyperventilation, mannitol administration, and intracranial pressure monitoring
- Treat seizures as necessary; status epilepticus occurs frequently and may require multiple anticonvulsants
- Antiviral treatment is only effective for HSV—begin treatment immediately in any suspected case of HSV (mortality is >70% if treatment is delayed more than 48 hrs)
- Antiviral treatment is generally not effective for other viral causes; however, other herpes viruses may respond to antivirals
- Consider empiric antibiotics until bacterial meningitis is ruled out
- Avoid fluid overload as this can exacerbate cerebral edema
- Antiviral therapy for West Nile virus is under investigation

Disposition

- All suspected cases require admission to ICU or monitored bed
- Frequent neurological exams allow rapid diagnosis and treatment of increased intracranial pressure
- Mortality is very high despite antiviral treatment and supportive care (especially in rabies and HSV encephalitis)
- Most patients will have some long-term complications, such as memory loss, partial paralysis, and affective disorders

76. Multiple Sclerosis and ALS

Etiology & Pathophysiology

- Multiple sclerosis
  - Demyelinating disease of young adults (onset 20–40)
  - Immune-mediated destruction of CNS myelin results in demyelination and inflammation of CNS white matter
  - Multiple plaques of demyelination of different ages and in different locations are seen (separated by both "time and space")
  - Residence in northern latitudes at or prior to puberty is a clear risk factor (southern migration prior to puberty lowers risk)
- Amyotrophic Lateral Sclerosis (Lou Gehrig's disease)
  - Degeneration of upper (pyramidal tract) and lower (anterior horn cells) motor neurons—the most common motor neuron disease
  - Uncertain etiology (may involve glutamate excitotoxicity, superoxide dismutase mutation, and free-radical neurotoxicity)
  - Progressive weakness and muscle wasting, eventually leading to respiratory failure and death

Differential Dx

- Multiple sclerosis
  - Demyelinating diseases (e.g., ALD, CPM)
  - Stroke, tumor, or trauma
  - Connective-tissue disease
  - Ischemic optic neuropathy
  - Infection (e.g., Lyme, HIV, encephalitis, neurosyphilis)
- ALS
  - Compressive myelopathy
  - Myasthenia gravis
  - Inflammatory myopathy
  - Hyperthyroidism
  - Multifocal motor neuropathy

Presentation

- Multiple sclerosis
  - Weakness, optic neuritis, visual disturbance, sensory loss or paresthesias, ataxia and incoordination, vertigo, and/or sphincter dysfunction
  - Increased reflexes and Babinski
  - Lhermitte sign (electric shocks down back upon neck flexion)
- ALS
  - Insidious onset of limb atrophy, weakness, and fasciculations
  - Slurred speech, dysphagia
  - Muscle aches and cramps
  - Dyspnea secondary to respiratory muscle weakness
  - Normal vision and sensation

Diagnosis

- Multiple sclerosis
  - A clinical diagnosis in a patient with 2 or more episodes of prolonged neurologic dysfunction
  - Eye exam demonstrating bilateral internuclear ophthalmoplegia (abnormal adduction and horizontal nystagmus) is pathognomonic for MS
  - MRI is the most sensitive indicator of inflammatory white matter disease (characteristic cerebral and brainstem plaques)
  - Slowed evoked responses (visual, brainstem, somatosensory)
  - Spinal fluid analysis reveals oligoclonal bands, elevated IgG
- ALS
  - Clinical finding of hyperreflexic deep tendon reflexes despite weak, wasted, fasciculating limb muscles is often diagnostic
  - CK is often normal (CK is elevated in myopathies)
  - EMG reveals acute and chronic motor nerve damage
  - Muscle biopsy shows denervation and excludes primary muscle diseases

Treatment

- Multiple sclerosis
  - No cure exists; existing therapies often decrease symptoms
  - Acute treatment: High-dose IV corticosteroids may shorten exacerbations, but have no long-term efficacy
  - Chronic treatment: Interferon β and copolymer-1 may diminish frequency of attacks
  - Optic neuritis: High-dose IV corticosteroids
  - Symptomatic treatment with physical therapy, prosthetics and orthotics, antispastic agents (i.e., baclofen, tizanidine, clonidine, benzodiazepines), antidepressants, analgesics
- ALS
  - No effective therapies exist—death generally occurs within 2–4 years from respiratory failure or pneumonia
  - Supportive, nursing, and spiritual care
  - Riuizole, a glutamate receptor antagonist, may prolong tracheostomy-free survival by 3–6 months
  - Antispastic agents may be beneficial
  - Tracheostomy to prevent aspiration, G-tube for feeding
  - Pulmonary toilet

Disposition

- Multiple sclerosis
  - Course is marked by exacerbations and remissions in most patients
  - Benign course in 30% of patients
  - Decision to admit relates to disability severity, such as inability to ambulate or blindness
  - Death from MS itself is rare; may predispose to pneumonia and decubitus ulcer formation with resulting morbidity and mortality
- ALS
  - Emergency room visits usually occur late in disease when respiratory failure is imminent or swallowing impossible, requiring ether ventilatory support, gastrostomy, or withdrawal of futile support
  - Admit for pneumonia, respiratory failure, or uncontrolled symptoms

77. Myasthenia Gravis

Etiology & Pathophysiology

- An autoimmune disease caused by the development of antibodies to acetylcholine receptors on the post-synaptic neuromuscular junction, which inhibit muscle membrane depolarization
- Results in interference of neuromuscular transmission, leading to an insidious onset of muscular weakness and disability
- Pathogenesis may revolve around the thymus tissue, which likely provides a milieu for autoantibody production in susceptible patients
- There is a 20% concurrent incidence of autoimmune hypothyroidism in MG patients, suggesting a more generalized autoimmune state
- Associated with thymic tumors (hyperplasia, thymoma), thyrotoxicosis, D-penicillamine therapy, rheumatoid arthritis, SLE
- Occurs in young adults (especially young females) and the elderly
- Myasthenic crisis: Respiratory muscle weakness causing respiratory failure

Differential Dx

- Cholinergic crisis (therapeutic drug overdose)
- Guillain-Barré syndrome
- Botulism
- Lambert-Eaton syndrome
- Paralytic medications
- Brainstem stroke
- Ocular myopathy
- Thyroid disease
- Idiopathic cranial neuropathy
- Tick paralysis
- Organophosphate poisoning
- Amyotrophic lateral sclerosis

Presentation

- Weakness
  - Ocular and facial muscles are most frequently involved (diplopia, ptosis, dysphagia, drooling, difficulty chewing)
  - Symmetrical limb weakness (proximal > distal)
  - May have respiratory failure due to respiratory muscle weakness
  - Weakness often fluctuates
  - Especially prominent following persistent activity
- Fatigue and exercise intolerance
- Symptoms may be so subtle as to suggest hysteria
- Normal reflexes, cerebellar, and sensory function

Diagnosis

- Subacute onset of fluctuating diplopia and ptosis with normal pupillary responses strongly suggests the diagnosis
- Anticholinergic challenge with edrophonium (Tensilon test) will rapidly and temporarily reverse symptoms in >70% of patients
  - Used for the initial diagnosis of MG
  - Also used to distinguish myasthenic crisis (worsening of disease) versus cholinergic crisis (supratherapeutic drug levels from MG medications)—edrophonium will reverse myasthenic crisis but have no effect on cholinergic crisis
- Acetylcholine receptor antibody assay is positive in 85%
- CBC, blood cultures, urinalysis, and CSF are normal
- TSH to rule out hyperthyroidism
- CT of mediastinum may be used to rule out tumor of thymus
- Repetitive nerve stimulation results in a decremental response in motor unit action potential amplitude
- Single-fiber EMG is very sensitive for MG

Treatment

- ED treatment
  - Symptomatic treatment with acetylcholinesterase inhibitors (e.g., neostigmine, pyridostigmine), which allow more time for acetylcholine to compete for binding at the neuromuscular junction
  - Intubate as necessary for respiratory failure (avoid paralytic agents during intubation, which may cause prolonged neuromuscular blockade)
- Additional inpatient and long-term treatments
  - Corticosteroids (30% chance of transient but severe symptom exacerbation)
  - Intravenous immunoglobulin (IVIG) or plasmapheresis for respiratory failure or severe limb weakness
  - Chemotherapy or immunosuppressives (e.g., azathioprine, methotrexate, cyclosporine) in refractory cases
  - Thymectomy may be curative; however, no accurate controlled trial data exist
- Avoid aminoglycosides, sedatives, β-blockers, and other medications that may cause or enhance weakness

Disposition

- With the appropriate use of supportive measures, MG is rarely fatal
- Observe for signs of restrictive pulmonary failure, such as agitation, diaphoresis, or rapid and shallow breathing (simple measurement of pO_2 and pCO_2 may fail to reveal significant respiratory distress)
- Patients with forced vital capacity <1 L usually require prophylactic intubation or BiPAP
- Admit patients with moderate to severe symptoms and/or any signs of respiratory compromise
- Discharge patients with mild disease on anticholinesterase inhibitors and with expeditious neurological follow-up
- Do not start steroids without direction from a neurologic consultant

78. Acute Neuropathy

Etiology & Pathophysiology

- Weakness, loss of sensation, and/or pain in the distribution of one or more nerves over hours to days
- Often due to compression by trauma, bleeding, or inflammation
- Bell's palsy is an idiopathic unilateral facial nerve palsy
- Guillain-Barré syndrome (GBS) is an autoimmune inflammatory polyneuropathy that damages myelin sheaths and is usually preceded by viral or *Campylobacter jejuni* infection
- Acute intermittent porphyria is an autosomal dominant defect in heme synthesis that causes episodic weakness, abdominal pain, and psychosis; medications or systemic illness cause exacerbations
- Brachial plexopathy is a benign idiopathic plexus inflammation
- Toxic chemotherapeutic agents may cause symmetrical neuropathy
- Other acute neuropathies include herpes zoster, acute diabetic lumbar plexopathy, and vasculitis

Differential Dx

- Bell's palsy: CVA, herpes zoster, acoustic neuroma, GBS, Lyme disease
- GBS: Myasthenia gravis, polio, botulism, tick paralysis, diphtheria, myositis, electrolyte abnormalities, spinal cord lesion, West Nile virus
- Bioterrorism
- Entrapment neuropathy
- Chronic neuropathy (e.g., diabetes, alcohol, drugs, HIV)

Presentation

- Note location of symptoms, symmetry of reflexes, strength, sensation, autonomic symptoms
- Bell's palsy: Unilateral facial *and* forehead muscle paresis
- GBS: Rapid onset of symmetric ascending paralysis that may involve facial or respiratory muscles (30%); areflexia; minimal sensory loss; may have autonomic symptoms
- Porphyria: Symmetrical decrease in strength, reflexes, and sensation; psychosis; abdominal pain
- Brachial plexopathy: Acute, severe shoulder, back, arm pain/weakness

Diagnosis

- Clinical diagnosis—Weakness and hypo- or areflexia is the most common presentation
- Bell's palsy: A clinical diagnosis in the presence of an otherwise normal neurologic exam and no evidence of zoster
- Guillain-Barré syndrome: Diagnosed clinically by a history of preceding viral illness followed by bilateral ascending paralysis with areflexia
  - CSF shows albuminocytologic dissociation (elevated spinal fluid protein with normal cell counts)
- Acute porphyria: Patient or family history of similar attacks of weakness; labs normal except for elevated serum porphobilinogen (PBG) and δ-aminolevulinic acid (ALA)
- Brachial plexopathy: CXR to rule out mass lesions
- Varicella-zoster: Dermatomal symptoms with vesicular skin lesions
- EMG and nerve conduction testing for diagnostic confirmation and prognosis (especially in cases of drug toxicities)

Treatment

- Bell's palsy
  - Eye lubricants
  - Systemic steroids for 10 days may shorten the recovery period and improve outcome
  - Acyclovir is sometimes used but is controversial
- Guillain-Barré syndrome
  - Intubate patients with respiratory muscle compromise
  - Intravenous immunoglobulins (IVIG) or plasmapheresis are equally effective
  - Steroids are ineffective
- Acute intermittent porphyria
  - Withdraw offending drugs or reverse offending conditions that may have precipitated the attack (e.g., dehydration)
  - Other therapies include glucose infusion (limits symptoms by preventing heme synthesis), vitamin B_6, or hematin
- Diabetes or vasculitis: Consider amitriptyline, gabapentin, or anticonvulsants to decrease neuropathic pain
- Herpes zoster: Acyclovir within 3 days of onset decreases the risk and severity of post-herpetic neuralgia

Disposition

- Inpatient versus outpatient disposition generally depends upon the perceived risk of respiratory compromise
- Guillain-Barré syndrome and acute porphyria require admission
- Bell's palsy: 80% recover within a few months
- >85% of patients with GBS recover with supportive care; however, patients may require prolonged hospital stays and 5% remain permanently disabled
- West Nile virus may present as GBS or a polio-like syndrome
- Brachial plexopathy usually resolves within 1–2 weeks
- Herpes zoster may cause a prolonged, painful post-herpetic neuralgia

79. Nerve Compression Syndromes

Etiology & Pathophysiology

- Nerve injury from compression can be divided into through-and-through lacerating injury (neurotmesis), crush injury affecting axons and myelin (axontmesis), and pure myelin injury (neuropraxia)
- Nerves most vulnerable to compression include the median nerve at the carpal tunnel, the ulnar nerve at the elbow, the common peroneal nerve at the head of the fibula, the radial nerve at the humerus, and the sciatic nerve at the piriformis muscle
- Common causes include pressure from surrounding structures in areas where minimal free space is available (e.g., carpal tunnel, lateral fibular head) and traumatic or inflammatory processes (e.g., hematoma due to stabbing or GSW, crush injury from falls, or MVC)
- Nerves may also be compromised at their respective nerve roots due to foraminal narrowing—C-7 and S-1 roots are commonly affected
- Metabolic diseases (e.g., diabetes mellitus, hypothyroidism, vasculitis) predispose to compression and damage

Differential Dx

- Tendon, muscle, and ligament tears
- Compartment syndromes
- Ischemic nerve injury
- Stroke
- Spinal cord injury
- Guillain-Barré syndrome
- Hysteria
- Chronic neuropathy (e.g., alcohol, diabetes, HIV)
- Bell's palsy
- Mononeuritis multiplex
- Lumbar plexopathy
- Brachial neuritis

Presentation

- Median nerve: Morning numbness and nighttime pain of the wrist, thumb, 2nd, and 3rd digits
- Ulnar nerve: Numbness of the 4th and 5th digits, elbow pain
- Radial nerve: Numbness over the lateral dorsal surface of the hand
- Peroneal nerve: Foot drop and lateral knee pain
- Sciatic nerve: Pain in the buttock radiating to lateral calf and sole; numbness of lateral foreleg/sole
- S-1 and C-7 root compression may mimic sciatic and radial nerve compression with back and neck pain, respectively

Diagnosis

- Diagnosis is suggested by history (see presentation box) and physical exam (below)
  - Entrapment/compression of any nerve is suspected by a positive Tinel's sign (tapping on the nerve elicits symptoms)
  - Median nerve: Phalen's sign (prolonged wrist flexion) provokes symptoms; thenar wasting; weak thumb opposition
  - Ulnar nerve: Hypothenar wasting; weakness of intrinsic hand muscles with decreased grip strength, finger abduction/adduction, and thumb adduction; claw hand in severe cases
  - Radial nerve: Extension weakness of wrist and fingers (triceps strength is generally preserved)
  - Peroneal nerve: Foot drop with poor dorsiflexion and eversion; preserved inversion and plantar flexion
  - Sciatic nerve: Weakness of the foot, lower leg, and hamstring
- Degree of nerve compression can generally be judged only by electromyography and nerve conduction testing performed several weeks after an anatomic insult

Treatment

- Acute nerve compression (e.g., spontaneous or provoked bleeding into nerve tissue due to trauma or coagulation abnormalities) necessitates emergent decompression
- If compartment syndrome is suspected, limb pressure measurements and appropriate compartment release is indicated
- General treatment with NSAIDs and rest of the affected area
- Chronic cases (e.g., carpal tunnel syndrome, ulnar, and peroneal neuropathies) rarely need urgent treatment; surgery or physical medicine referral is generally appropriate
  - Carpal tunnel syndrome: Wrist splinting, physical therapy, surgical release if conservative measures fail
  - Radial neuropathy: Wrist splinting, physical therapy
  - Ulnar neuropathy at the elbow: Elbow pad and cessation of traumatic activity
  - Peroneal neuropathy: Ankle-foot orthosis, physical therapy
  - Nerve root compression: Physical therapy, analgesia, and possible surgery

Disposition

- Admit patients with acute nerve compression or possible compartment syndromes
- Follow-up care and EMG/nerve conduction velocity is generally required to determine prognosis and need for surgical intervention in persistent nerve compressions
- Presence of chronic symptoms, muscle weakness, or muscle wasting requires surgical referral for possible decompressive surgery

80. Spinal Cord Compression Syndromes

Etiology & Pathophysiology

- Spinal cord compression is a medical emergency in which pressure causes bilateral loss of motor and sensory function below the lesion
- Red flags (high-risk criteria) for cord compression
  - Medical history: Cancer, age >50, conditions predisposing to hemorrhage or infection, weight loss, bone disease, elevated ESR
  - HPI: Trauma, pain upon lying down, bilateral symptoms, fever, bowel/bladder dysfunction, unexplained or progressive weakness
- Disc herniation may cause root or cord compression
- Metastatic cord compression is due to impingement by pathologically fractured bone or due to direct tumor extension
- Epidural abscess: Infection of the spinal epidural space due to hematogenous or contiguous spread of organisms
- Epidural hematoma: Bleeding into the epidural space
- Radiculopathy is a non-urgent compression of nerve roots resulting in pain, parestheias, and weakness in the nerve root distribution

Differential Dx

- Herniated intervertebral disc
- Neoplastic cord compression
- Epidural abscess
- Spinal cord abscess
- Epidural spinal hemorrhage
- Post-traumatic compression
- Osteoporotic compression
- Cervical spondylosis
- Spinal cord AVM
- Transverse myelitis
- Multiple sclerosis
- Syringomyelia
- Vitamin B_{12} deficiency

Presentation

- Symptoms of cord compression may include back pain; motor, reflex, or sensory losses below the level of the lesion; and bowel or bladder dysfunction
- Disc herniation: Pain, usually with radicular symptoms; <10% have cord compression
- Metastatic pain is often worse with recumbancy
- Epidural abscess: Pain, fever, progressive weakness
- Epidural hematoma: Pain and progressive weakness
- Spinal subarachnoid: Sudden onset of back pain with meningeal signs

Diagnosis

- Imaging of suspected cord compression
  - Low-risk patients (back pain only, no red flags) do not require imaging
  - Medium-risk patients (back pain or abnormal exam plus any red flag) require MRI of the spine within 24 hours
  - High-risk patients (exam suggesting cord or cauda equina lesion or suspicion of epidural abscess) require emergent MRI
- MRI is the gold standard to identify compression—very high sensitivity for cord impingement
- CT myelogram is used if MRI cannot be performed or is unavailable
- Plain X-rays may show metastatic disease but do not rule out compression and should not delay more definitive studies
- ESR is elevated in metastatic or epidural abscess (100% sensitive for abscess)
- CBC is insensitive for epidural abscess
- Check PT/PTT in cases of spinal cord hemorrhage

Treatment

- Metastatic compression
  - Steroids: IV dexamethasone improves outcomes
  - Radiotherapy (if done emergently) may improve pain and decrease the incidence of paraplegia
  - Surgery is often not an option in patients with advanced cancer, but may provide stabilization of unstable bony structures
- Epidural abscess
  - IV antibiotics to cover *Staphylococcus* and gram negative organisms
  - Emergent neurosurgical consultation for emergency decompressive laminectomy and drainage in most patients
- Epidural hematoma requires correction of any coagulation abnormalities and emergent decompressive laminectomy with clot evacuation
- Disc herniation should be treated with NSAIDs, IV steroids, and surgical consultation if motor symptoms are present

Disposition

- Early diagnosis of compression is the factor that most significantly improves outcomes
- Duration of pretreatment paralysis is the main predictor of paraplegia
- The key differential is between actual spinal cord compression, which requires emergent diagnosis and intervention, and radiculopathy, which does not require urgent therapy
- Cauda equina syndrome presents with lower extremity weakness, bowel or bladder dysfunction, and decreased perianal sensation
- Epidural abscess is often present in patients without risk factors for infection (20–60%) and may present prior to development of neurologic symptoms—consider the diagnosis in any patient with fever and back pain

Renal and Genitourinary Emergencies

ADAM COHEN, MD

81. Acute Renal Failure

Etiology & Pathophysiology

- A rapid decline in renal function (GFR) over hours to days
- Prerenal failure (40% of cases): Due to conditions that reduce renal blood flow/perfusion, such as decreased circulating volume (e.g., dehydration, hemorrhage, excessive diuresis, GI/renal losses), decreased cardiac output (e.g., CHF, cardiogenic shock), 3rd spacing (e.g., sepsis, cirrhosis, pancreatitis), ACE-inhibitor or NSAID use
- Intrinsic (parenchymal) failure (50%): Due to disease of the glomerulus or tubule (e.g., ATN due to ischemia secondary to poor renal perfusion, drugs, or contrast agents), renal artery obstruction, glomerulonephritis, TTP, vasculitis, post-streptococcal, SLE, interstitial nephritis (e.g., drug, infection, idiopathic), drug nephrotoxicity, rhabdomyolysis, myeloma, or atheromatous emboli
- Postrenal failure (10%): Due to processes that increase tubular pressures by blocking urine outflow (e.g., enlarged prostate, urethral stricture, pelvic mass, urolithiasis, surgery, or neurogenic bladder)

Differential Dx

- Chronic renal failure
- Diabetic or alcoholic ketoacidosis
- CHF
- Pulmonary edema
- Anemia
- Abdominal aneurysm
- Hemolytic-uremic syndrome
- Hypertensive crisis
- Urolithiasis
- Ureteral transection
- Traumatic kidney laceration with urinary extravasation

Presentation

- Symptoms of renal failure include nausea/vomiting, metallic taste, abdominal pain, lethargy
- Oliguria or anuria may be present
- Symptoms of volume overload
- History or symptoms of specific etiologies may be apparent
  - Prerenal: Vomiting, diarrhea, poor oral intake, edema, CHF, use of diuretics/NSAIDs/ACE-inhibitors
  - Intrinsic: Diabetes, SLE, HTN, recent nephrotoxic drug or contrast exposure, strep infection, crush injury
  - Postrenal: BPH, recent surgery, recurrent UTIs, kidney stones

Diagnosis

- Increasing serum BUN and creatinine
- Abnormal urine output
  - Anuria (<100 mL/d) suggests postrenal obstruction, severe intrinsic renal injury, or renal artery occlusion
  - Oliguria (100–400 mL/d) suggests prerenal disease
  - Non-oliguria (>400 mL/d) is typical of intrinsic processes
- Electrolytes: Hyperkalemia, increased phosphate, and metabolic acidosis in most cases (may have elevated or normal anion gap)
  - Prerenal: Serum BUN/Cr ratio >20, contraction alkalosis, elevated uric acid, low urine Na^+ (<20 meq/L), high urine creatinine and osmoles, normal urine microscopy, $Fe_{Na} = [(U_{Na}/P_{Na})*(P_{Cr}/U_{Cr})*100]$ is <1
  - Intrinsic: Fe_{Na}>1; microscopy shows casts (granular, WBC, or RBC), high urine Na^+ (>20 meq/L), low urine Cr, proteinuria
  - Postrenal: Urine electrolytes and Fe_{Na} vary
- Serologies may help to identify causes of intrinsic disease
- Renal ultrasound may be used to exclude postrenal obstruction

Treatment

- Place a Foley catheter in all patients to rule out potential urethral/bladder outlet obstruction and monitor urine output
- Discontinue all nephrotoxic drugs
- Prompt treatment of hypovolemia in prerenal disease
- Diuresis with loop diuretics does not improve renal function but may decrease volume overload, preventing the need for hemodialysis
- Low-dose ("renal") dopamine may transiently improve urine output but has not been shown to improve outcome or renal function
- In prerenal states, afterload reducers and positive inotropes to increase cardiac output may improve renal perfusion
- Administer bicarbonate to counter severe acidosis
- Treat hyperkalemia appropriately and monitor closely
- Dialysis or continuous hemodiafiltration is indicated for symptoms of uremia (e.g., encephalopathy), fluid overload (e.g., pulmonary edema), or severe electrolyte/acid-base abnormalities (e.g., severe hyperkalemia, acidosis)
- Treat underlying etiologies as appropriate

Disposition

- Mortality from ARF is approximately 50%, regardless of age
- Prognosis depends on etiology, co-morbid conditions, preexisting renal disease, and degree of oliguria
- 20–60% require hemodialysis at some point during the course of disease
- Admit all patients
- Nephrology consultation is indicated for cases of intrinsic renal failure of undetermined etiology and if urgent dialysis is required
- Drug dosages must be adjusted based on the patient's new GFR

82. Urinary Retention

Etiology & Pathophysiology

- Caused by physical obstruction of the urinary tract or failure of neurologic control mechanisms
- May occur at any level from the renal pelvis to the distal urethra
- Results in increasing tubular pressures, leading to a progressive decrease in GFR and, eventually, compromised renal perfusion
- Causes of physical obstruction include benign prostatic hypertrophy, urolithiasis, pelvic surgery, pelvic malignancy, prostate cancer, pregnancy, trauma, blood clots, phimosis or meatal stenosis, and infection
- Neurogenic causes include diabetes, herniated disc, spinal cord injury or compression, medications (e.g., α-agonists, β-agonists, antihistamines, dicyclomine, diazepam, tricyclics, anticholinergics), multiple sclerosis, myasthenia gravis, Parkinson's disease, brain tumor, and CVA
- Common post-operatively

Differential Dx

- Urolithiasis
- Intravascular volume depletion
- Acute renal failure
- Phimosis
- Meatal stenosis
- Aortic aneurysm
- Cauda equina syndrome
- Pregnancy
- Pelvic or renal malignancy
- Uterine leiomyoma

Presentation

- Inability to void
- Change in urinary patterns (e.g., nocturia, polyuria, hesitancy, urgency, or difficulty starting stream)
- Abdominal pain may be present secondary to distension of bladder, ureter, or collecting system
- Slowly progressive processes (e.g., tumors, BPH) may present without pain
- Palpable bladder on abdominal exam
- Rectal or pelvic exam may demonstrate enlarged pelvic structures, especially the prostate

Diagnosis

- Often presents with renal failure and concomitant electrolyte and blood pressure disturbances
  - Hyponatremia
  - Hyperkalemia
  - Acidosis (anion gap may be normal or increased)
  - Azotemia (elevated BUN and creatinine) in advanced states
- Urinalysis may reveal hematuria, pyuria, or crystalluria and will also rule out infection
- Post-void residual is a good measure of adequacy of bladder emptying (abnormal is >125 cc residual urine)
- Imaging studies (helical CT scan, renal ultrasound, and/or intravenous pyelography) may be used to rule out causes of obstruction

Treatment

- Immediate catheter drainage of bladder contents
  - Foley or coudé catheter is preferred
  - Place suprapubic catheter if unable to pass a Foley
  - Maintain catheter drainage until definitive therapy is possible
- Correct electrolyte and volume disturbances
- Treat UTIs with appropriate antibiotics
- Medications may include α-1 antagonists (e.g., tamsulosin) for BPH, oxybutynin to prevent spasm of urinary bladder muscle, and bethanechol to induce urinary bladder muscle contraction
- Definitive therapy may require prostate surgery, percutaneous nephrostomy tube (for obstruction proximal to the mid-ureter), or cystoscopy with ureteral stent placement (for distal ureteral obstructions)

Disposition

- Discharge with close follow-up is acceptable for simple distal bladder/urethral obstructions relieved by catheter placement (the catheter should be left in place and attached to a leg bag)
- Inpatient management for renal failure, surgical drainage, severe volume or electrolyte disturbances, and any evidence of post-obstructive diuresis
- Complications include acute renal failure, transient gross hematuria, and post-obstructive diuresis
- Post-obstructive diuresis involves the loss of up to 20 L of fluid after relief of chronic obstruction (due to transient tubule dysfunction) and often results in volume, blood pressure, and electrolyte imbalances

83. Nephrolithiasis

Etiology & Pathophysiology

- Most often due to increased concentrations of stone-forming material in urine, either from increased excretion or decreased urinary volume
- Calcium oxalate/phosphate stones (80%): Due to idiopathic hypercalciuria, hyperuricosuria, hyperoxaluria, primary hyperparathyroidism, low urine citrate, and type I RTA
- Uric acid stones (10%): Associated with low urine pH and hyperuricosuria
- Struvite stones (magnesium ammonium phosphate): Associated with UTIs with urea-splitting organisms (e.g., *Proteus, Klebsiella*)
- Cystine stones (<1%): Associated with cystinuria
- Risk factors include male gender, high protein diet, low water intake, HTN, malignancy, post-vasectomy, immobilization, gout, short-bowel syndrome, spinal cord injuries, protease inhibitors, allopurinol, and family history
- May result in obstruction with eventual irreversible renal damage

Differential Dx

- Ectopic pregnancy
- Pelvic inflammatory disease
- Mittelschmertz
- Pyelonephritis
- Renal infarct/vein thrombosis
- Acute papillary necrosis
- Renal cancer with obstruction
- Common causes of abdominal pain (e.g., appendicitis, biliary colic, diverticulitis, AAA, pancreatitis, obstruction)
- Mesenteric ischemia
- Herpes zoster (shingles)
- Factitious/malingering

Presentation

- Sudden onset of severe, colicky, unilateral flank pain (may radiate to the lower abdomen, groin, testicles, or perineum)
- Pain occurs in paroxysms lasting 20–60 minutes; may have complete resolution between episodes
- Nausea, vomiting, and diaphoresis are common
- Urinary symptoms may include dysuria and frequency
- Severe acute urethral pain may signal the passage of a stone
- Hematuria
- History of prior urolithiasis
- Fever suggests concurrent infection

Diagnosis

- Characteristic clinical presentation is highly predictive, especially in patients with a past history of urolithiasis
- Urinalysis reveals hematuria in >90% of cases; however, its absence does not exclude the diagnosis; also used to evaluate for the presence of infection
- Strain urine for stones and send to lab for analysis
- Renal function tests (BUN/creatinine) are usually normal
- Non-contrast helical CT is the gold standard for detecting stones and signs of obstruction (e.g., ureteral and collecting system dilatation, perinephric stranding); will also differentiate urolithiasis from other diagnoses (e.g., aortic aneurysm, tumor)
- Intravenous pyelogram and ultrasound are now used less frequently and are less sensitive than CT, but may diagnose radiolucent stones, better localize stones, and detect obstruction

Treatment

- Most stones are smaller than 5 mm and will pass on their own; thus, treatment for a first-time stone is generally supportive (stone passage depends on size, location, and presence of obstruction)
  - Analgesia (NSAIDs, especially IV/IM ketorolac, are probably as effective as opiates)
  - Hydration (1–2 L bolus of normal saline)
  - Antiemetics as needed for nausea/vomiting
- IV antibiotics if infection is present (usually ampicillin plus gentamycin or a fluoroquinolone alone)
- Stones too large to pass are treated with endoscopic lithotripsy, extracorporeal shock wave lithotripsy, open pyelolithotomy, or percutaneous nephrolithotomy
- Type of stones may indicate further outpatient treatment
  - Calcium: Limit sodium intake, thiazide diuretics for hypercalciuria, allopurinol for hyperuricosuria, potassium citrate for hypocitraturia
  - Uric acid: Alkalinize urine, allopurinol
  - Cystine: High fluid intake, alkalinize urine

Disposition

- Most patients can be managed as outpatients with oral hydration (>2 L water per day) and NSAIDs
- Instruct patients to strain their urine and submit stones for further analysis
- Urgent urology consultation for renal failure, urosepsis, or solitary kidney
- Criteria for admission include inability to tolerate oral intake, refractory severe pain, concurrent infection, or single kidney with obstruction
- Consider admission for patients with large (>5 mm) stones that are unlikely to pass or with severe co-morbid diseases
- Patients with recurrent stones should be referred for more detailed metabolic and radiologic evaluation
- Ironically, high dietary calcium may decrease the risk of stones by forming ligands with oxalate and phosphate

84. Urinary Tract Infections

Etiology & Pathophysiology

- Infection of the lower urinary tract (cystitis) and/or upper tract (pyelonephritis)
- Complicated UTIs may result in systemic illness, bacteremia, and/or treatment failure—complicating factors include male sex, old age, hospital-acquired infection, indwelling catheter, recent urinary tract instrumentation, functional or anatomic abnormality, recent antibiotic use, symptoms >7 days, diabetes, neurogenic bladder, and immunosuppression
- Uncomplicated UTIs are generally due to *E. coli* (80–90%), *Staphylococcus saprophyticus* (20%), *Proteus, Klebsiella, Enterococcus, Chlamydia*
- Complicated UTIs are often due to antibiotic resistant organisms, including *E. coli, Pseudomonas, Proteus, Klebsiella, S. aureus, Enterococcus, Serratia*, and *Enterobacter*

Differential Dx

- Vulvovaginitis (*Candida, Trichomonas, Gardnerella*)
- Urethritis
- Cervicitis
- Pelvic inflammatory disease
- Prostatitis
- Epididymitis
- Urolithiasis
- Various causes of abdominal pain (e.g., pregnancy/ectopic pregnancy, diverticulitis, appendicitis)
- Interstitial cystitis

Presentation

- Dysuria
- Urinary frequency/urgency
- Suprapubic pain/tenderness
- Sense of incomplete voiding
- Hematuria may be present
- Pyelonephritis will additionally present with fever, nausea, vomiting, flank pain, and CVA tenderness
- Infants most commonly present with fever and irritability
- Elderly may present with mental status change, fever, abdominal pain, or without symptoms

Diagnosis

- Midstream voiding specimen (large numbers of epithelial cells suggest contamination and need for a catheter specimen) or catheter specimen
- Urinalysis with >5 leukocytes/HPF suggests UTI
- Urine dipstick is generally considered positive if either leukocyte esterase or nitrites are present
  –Leukocyte esterase has >75% sensitivity and 95% specificity
  –Nitrites are highly specific (>90%) but not sensitive (50%)
  –Symptomatic patients with a negative dipstick require a more sensitive microscopic examination for pyuria
- Urine culture is only required for complicated UTIs (positive culture is >100,000 organisms/mL)
- Consider CT or renal ultrasound for UTIs that are refractory to treatment; may reveal renal abscess, obstruction, or stone

Treatment

- Antibiotic choice depends on local drug resistance patterns (e.g., up to 35% of *E. coli* are resistant to TMP-SMX but only 2% are resistant to fluoroquinolones)
- Uncomplicated cystitis
  –First Line: TMP/SMX or fluoroquinolone for 3 days
  –Second Line: Nitrofurantoin or β-lactam for 7 days
  –Pregnancy: Amoxicillin, cephalexin, or nitrofurantoin
  –Children: Cefixime, ampicillin/sulbactam, or TMP/SMX
- Complicated cystitis: Fluoroquinolone, aminoglycoside, or ceftriaxone for 7–14 days
- Uncomplicated pyelonephritis
  –First Line: Oral fluoroquinolone for 10–14 days
  –Second Line: TMP/SMX or cefixime for 14 days
  –Consider initial IV dose in the ED, then begin oral therapy
- Complicated pyelonephritis: Fluoroquinolone, ampicillin plus gentamicin, or penicillin/anti-penicillinase (start IV then change to oral when improving) for 14 days
- Phenazopyridine may be used as analgesia for dysuria

Disposition

- Patients with cystitis can be discharged
- Admit all patients with complicated pyelonephritis for IV antibiotics
- Admit patients with uncomplicated pyelonephritis who cannot tolerate oral intake, have severe illness or high fever, are pregnant, or have questionable compliance
- Urology referral for any upper UTI that remains symptomatic after 72 hours of therapy, recurrence of pyelonephritis, and men with recurrent UTIs
- Urology/PCP follow-up in all children
- Obtain cultures in all pregnant women and follow up in 2–3 days

85. Male Urethritis

Etiology & Pathophysiology

- Infectious or traumatic inflammation of the urethra
- Sexually transmitted organisms are the most common infectious causes
  - Gonococcal urethritis
  - Nongonococcal urethritis: Commonly *Chlamydia, Ureaplasma, Mycoplasma,* or *Trichomonas*; less commonly HSV, lymphogranuloma venereum or gram negatives
- Post-traumatic urethritis may occur following catheterization
- Urethritis may also be associated with epididymitis, orchitis, prostatitis, Reiter's syndrome, pneumonia, and otitis media

Differential Dx

- Urethral foreign body
- Reiter's syndrome
- Prostatitis
- Epididymitis
- Orchitis
- Cystitis

Presentation

- Patients may present with common STD symptoms
  - Dysuria
  - Urethral discharge
  - Arthritis
  - Conjunctivitis/uveitis
  - Proctitis
- Patients may have a history of STDs, partner with STD, promiscuous or unprotected intercourse, urethral stricture, or recent urethral instrumentation

Diagnosis

- Palpate along the urethra to exclude abscess or foreign body and to determine if there is an expressible purulent discharge
- Examine the testes and prostate to exclude epididymitis, orchitis, or prostatitis
- Examine the genitals for evidence of other STDs, such as herpes, syphilis, or condyloma
- Laboratory studies
  - Gram stain and culture of urethral discharge for *N. gonorrheae* and *Chlamydia*
  - Test a first void specimen for leukocyte esterase or WBCs (presence may indicate simple urethritis or UTI)
  - Syphilis serology (VDRL or RPR)
- Urethritis is suggested by a mucopurulent or purulent discharge, gram stain demonstrating >5 WBC/hpf, or presence of intracellular gram-negative diplococci, and first void urine containing leukocyte esterase or >10 WBC/hpf

Treatment

- Urethritis should be confirmed before treatment is initiated
- Empiric treatment prior to identification of pathogens should be administered in all patients with a clinical presentation consistent with urethritis
- All patients with potential STDs must be treated for both gonococcus and chlamydia; cover with both gonococcal and non-gonococcal antibiotics
- Gonococcal urethritis
  - Single dose IM 3rd generation cephalosporin (add probenicid to the shorter acting cephalosporins)
  - Single dose oral cefixime
  - Single dose oral ofloxacin or levofloxacin
- Non-gonococcal urethritis
  - Single dose oral azithromycin
  - Doxycycline, ofloxacin, or levofloxacin for 7 days

Disposition

- Instruct patients to return if symptoms persist or recur after completion of therapy
- Instruct patients to abstain from intercourse for seven days after therapy is initiated and until all partners have been appropriately treated
- All sexual partners who had contact with the patient within the past 60 days should be referred for evaluation and treatment
- Pregnant women and adolescents should be referred for re-screening 3 weeks after completion of therapy
- STDs must be reported to the local health department

86. Penile Disorders

Etiology & Pathophysiology

- Balanitis: Inflammation of the glans, often due to fungal infection secondary to poor hygiene
- Phimosis: Inability to retract the foreskin proximally over the glans
  - May be congenital (physiologic in young boys and resolves spontaneously by age 11–12) or acquired (due to poor hygiene, balanitis, or repeated forced retraction of a congenital phimosis)
- Paraphimosis is a true emergency with entrapment and inability to reduce the retracted foreskin over the proximal glans
  - Etiologies include frequent catheterizations, poor hygiene, skin piercing, and chronic balanoposthitis leading to phimosis
  - Blood supply to the glans may be compromised, causing necrosis
- Penile tourniquet occurs when an object (e.g., hair, rubber band) wraps around the penis, causing ischemia
- Penile fracture: Blunt trauma (often during intercourse) may tear the tunica albuginea, corpora cavernosa, and/or the urethra

Differential Dx

- Balanitis
- Cellulitis
- Penile tourniquet
- Penile cancer
- Prostatitis
- Urethritis
- Urethral foreign bodies
- Epididymitis
- Fournier's gangrene

Presentation

- Balanitis: Erythematous, tender, and itchy glans; penile discharge; difficulty with urination
- Phimosis: Inability to retract the foreskin over the glans; concerning symptoms include pain, decreased urinary stream, and hematuria
- Paraphimosis: Tender, edematous, erythematous glans with foreskin edema and flaccidity of the proximal penile shaft
- Penile tourniquet: Swollen penis in the presence of a constricting agent
- Penile fracture: Penile pain, edema, and ecchymoses or hematoma following an audible "crack"

Diagnosis

- History and characteristic physical findings are often diagnostic
- If there is a high suspicion of urethral injury (e.g., blood at the urethral meatus), a retrograde urethrogram should be obtained to rule out urethral involvement
- Check glucose in persistent cases of balanitis to rule out diabetes mellitus
- Penile ultrasound for suspected cases of penile fracture

Treatment

- Balanitis: Topical antifungals; ensure good personal hygiene
- Phimosis
  - Asymptomatic cases do not require ED treatment
  - Patients with severe, concerning symptoms may require semi-urgent foreskin opening (preferably by urology)
  - Urinary catheter for urinary retention
- Paraphimosis and penile tourniquet require emergent reduction
  - First, ensure that there is no foreign material (e.g., rings, hair, clothing, rubber bands) causing the problem
  - Prior to reduction, consider maneuvers to reduce glans edema (e.g., ice, direct digital pressure, wrapping the glans with gauze)
  - Manual reduction may be attempted prior to urologic referral by applying pressure over the glans with both thumbs while simultaneously pulling the retracted foreskin over the glans with the index fingers
- Penile fractures require surgical repair; administer pain control, cold compresses, and a Foley catheter in the ED

Disposition

- Balanitis: Urology outpatient referral to screen for penile cancer; may be the initial presentation of diabetes mellitus
- Phimosis: Non-emergent urologic referral for elective circumcision if accompanied by decreased urinary stream, hematuria, or preputial pain
- Paraphimosis: If reduction is successful, outpatient referral to urology is indicated for elective circumcision as recurrence is likely
- Penile tourniquet: Emergent urologic referral if tourniquet cannot be removed

87. Priapism

Etiology & Pathophysiology

- A persistent erection (>6 hours) despite orgasm or end of sexual desire
- A urologic emergency due to deregulation of detumescence with persistently elevated pressure in the corpora cavernosa
- Low flow (ischemic) priapism: Venous occlusion/obstruction of corpora cavernosal outflow results in persistent venous engorgement, decreased blood flow, persistent erection, and, eventually, penile ischemia (after 6 hours)
- High flow (non-ischemic) priapism: Increased cavernosal arterial inflow exceeds venous outflow, usually due to trauma that results in an arterial fistula in the penis—ischemia is less common
- Impotence is the most feared complication—risk of impotence increases with duration of priapism (especially if >24 hr)
  - Up to 50% of low flow cases result in impotence
  - 20% of high flow cases result in impotence

Differential Dx

- Medication or injection therapy for erectile dysfunction
- Sickle cell disease/thalassemia
- Drugs (e.g., antihypertensives, phenothiazines, anticoagulants)
- Illicit drugs (e.g., cocaine, MDMA, marijuana)
- Ethanol
- Spinal cord injury
- Leukemia/polycythemia
- Amyloidosis
- Snake/scorpion bite
- Penile/perineal trauma

Presentation

- Low flow priapism
  - Extremely painful erect or semi-erect penis
  - Soft glans
  - Erection may be present for hours to days
- High flow priapism
  - Usually presents with a lesser degree of pain and tumescence
  - Glans is usually firm
  - Soft corpora cavernosa
  - Penile bruit may be present
  - There may be a significant delay between the traumatic incident and onset of erection

Diagnosis

- History and physical is usually sufficient to make the diagnosis—presence of persistent tumescence in the absence of sexual stimulation and predisposing conditions or drug use
- Spinal cord injury must be ruled out in any trauma victim with priapism
- Laboratory evaluation should include CBC (rule out sickle cell and leukemia), coagulation profile, and urinalysis (rule out infection)
- Corporeal blood gas analysis distinguishes high flow from low flow priapism: Dark blood with pH <7.25, pO_2 <30, and pCO_2 >60 indicates a low flow, ischemic state
- Penile Doppler ultrasound testing may also distinguish high flow from low flow priapism
- Angiogram may be necessary in high flow disease to localize the fistula

Treatment

- Foley catheter may be necessary as some patients are unable to urinate
- Discontinue and avoid offending drugs
- Perineal ice packs and ice water enemas may be tried
- Subcutaneous terbutaline (β-agonist) causes detumescence in up to 30% of patients
- Corporeal aspiration and vasoconstrictor injection is nearly 100% effective
  - Aspirate blood from the corpora cavernosa using a butterfly needle (penile nerve block may be used)
  - Follow with a corporeal injection of 250 mcg of diluted phenylephrine
- High flow priapism usually cannot be treated in the ED; arterial embolization may be required
- Sickle cell patients require hydration, analgesia, and supplemental O_2; consider exchange transfusion if conservative measures fail
- Complications of therapy may occur due to vasoactive substances (HTN, headache, palpitations, arrhythmia), or due to needle puncture (bleeding, infection, urethral injury)

Disposition

- Risk of impotence increases with duration of priapism, especially after 24 hours
- Patients who respond to ED management may be discharged with urology follow-up in 24 hours
- Discharged patients should be instructed to return as needed and should understand the potential consequences of prolonged priapism (i.e., impotence)
- Any patient refractory to ED management should have an urgent urological evaluation
- Urethral obstruction may occur in high or low flow disease

88. Acute Scrotal Pain

Etiology & Pathophysiology

- 90% of cases are due to testicular torsion, appendage torsion, or acute epididymitis
- Testicular torsion (peak ages 1 year and mid-teens)
  - Congenitally abnormal attachment of testicle to scrotum ("bell-clapper deformity") is present in up to 12% of males, allowing rotation of the testicle around the spermatic cord
  - Venous and arterial supply is compromised, causing ischemia
  - Some cases present after trauma
- Acute epididymitis (peak ages 20s–30s)
  - Infection or inflammation of the epididymis due to retrograde spread of bacteria through the urethra and bladder
  - *Chlamydia* and *Gonorrhoeae* are the most common causes in young males; *E. coli, Klebsiella,* or *Pseudomonas* in older patients
- Appendage torsion (ages 3–13): Appendix of the testis or epididymis twists on its own axis

Differential Dx

- Acute hydrocele/varicocele
- Orchitis (either extension of epididymitis to the testicle or isolated orchitis due to mumps or other viral infections)
- Testicular trauma
- Testicular cancer
- Renal colic
- Scrotal abscess
- Fournier's gangrene
- Henoch-Schönlein purpura
- Inguinal hernia
- Abdominal aortic aneurysm

Presentation

- Testicular torsion
  - Sudden onset of severe pain, independent of position
  - Vomiting is common
  - Testicle is elevated, enlarged, horizontally oriented, and diffusely tender
- Epididymitis
  - Gradual onset (>24 hours)
  - Worse when standing
  - Scrotal elevation deceases pain
  - Fever, dysuria (vomiting is rare)
  - Tenderness is usually limited to epididymis +/− prostate
- Appendage torsion: Sudden onset; N/V, dysuria, fever are uncommon; small "blue dot" on scrotum

Diagnosis

- Urinalysis is usually normal in torsions but positive (for WBCs) in epididymitis
- Serum leukocytosis is unreliable (elevated in up to 60% of torsions)
- Obtain urethral swab for culture and gram stain in epididymitis
- HIV and syphilis testing is often advised in epididymitis
- Handheld bedside Doppler may be used to assess for absent pulses in the testicle indicating torsion
- Color-flow Doppler is highly sensitive and specific to differentiate torsion from epididymitis by showing decreased flow in torsion
- If suspicion for torsion is high, immediate surgical exploration is indicated—studies should not delay surgical evaluation

Treatment

- Testicular torsion
  - Attempt manual detorsion while awaiting urological consultation: Rotate the testicle away from the midline using subjective relief from pain (and Doppler if available) as a guide
  - Cooling with ice packs will preserve function if care is delayed
  - Surgical repair is the definitive treatment
- Epididymitis
  - Administer antibiotics against the most common pathogens for each age group
  - Sexually active young adults: Cover *Gonorrhoeae* and *Chlamydia* with either ofloxacin (10–21 days) or single dose IM ceftriaxone plus either doxycycline (10 days) or single dose azithromycin
  - Age >35: Ofloxacin or ciprofloxacin for 10–21 days
- Appendage torsion requires no acute intervention; conservative management with analgesia and scrotal elevation is sufficient until degeneration occurs

Disposition

- Testicular torsion
  - Urgent urologic referral is indicated for any suspected testicular torsion
  - Testicular salvage is nearly 100% if detorsed within 4–6 hours but just 20% at 24 hours
- Epididymitis: Inpatient management is only indicated for testicular or scrotal abscess or for generalized systemic symptoms
- Appendage torsion
  - Outpatient conservative management is indicated once the diagnosis has been definitively established
  - Any suspicion of testicular torsion should prompt immediate surgical evaluation

89. Rhabdomyolysis

Etiology & Pathophysiology

- Muscle injury and necrosis causes Na^+/K^+ pump dysfunction, disruption of the normal calcium balance, and release of intracellular contents (particularly myoglobin)
- Serious associated morbidity and mortality; thus, a high degree of suspicion for the diagnosis must be maintained
- Etiologies include trauma, immobilization, muscle overactivity (e.g., sports, exercise, seizures, dystonia), infections, drugs of abuse, medications, poly/dermatomyositis, ischemia (e.g., compartment syndrome, vasculitis, vascular occlusion), electrolyte abnormalities, endocrine disturbances (e.g., DKA, thyroid), temperature extremes, electrical/lightning injury, hemolysis, toxins, venomous bites (e.g., snake, spider), and hereditary myopathies
- Diagnosis and treatment are aimed at preventing further muscle injury and minimizing complications (most commonly renal failure due to precipitation of nephrotoxic substances in renal tubules)

Differential Dx

- Polymyositis
- Dermatomyositis
- Connective tissue disease
- Vasculitis
- Traumatic injury (e.g., crush, fall, MVC, electrocution)

Presentation

- General symptoms include malaise, low-grade fever, tachycardia, nausea, and vomiting
- Muscle symptoms include pain and tenderness, weakness, stiffness, and swelling (which usually occurs after hydration has been initiated, due to vigorous myocyte uptake)
- Dark, brownish urine and decreased urine output
- Symptoms of the inciting process may be present

Diagnosis

- Urinalysis is positive for blood (due to heme contained in the myoglobin) in the absence of RBCs
- Elevated serum CPK (CK-MB remains <5% of total CPK), myoglobin, and aldolase (degree of elevation correlates with severity of injury)
- Electrolyte abnormalities may include hyperkalemia, hyperphosphatemia, and hypocalcemia (early) or hypercalcemia (late)
- Elevated creatinine with decreased BUN/creatinine ratio if acute renal failure has occurred
- Elevated LDH and uric acid
- CBC and PT/PTT should be ordered to screen for DIC

Treatment

- Cardiac monitoring and frequent electrolyte checks
- IV fluid administration is the most important management
  - Goal is a urine output of 200–300 cc/hr (increasing glomerular filtration facilitates clearance of myoglobin and other toxins and helps to prevent acute renal failure)
  - IV diuretics (loop diuretics or mannitol) are often added to maintain volume status and promote urine output
  - In the face of renal failure or co-morbid conditions, invasive monitoring of volume status may be necessary
- Urinary alkalinization via sodium bicarbonate infusion may limit renal damage
  - Recommended for CPK values >1000
  - Goal is a urine pH >6.5 and serum pH 7.40–7.45
- Treat electrolyte disturbances as necessary
- Treat underlying etiologies

Disposition

- All patients require admission for intensive electrolyte monitoring, hydration, serial enzyme measurements, and monitoring for complications
- Complications include acute renal failure (usually reversible), electrolyte abnormalities (may result in cardiac arrhythmias), DIC, compartment syndrome, and compression neuropathy
- Outcome depends on the reversibility of the original insult, the degree of CPK elevation at presentation, the presence of complications, and the adequacy of therapy
- Mortality is approximately 5%

Electrolyte Abnormalities

JACK PERKINS, MD

90. Hyponatremia

Etiology & Pathophysiology

- Plasma Na^+ concentration <135 mmol/L
- Classified based on serum tonicity and volume status
- Hypertonic hyponatremia: Increased serum osmolality (e.g., due to hyperglycemia—decrease in Na^+ of 1.6 for every 100 mg/dL increase in glucose)
- Isotonic: Normal serum osmolality (e.g., pseudohyponatremia—lab artifact resulting in a falsely decreased sodium secondary to hyperlipidemia or hyperproteinemia)
- Hypotonic hyponatremia (majority of cases)
  - Hypovolemic: Loss of both Na^+ and H_2O results in a total body water deficit plus a larger total body Na^+ deficit
  - Euvolemic (e.g., SIADH, excess free water intake): Normal ECF volume with slightly decreased total body Na^+
  - Hypervolemic: Excess total body Na^+ plus a larger excess total body H_2O due to an impaired ability to excrete H_2O

Differential Dx

- Hypertonic: Hyperglycemia, iatrogenic hypertonic infusions
- Isotonic: Hyperlipidemia, hyperproteinemia
- Hypotonic
  - Hypervolemic: Cirrhosis, CHF, nephrosis, pregnancy
  - Isovolemic: SIADH, renal failure, hypothyroidism, psychogenic polydipsia, drugs
  - Hypovolemic: Vomiting, diarrhea, burns, 3rd spacing (e.g., pancreatitis), Addison's, RTA, renal losses (e.g., diuretics, renal disease)

Presentation

- Severity of clinical presentation depends both on the rapidity and magnitude of the fall in serum Na^+
- Symptoms and clinical signs become most apparent when serum Na^+ <120 mEq/L
- Early clinical symptoms
  - Change in mental status
  - Apathy
  - Agitation
  - Headache
  - Ataxia
  - Focal weakness or hemiparesis
  - Altered level of consciousness
- May progress to seizures and coma

Diagnosis

- History and physical will often narrow the diagnosis
- Check plasma and urine electrolytes, plasma and urine osmolality
- Hypertonic (plasma osmolality >295): Check serum glucose
- Isotonic (plasma osmolality 275–295): Check protein and lipids
- Hypotonic (plasma osmolality <275): Assess volume status and check BUN/creatinine ratio, urine Na^+, and urine osmoles
  - Hypervolemic: Urine Na^+ will be <10 mmol/L in CHF, cirrhosis, nephrosis; urine Na^+ >20 mmol/L in renal failure
  - Hypovolemic: Urine Na^+ <10 mmol/L in extrarenal losses (e.g., GI, 3rd spacing, hypotonic fluids); urine Na^+ >20 mmol/L in renal losses (e.g., diuretics, Addison's disease, salt wasting nephropathy)
  - Isovolemic: Urine Na^+ is usually >20 mmol/L; in SIADH, urine osmoles >300 mOsm/L; in psychogenic polydipsia, urine osmoles <50 mOsm/L

Treatment

- Correct serum Na^+ gradually (especially in chronic cases) so as not to precipitate seizures, cerebral edema, or central pontine myelinolysis (CNS demyelination due to paradoxical dehydration of neurons)
- Serum Na^+ should not rise faster than 1–2 mEq/L/hr or 12 mEq/L in 24 hours (even if patient is symptomatic)
- Calculate Na^+ deficit = (desired Na^+ – actual Na^+)×(0.6 × wt)
- Isotonic and hypertonic hyponatremia: Correct glucose, lipids, and protein abnormalities as necessary
- Hypotonic, isovolemic hyponatremia: Treat by restricting fluids or administer saline plus a loop diuretic
- Hypotonic, hypovolemic hyponatremia: Administer normal saline (0.9%)
- Hypotonic, hypervolemic hyponatremia: Restrict Na^+ and H_2O; administer loop diuretics
- Treat severe hyponatremia (defined as serum Na^+ <120 mEq/L OR rapidly developed hyponatremia OR hyponatremia with serious CNS symptoms) with 3% saline at 25–100 mL/hr

Disposition

- Hyponatremia is a manifestation of an underlying disorder—disposition depends on the underlying etiology and magnitude of the patient's hyponatremia
- Most patients are admitted
- Consider ICU admission in cases of severe hyponatremia
- SIADH is a common cause of hyponatremia; 6 criteria must be present for diagnosis
  - Euvolemia
  - Hypotonic hyponatremia
  - Urine osmolality >200 mEq/L
  - Urine Na^+ >20 mmol/L
  - Normal organ function (e.g., kidney, heart)
  - Corrects with H_2O restriction

91. Hypernatremia

Etiology & Pathophysiology

- Plasma Na^+ >145 mmol/L
- Majority of cases are due to free water deficit (not sodium excess)
  - Increased H_2O loss: Vomiting, diarrhea, sweating, fever, diuretics, hyperventilation, diabetes insipidus, severe burns, alcohol, osmotic diuresis due to hyperglycemia, drugs (e.g., lithium, phenytoin), thyrotoxicosis, hyperthermia, adrenal or renal failure
  - Decreased H_2O intake: Impaired thirst, poor oral intake (e.g., in the elderly), coma, CVA, infants, ventilated patients
  - Increased Na^+: $NaHCO_3$ administration, hypertonic saline, renal salt retention (e.g., mineralocorticoid excess—Conn's, Cushing's, congenital adrenal hyperplasia)
- Diabetes insipidus (DI): Inappropriate loss of urine concentrating ability, resulting in huge losses of free water
  - Central DI: Failure of ADH secretion
  - Nephrogenic DI: Renal insensitivity to ADH

Differential Dx

- Differential diagnosis of mental status change:
  - Infection
  - Hyponatremia
  - Medication effect
  - Urinary retention
  - Fecal impaction
  - CVA
  - Renal failure
  - Liver failure
  - Thyroid dysfunction
  - Hypercalcemia
  - Hypoglycemia
  - Acute MI/CHF

Presentation

- Clinical signs and symptoms generally do not appear until serum Na^+ >158 mEq/L
- Severity of symptoms relates to both the acuity and magnitude of rise in Na^+
- Weakness, hypertonia, ataxia, restlessness, tremulousness, irritability, confusion, and lethargy
- Dry mucous membranes, poor skin turgor
- May progress to change in mental status, focal neurologic deficits, seizures, coma, and even cerebral hemorrhage (due to severe neuronal dehydration—most often in infants)

Diagnosis

- Electrolytes, renal function, serum osmolarity, urine Na^+, and urine osmolarity
- BUN/creatinine ratio may provide a clue to the etiology
  - Elevated in diuretic use, glycosuria, fluid loss (e.g., GI, respiratory, skin), impaired thirst, adrenal insufficiency, and diabetes insipidus
  - Normal in hyperaldosteronism (e.g., Conn's, Cushing's, CAH)
- Urine Na^+ is elevated in renal losses (>20 meq/L); decreased in GI, respiratory, and skin losses or poor intake (<10 mEq/L); and normal in hyperaldosteronism
- Urine osmolarity is decreased in renal losses (e.g., diuretics and DI); increased in GI, respiratory, and skin losses or poor intake
- Serum Na^+ between 150–170 is usually due to dehydration, 170–190 is usually due to DI, >190 is usually due to chronic salt ingestion
- DI is diagnosed by polyuria and hypotonic urine (urine osmoles <250 mOsm/L)

Treatment

- Patients with severe dehydration and hypotension should be treated emergently with IV fluids (LR or NSS)
- Calculate free water deficit
  0.6 * weight * [(Na measured / Na normal) -1)]
- Correct the free water deficit over 48–72 hrs while making sure that the patient receives maintenance fluids and replacements for ongoing losses as well
- Serum Na^+ should be reduced by no more than 10–15 mEq/L per day (0.5 mEq/L per hr) in chronic hypernatremia and 1 mEq/L/hr in acute hypernatremia
- Overly rapid correction of serum Na^+ can precipitate seizures or cerebral edema with ensuing herniation
- Isovolemic hypernatremia: Replace fluid with D_5W (replace ½ of fluid deficit in the first 24 hrs)
- Hypovolemic hypernatremia: Replace fluid with NSS
- Hypervolemic hypernatremia: Administer D_5W and loop diuretics both to decrease hypertonicity by increasing Na^+ excretion and to add free H_2O while removing volume
- DI: Exogenous vasopressin administration in central DI

Disposition

- Overall mortality is 10%
- Very young children with hypernatremia have a high risk of developing chronic neurologic deficits
- Very young and very old patients require close monitoring when correcting hypernatremia (the young for neurologic sequelae and the old for difficulties in administering large volumes of fluid)
- Most patients will be admitted—decision to discharge depends on the magnitude of hypernatremia, the underlying cause, the age of the patient, and co-morbid conditions

92. Hypokalemia

Etiology & Pathophysiology

- Serum K^+ <3.5 mmol/L
- Potassium is the major intracellular cation; responsible for facilitating muscular contraction, including cardiac muscle
- Serum potassium concentration is primarily mediated by aldosterone
- Etiology can be divided into the following categories:
    - Increased renal or GI potassium loss: Drugs (e.g., diuretics, penicillin, aminoglycosides, steroids), RTA types 1 or 2, DKA, Mg^{3+} deficiency, Bartter's syndrome, hyperaldosteronism, Cushing's syndrome, vomiting, diarrhea, laxative abuse, GI fistula, NG suction, excess sweating, kayexelate administration
    - Intracellular redistribution of potassium: Insulin excess, β-agonists, alkalosis, caffeine, hypokalemic periodic paralysis (familial disorder with recurrent acute hypokalemia and weakness), Digibind therapy, barium or toluene ingestion
    - Decreased potassium intake: Starvation, malabsorption

Differential Dx

- Differential diagnosis of muscle weakness:
    - Hypercalcemia
    - Hyponatremia
    - Bacterial infection
    - Myositis
    - Hypothyroidism
    - Steroid myopathy
    - Myasthenia gravis
    - Diabetes
    - Guillain-Barré syndrome
    - Botulism
    - Uremia

Presentation

- Symptoms usually begin at K^+ <2.5 mEq/L
- Common initial symptoms include fatigue, weakness, myalgias, muscle cramps, constipation, respiratory muscle weakness or paralysis
- Cardiac abnormalities may include hypertension, life-threatening arrhythmias (e.g., Vtach, Vfib), potentiation of digoxin, and heart block
- Other complications may include rhabdomyolysis, dehydration, hyperglycemia, ileus, hepatic encephalopathy, nephrogenic diabetes insipidus

Diagnosis

- Labs should include electrolytes (may reveal associated hypomagnesemia or hypophosphatemia), glucose (rule out DKA), and CBC
- Urine K^+ is increased in renal potassium wasting
- Check ABG (every 0.1 increase in pH causes a decrease in plasma K^+ of 0.5 mmol/L)
- Progressive ECG changes occur as serum potassium levels fall (however, ECG changes do not correlate well with plasma K^+)
    - Low voltage QRS complexes
    - Flattening of T-waves occurs first
    - Depressed ST segments
    - Prominent P and U waves (U waves follow the T wave)
    - Prolonged PR and QT intervals
    - Wide QRS complexes
    - Ventricular arrhythmias
- Pseudohypokalemia may occur with massive leukocytosis (e.g., leukemia)

Treatment

- Treat underlying causes of potassium deficiency
- Replete potassium
    - Oral replacement may be attempted in patients who have minimal symptoms and can tolerate oral intake
    - IV replacement if severe sequelae (e.g., cardiac manifestations) are present; do not administer the K^+ in a dextrose solution (may worsen the hypokalemia by increasing insulin output)
    - Each 10 mEq of K^+ should increase serum K^+ by 0.1
    - It is important to replete Mg^{3+} and Ca^{2+} concurrently, especially if the patient is on digitalis
- Continuous ECG monitoring
- Volume depleted patients require IV rehydration with NSS plus K^+
- It is easy to under- or overestimate the actual K^+ deficit depending on the amount of K^+ redistribution that has occurred; as a result, frequently recheck the plasma K^+ as it is being corrected

Disposition

- Admission is required for patients with severe hypokalemia (<2.5) or those who exhibit cardiac toxicity
- Discharge asymptomatic patients with mild hypokalemia
- Adjust home medications and add potassium supplementation as necessary (e.g., decrease loop diuretic dose, add K^+ sparing diuretic, or increase oral K^+ supplementation)

93. Hyperkalemia

Etiology & Pathophysiology

- Plasma K^+ >5.0 mmol/L
- Normally, potassium is excreted almost exclusively (90%) by the kidney, with some excretion by the colon
- K^+ is the major intracellular cation and is the significant factor in determining resting membrane potential and thus determining muscle and nerve excitability/contractility
- Net K^+ absorption or excretion is determined by the actions of aldosterone and the effective plasma K^+ level on the collecting duct
- Hyperkalemia may be due to laboratory artifact, excess total body K^+ (e.g., due to renal disease or excess oral intake), or redistribution between intracellular and extracellular compartments (e.g., acidosis shifts K^+ out of cells, insulin shifts K^+ into cells)

Differential Dx

- Pseudohyperkalemia: Lab artifact due to hemolysis, or elevated WBC/platelets
- Excess total body K^+ due to decreased renal excretion: Renal failure/insufficiency, hypoaldosteronism, RTA type 4, spironolactone, β-blocker, ACE inhibitor, NSAIDs
- Excess intake of K^+: Dietary, oral K^+ replacement
- Redistribution: Acidosis, excess insulin, rhabdomyolysis, hemolysis, succinylcholine, periodic paralysis

Presentation

- May be completely asymptomatic
- Numbness
- Weakness (possibly leading to paralysis)
- Decreased reflexes
- Irritability
- Cardiac arrhythmias
- Hypoventilation is a late finding associated with weakness of the respiratory muscles
- Cardiac toxicity most likely will *only* be detected via ECG, unless the patient is hemodynamically unstable

Diagnosis

- Rule out spurious hyperkalemia (e.g., hemolysis) by repeat measurement
- ECG shows classic progressive changes:
  - Peaked T-waves occur first
  - Prolonged PR and QT intervals
  - Flattening of the p waves and ST depression
  - QRS widening progressing to a sine wave pattern
  - Ventricular fibrillation may follow
- Electrolytes, Ca, Mg, PO_4: May show acidosis or abnormalities contributing to the hyperkalemia
- BUN/Cr to determine renal function
- Consider cortisol, renin, and aldosterone levels
- Rule out pseudohyperkalemia (e.g., presence of hemolysis, leukocytosis >70,000/cm^3, or thrombocytosis >1,000,000/cm^3)

Treatment

- IV calcium is indicated for severe hyperkalemia (>7.5 mmol/L) or if ECG changes are present; will stabilize cardiac cell membranes, but does not treat the hyperkalemia itself
- Insulin is administered to force K^+ into cells; usually given with glucose as an IV drip or SQ
- Kayexalate (sodium polystrene sulfonate) is given orally or rectally to exchange Na^+ for K^+ in the GI tract
- Loop diuretics may be helpful to increase renal excretion in patients with intact renal function
- $NaHCO_3$ should be administered to correct acidosis, thereby driving K^+ back into cells
- β-agonists via IV or nebulizer will increase cellular K^+ uptake
- Hemodialysis is indicated in patients who do not respond to treatment, those who have underlying renal failure, or those with life-threatening complications
- Replace magnesium
- Discontinue offending drugs (e.g., K^+ tablets, potassium sparing diuretics)

Disposition

- Admit all patients with hyperkalemia and associated ECG changes to a monitored bed
- Otherwise, admission depends on etiology of the hyperkalemia
- Inciting events must be identified prior to discharge

94. Hypocalcemia

Etiology & Pathophysiology

- The regulation of calcium is described in the Hypercalcemia entry
  - Lack of PTH may be due to primary hypoparathyroidism, acquired/secondary hypoparathyroidism (e.g., surgery, autoimmune disease), or hypomagnesemia
  - Ineffective PTH occurs in pseudohypoparathyroidism (end organ PTH resistance) and vitamin D deficiency
  - PTH action is overwhelmed (bony deposition of Ca^{++} is elevated despite high PTH) in cases of shock, sepsis, burns, pancreatitis, acute renal failure, or osteoblastic metastases
- Vitamin D levels are affected by malabsorption, poor intake, decreased production, liver failure, and anticonvulsants
- Hypoalbuminemia results in decreased total serum Ca^{++}, but normal free, ionized (active) Ca^{++}; it does not cause sequelae of hypocalcemia

Differential Dx

- Hypoalbuminemia
- Hypoparathyroidism
- Pseudohypoparathyroidsim
- Vitamin D deficiency (poor intake, malabsorption, hepatic or renal failure, decreased production, anticonvulsants)
- Pancreatitis
- Alkalosis
- Shock/sepsis/burns
- Hypermagnesemia
- Hyperphosphatemia
- Transfusion with citrated blood
- Drugs (e.g., cimetidine, heparin, glucagon, phosphates)

Presentation

- Severity of symptoms depends on rapidity of fall in serum calcium
- Weakness, fatigue
- Paresthesias (perioral or fingertip)
- Neuromuscular irritability (Chvostek's or Trousseau's sign, muscle spasm, cramping, tetany)
- Dry skin, hyperpigmentation
- Irritability, psychosis, seizures
- Bony osteodystrophy, osteomalacia
- Cardiac arrhythmias, decreased myocardial contractility (may lead to CHF), hypotension

Diagnosis

- Serum Ca^{++} <8.5 mg/dL
- Electrolytes, albumin, PTH levels, ionized calcium level, vitamin D levels (25- and 1,25-vitamin D), renal function, CBC, and amylase/lipase
- Correct calcium for hypoalbuminemia: Decrease serum Ca^{++} by 0.8 for each 1 g/dL drop in albumin; ionized calcium is normal
- Hypoparathyroidism: ↓ intact PTH, ↑ phosphorus
- Pseudohypoparathyroidism: ↑ intact PTH, ↑ phosphorus
- Vitamin D deficiency: ↑ intact PTH, ↓ phosphorus
- ECG: May show QT prolongation
- X-rays: Sometimes show cortical thinning, bone demineralization, or fractures of extremities
- Chvostek's sign: Twitching of the corner of the mouth or eyelid after tapping on the facial nerve in the pre-auricular area
- Trousseau's sign: Inflate a BP cuff on the upper arm and maintain pressure for 3 minutes; positive test is extension at the IP joints, flexion at the MCP joints, and flexion of the wrist

Treatment

- Calculate corrected serum calcium:
  [(normal albumin − serum albumin) * 0.8] + serum Ca^{++}
- Asymptomatic: Oral calcium supplements (e.g., calcium carbonate, citrate, lactate, or gluconate)
- Symptomatic: IV calcium gluconate bolus over 15 minutes, follow by an IV drip of calcium chloride or gluconate
- Thiazide diuretics to decrease renal Ca^{++} excretion may be used in patients with a history of nephrolithiasis
- Vitamin D supplementation in patients with deficiency to increase Ca^{++} absorption; however, this is not effective for short term management of hypocalcemia
- Hypoalbuminemia may improve with adequate nutrition; however, there is no need to correct serum Ca^{++} since the ionized calcium is normal
- Continuous ECG monitoring for those exhibiting ECG changes
- Correct other electrolyte abnormalities (e.g., hypomagnesemia)

Disposition

- Admit symptomatic patients, those with ECG changes, and those with pancreatitis
- Discharge mild or asymptomatic cases

95. Hypercalcemia

Etiology & Pathophysiology

- Serum Ca^{++} >10.5 mg/dL
- Calcium is the most abundant mineral in the body, with 99% stored in bone; Ca^{++} in the plasma is either protein-bound (mostly to albumin) or is ionized and readily available for use
- Decreased plasma Ca^{++} stimulates parathyroid hormone (PTH) release; PTH counteracts the decreased serum Ca^{++} by stimulating Ca^{++} resorption from bone, renal PO_4^- excretion, and renal activation of vitamin D
- Vitamin D is made in the skin and converted to its active (1,25) form in the kidney; vitamin D increases Ca^{++} absorption from the GI tract
- Hypercalcemia stimulates calcitonin release from the thyroid, which decreases bone resorption and increases renal Ca^{++} excretion
- 90% of cases of hypercalcemia are secondary to an underlying malignancy (via bone metastases or PTH-related peptide secretion) or hyperparathyroidism (especially parathyroid adenoma)

Differential Dx

- Malignancy (e.g., myeloma, breast, kidney, lung, leukemia)
- Primary hyperparathyroidism
- Vitamins D or A toxicity
- Drugs (e.g., thiazides, lithium)
- Hyperthyroidism
- Addison's disease
- Pheochromocytoma
- Paget's disease
- Immobilization
- Familial hypercalcemia
- Granulomatous disease (e.g., sarcoidosis, tuberculosis)
- Milk-alkali syndrome

Presentation

- Most cases are relatively asymptomatic (fatigue and other non-specific symptoms present)
- *"Stones, bones, abdominal groans, and psychic overtones"* is the classic presentation; however, these rarely present concurrently
  - *Stones:* Renal stones in 50%
  - *Bones:* Bone pain, weakness, osteoporosis
  - *Groans:* Abdominal pain, N/V, constipation, PUD, pancreatitis
  - *Psychic overtones:* Psychosis, depression, anxiety
- CNS: Confusion, mental status changes, hyporeflexia, coma
- Cardiac: HTN, arrhythmias

Diagnosis

- Electrolytes and renal function may rule out other abnormalities
- Correct calcium level for serum albumin
- $[0.8 \times (\text{normal albumin} - \text{serum albumin}) + \text{serum } Ca^{++}]$
- PTH is elevated in primary hyperparathyroidism; decreased in non-parathyroid causes
- PO_4^- is elevated or normal in vitamin D-mediated diseases; decreased in parathyroid-mediated disease and malignancy
- PTH-related peptide (PTHrp) is secreted by certain cancers
- 1,25-vitamin D (active form) is elevated in granulomatous diseases
- 25-vitamin D is elevated in exogenous vitamin D intoxication
- Alkaline phosphatase is elevated in etiologies that cause bone resorption (e.g., hyperparathyroidism)
- ECG may show ST depression, wide T waves, short ST segments, QT shortening, bradyarrhythmias, and heart block
- Other lab tests/imaging are directed towards specific etiologies or complaints (e.g., CT scan to rule out nephrolithiasis)

Treatment

- Calculate the corrected serum Ca^{++}
- Patients are often dehydrated; repletion of blood volume may correct the hypercalcemia
- Severe hypercalcemia (calcium >13 mg/dL or symptoms) requires immediate intervention to prevent cardiac sequelae
  - IV rehydration with large volumes of normal saline
  - Loop diuretics to prevent volume overload and augment renal Ca^+ excretion
  - Bisphosphonates (e.g., IV pamidronate) inhibit bone resorption; full effect may not occur for 1–5 days
  - Calcitonin and mithramycin decrease bone resorption via osteoclast inhibition (mithramycin is cytotoxic and causes renal toxicity)
  - IV steroids may be used in vitamin D disorders, granulomatous diseases, and malignancy
  - Correct other electrolyte abnormalities as necessary

Disposition

- PTH-mediated hypercalcemia rarely increases Ca^{++} above 13 mg/dL and is generally asymptomatic
- The higher the plasma Ca^{++}, the more likely it is due to a malignancy and is generally more difficult to correct
- Admit anyone with severe or symptomatic hypercalcemia
- Patients with hypercalcemia require a thorough diagnostic workup to rule out malignancy
- Prognosis depends on etiology (e.g., parathyroid adenomas are usually benign, malignant hypercalcemia usually indicates an advanced cancer)

96. Metabolic Acidosis

Etiology & Pathophysiology

- Characterized by an arterial pH <7.40 and serum HCO_3 <24
- Caused by a loss of bicarbonate (non anion gap acidosis) or an increase in endogenous acids (anion gap acidosis)
- The anion gap is an estimate of unmeasured serum anions; increased AG indicates the presence of additional serum acids
- To compensate for metabolic acidosis, ventilation increases to blow off CO_2 (compensatory respiratory alkalosis)
- Acidosis causes decreased cardiac contractility, arrhythmias (including Vfib), hypokalemia, and hypoxia
- Mixed acid/base disorder may occur (e.g., metabolic acidosis with concurrent metabolic alkalosis, respiratory alkalosis, or respiratory acidosis; anion gap acidosis with concurrent non anion gap acidosis)
- Lactic acidosis is a common cause of anion gap acidosis; some causes include poor tissue perfusion (e.g., shock, CHF, sepsis, anemia), carbon monoxide, liver failure, salicylate, alcohol, isoniazid

Differential Dx

- Increased anion gap
  - Methanol
  - Uremia
  - DKA
  - Paraldehyde
  - Iron, isoniazid
  - Lactic acidosis
  - Ethanol, ethylene glycol
  - Salicylates, starvation
- Normal anion gap: GI losses (e.g., diarrhea, small bowel fistula) and renal losses (e.g., uremia, RTA, adrenal or aldosterone insufficiency, acetazolamide, spironolactone)

Presentation

- General symptoms include headache, N/V, abdominal pain, tachypnea, Kussmaul's respiration, peripheral vasodilation, lethargy, stupor, coma
- Cardiac depression may occur with CHF, shock, or arrhythmias
- Acidosis-induced hypokalemia may occur with associated symptoms of hypokalemia (e.g., weakness)
- Presentation depends heavily on the underlying etiology of the acidosis (e.g., a patient with DKA will be dehydrated and lethargic, a patient with methanol poisoning may complain of blindness due to the formaldehyde byproduct)

Diagnosis

- Confirm metabolic acidosis: pH <7.40, HCO_3 <24
- Calculate anion gap: $Na^+ - (Cl^- + HCO_3^-)$; normal AG <12 mEq/L
- Examine the appropriateness of respiratory compensation: pCO_2 should equal $(1.5*HCO_3) + 8 +/-2$ (if not, a primary respiratory disorder also exists)
- Calculate the delta-delta: In anion gap acidosis, the AG should increase by 1 for each 1-point decrease in serum HCO_3 (if not, a non anion gap acidosis is also present)
- Search for the underlying cause
  - Labs may include: Lytes, lactate, serum osmolarity, and U/A
  - DKA: Ketones and glucose in urine; elevated serum glucose
  - Starvation or alcohol ketoacidosis: Ketones; normal glucose
  - Lactic acidosis: Elevated serum lactate
  - Methanol/ethylene glycol: Elevated serum osmolar gap
  - Ethlyene glycol: Urine calcium oxalate crystals
  - Salicylate poisoning: AG acidosis with respiratory alkalosis; normal osmolar gap; positive urine dip for ferric chloride

Treatment

- Ensure airway and breathing, especially to ensure maximum respiratory compensation; intubation may be necessary
- Treat the underlying cause
  - Restore tissue perfusion with IV fluids +/- inotropic medications
  - Hemodialysis and IV ethanol or fomepizole for methanol and ethylene glycol poisoning
  - Hemodialysis for uremia
  - Deferoxamine or hemodialysis for iron intoxication
- Administer IV bicarbonate in non anion gap acidosis
- Bicarbonate administration is controversial in anion gap acidosis
  - Generally used if serum HCO_3 <8 or pH <7.1 with refractory shock or arrhythmia
  - Side effects may occur due to bicarbonate breakdown into CO_2 and H_2O, including worsening of intracellular acidosis (acidic CO_2 diffuses into cells faster than HCO_3) and worsening respiratory failure (increased serum CO_2 needs to be blown off)

Disposition

- Disposition depends on the underlying etiology
- Most patients require admission
- Patients should be monitored for possible respiratory failure due to the ongoing high ventilatory demands as the body attempts to blow off CO_2 to normalize the pH
- Frequent labs should be obtained to ensure progressive resolution of the acidosis with therapy

97. Metabolic Alkalosis

Etiology & Pathophysiology

- Arterial pH >7.40 with a bicarbonate level >26 mEq/L
- Due to bicarbonate gain, acid loss (e.g., vomiting), or acid redistribution (e.g., H^+ is forced into cells during hypokalemia)
- The physiologic compensation to alkalosis is hypoventilation to retain CO_2; however, since the amount of compensation is limited by hypoxemia, the $PaCO_2$ will rarely rise higher than 50–55 mmHg.
- Divided into chloride-responsive and chloride-resistant forms
  - Chloride-responsive alkalosis is usually due to volume loss +/− acid loss; the volume depletion stimulates aldosterone release, resulting in Na^+ retention with HCO_3^- and K^+ loss; the urine is alkaline and contains little chloride
  - Chloride-resistant alkalosis is due to inappropriate aldosterone activity with the same results as above (there is no hypovolemia, so urine chloride is normal and NSS does not cure the alkalosis)

Differential Dx

- Chloride-responsive
  - Vomiting
  - Dehydration
  - Diuretics   – Diarrhea
  - Antacids   – NG suction
- Chloride-resistant
  - Excess mineralocorticoids (e.g., hyperaldosteronism, Cushing's syndrome, licorice, renin-producing tumor)
  - Excess citrate (e.g., massive blood transfusion) or lactate (e.g., large infusion of LR)
  - Hypokalemia
  - Gitelman or Bartter syndrome
  - Liddle syndrome

Presentation

- Hypoventilation and hypoxemia, resulting in mental status changes
- Seizures
- Volume depletion in some cases
- Tachyarrhythmias secondary to associated hypokalemia or hypocalcemia
- Weakness
- Ileus
- Neuromuscular irritability
- Cardiovascular dysfunction
- Signs and symptoms of the primary disease process will also be present

Diagnosis

- Determine the primary alkalosis disorder by evaluating the pH, pCO_2, and HCO_3^- (metabolic alkalosis has elevated pH and serum bicarbonate >26 mEq/L)
- Examine the appropriateness of respiratory compensation: pCO_2 should equal [0.6* (serum bicarbonate – normal bicarbonate)] (if not, a primary respiratory disorder also exists)
- Alkalosis causes a secondary hypokalemia, hypocalcemia, hypophosphatemia, and hypomagnesemia
- Urine chloride levels (not accurate in patients taking diuretics) should be measured
  - Chloride-responsive: Urine chloride <10 mEq/L; alkalosis will be responsive to normal saline alone
  - Chloride-resistant: Urine chloride >20 mEq/L; correction of alkalosis will require more than just normal saline

Treatment

- Correct the underlying cause
- Ensure adequate respiratory support
- Rehydrate as necessary
- Chloride-responsive alkalosis responds well to administration of normal saline
  - Determine the chloride deficit and replace appropriately
  - Chloride deficit = (weight in kg × 20%) × (normal Cl^- − serum Cl^-)
  - Administer half the chloride over the initial 4–12 hours
  - Administer ¾ of the chloride as sodium chloride and ¼ as potassium chloride
- Chloride-resistant alkalosis typically requires significant infusions of potassium to correct the alkalosis (potassium is excreted in the renal collecting ducts in exchange for H^+ retention to correct the alkalosis)
- Severe alkalosis (pH >7.55) may necessitate the use of acidifying agents (e.g., NaCl, acetazolamide, ammonium chloride, IV hydrochloric acid, arginine-hydrochloride)

Disposition

- Minor alkalosis with known etiology may be discharged
- Admit patients with severe symptoms or significant co-morbidities or patients with volume depletion from any cause who are unable to rehydrate themselves

98. Respiratory Acidosis and Alkalosis

Etiology & Pathophysiology

- Respiratory alkalosis is defined as pH >7.40 and pCO_2 <40 mmHg
  - Caused by alveolar hyperventilation
  - Results in cerebral vasoconstriction and diminished oxyhemoglobin dissociation; this may cause peripheral and cerebral hypoxia (may lead to paradoxical cerebral acidosis, which worsens the respiratory alkalosis by causing hyperventilation)
- Respiratory acidosis is defined as pCO_2 >45 with pH <7.40
  - Caused by alveolar hypoventilation
  - The kidney compensates for elevated pCO_2 by increasing reabsorption of HCO_3^-; however, the compensatory mechanism takes up to 24 hrs for full effect, so a precipitous drop in pH may occur in a patient with acute respiratory acidosis
  - Chronic respiratory acidosis is frequently seen in those with COPD or Pickwickian syndrome (obesity-hypoventilation)

Differential Dx

- Respiratory alkalosis
  - Shock   –Sepsis
  - Trauma   –PE
  - Anxiety/pain   –Altitude
  - Nicotine, aspirin –Asthma
- Respiratory acidosis
  - Sedatives
  - Narcotics
  - COPD/asthma   –CHF
  - Head trauma   –CVA
  - Interstitial lung disease
  - Neuromuscular disease (e.g., myasthenia gravis, botulism, hypokalemia, Guillain-Barré)
  - Airway obstruction

Presentation

- Respiratory alkalosis
  - Hyperventilation
  - Mental status changes, anxiety
  - Syncope
  - Electrolyte disturbances may cause neuromuscular irritability, ileus, cardiovascular dysfunction, and arrhythmias
- Respiratory acidosis
  - Decreased/altered respirations
  - Headache
  - Anxiety, confusion, coma
  - Sleep disturbances
  - Psychosis
  - Myoclonic jerks, tremor, and hyperreflexia

Diagnosis

- Determine the primary acid-base disorder; then determine if a secondary disorder is present by evaluating the appropriateness of the compensatory response
- Compensatory response to respiratory disorders is performed by the kidney; appropriate compensation depends on the acute or chronic nature of the respiratory process (the kidney takes time to react to acid-base changes completely)
- Respiratory alkalosis
  - Workup suspected causes as appropriate
  - Check CBC, electrolytes (e.g., hypocalcemia, hypomagnesemia, hypophosphatemia), CXR, ABG, and ECG
- Respiratory acidosis
  - Workup suspected causes as appropriate
  - Check CBC, electrolytes, ABG, U/A, and CXR
  - Head CT is generally indicated if the patient presents with altered mental status

Treatment

- Respiratory alkalosis
  - Treat the underlying cause; maintain a high suspicion for life-threatening disorders (e.g., sepsis, pulmonary embolus)
  - Rebreathing via a face mask is recommended to increase pCO_2
  - Some patients may require intubation in order to manipulate the ventilatory rate without causing hypoxemia
- Respiratory acidosis
  - Increase minute ventilation (rate and/or tidal volume) to blow off excess CO_2
  - Many patients require ventilatory assistance via intubation or noninvasive positive pressure ventilation (CPAP or BiPAP)
  - Patients with chronic respiratory acidosis require a gradual decrease in pCO_2 to avoid a combined metabolic and respiratory alkalosis and ensuing arrhythmias
  - Treat the underlying cause (e.g., bronchodilators for COPD, diuretics for CHF)

Disposition

- Respiratory alkalosis: Discharge patients with benign causes (e.g., anxiety) and those with resolution of symptoms; others require admission
- Respiratory acidosis: Disposition depends on the underlying etiology and chronicity of symptoms; many patients will progress to respiratory failure
- "Normal" pCO_2 in some patients may actually reflect impending respiratory acidosis and failure (e.g., tachypneic asthma patients should have decreased pCO_2; a normal pCO_2 in these patients signifies tiring respiratory effort)
- CO_2 diffuses better across the blood-brain barrier than HCO_3^-, resulting in greater cerebral acidosis than serum acidosis; this explains the preponderance of CNS symptoms in respiratory acidosis

Infectious Disease Emergencies

NATHAN W. MICK, MD
RICHARD R. WATKINS, MD, MS

99. Sepsis

Etiology & Pathophysiology

- Systemic inflammatory response syndrome (SIRS) describes a systemic response to infectious or non-infectious illnesses (e.g., pancreatitis, trauma), which may result in compromised organ perfusion and multi-organ failure
- Sepsis: SIRS secondary to infection
- Severe sepsis: Sepsis associated with organ dysfunction, hypotension, or hypoperfusion
- Septic shock: Sepsis plus hypotension despite fluid resuscitation
- Multisystem organ dysfunction syndrome (MODS) is the final common pathway of sepsis and SIRS; characterized by renal failure, altered mental status, metabolic acidosis, and hepatic dysfunction
- Sepsis is associated with systemic vasodilation, increased cardiac output, and hypotension ("warm shock")

Differential Dx

- Pneumonia
- Pyelonephritis
- Meningitis
- Cholangitis
- Endocarditis
- Pancreatitis
- Trauma
- Fasciitis
- Other causes of shock (cardiogenic, neurogenic, hypovolemic, anaphylaxis)

Presentation

- Extremes of temperature (fevers/chills or hypothermia)
- Hyperventilation
- Mental status changes
- Hypotension and tachycardia may be present
- Local signs of infection may include cough, SOB, dysuria, diarrhea, heart murmur, signs of cellulitis, or abdominal pain depending on initial cause of infection
- End organ failure may ensue (e.g., lung, kidney, heart)

Diagnosis

- Generally a clinical diagnosis supported by microbiologic data
- SIRS is defined as the presence of 2 or more of the following: Temperature <36°C or >38°C, heart rate >90, respiratory rate >20 or $PaCO_2$ <32 mmHg, and WBC >12,000 or <4000 cells/mm^3
- Sepsis is diagnosed when SIRS occurs secondary to infection
- Draw blood for CBC, chemistries, coagulation studies, DIC panel, CK, lactate, and culture
- Workup should be directed to find the infectious focus and may include blood cultures, urinalysis and culture, chest X-ray, CT scans of potentially affected areas, culture of infected lines or indwelling devices, and LP (if CNS infection is suspected)
- ABG may reveal respiratory alkalosis due to tachypnea and metabolic acidosis due to hypoperfusion
- Swan-Ganz catheter will reveal decreased SVR (due to vasodilatation) with increased cardiac output (however, cardiac output may be decreased in severe cases)

Treatment

- Intubation may be required to maintain oxygenation
- Hypotension must be aggressively corrected
  - First, administer large volumes (4–6 L) of IV crystalloid (normal saline or lactated Ringer's solution) to compensate for increased intravascular space caused by vasodilation
  - Vasopressors for refractory hypotension (e.g., norepinephrine, dopamine, or phenylephrine)
  - Central venous access and arterial blood pressure monitoring may be indicated to guide therapy in severe cases
- Once blood, urine, and sputum have been obtained for culture, begin empiric broad-spectrum IV antibiotic therapy
- Activated protein C (droctrecogin alfa) has been proven to decrease mortality in severely ill patients with sepsis
- If anemia complicates the illness, transfusion with packed red blood cells is indicated to achieve a hematocrit >30 in order to increase the oxygen carrying capacity of the blood

Disposition

- All patients with presumed sepsis or SIRS should be admitted to an ICU for hemodynamic and respiratory monitoring
- Early aggressive volume resuscitation, antibiotic therapy, and hemodynamic support improves mortality
- Complications include ARDS, cardiac ischemia, mesenteric ischemia, acute renal tubular necrosis with renal failure, acute liver injury, DIC, and cerebral hypoperfusion

100. Upper Respiratory Infections

Etiology & Pathophysiology

- Viral upper respiratory tract infections (URI) are common illnesses caused by many different viruses (e.g., respiratory syncytial virus, parainfluenza virus, influenza virus, adenovirus, rhinoviruses, and coronaviruses)
- Sinusitis: Acute infection of the frontal, ethmoid, sphenoid, or maxillary sinuses
  - Many cases begin with a viral upper respiratory tract infection with subsequent bacterial superinfection
  - Common organisms include *Streptococcus pneumoniae, Moraxella catarrhalis,* and *Haemophilus influenzae*
- Acute bronchitis: Infection of the upper bronchial tree (lung parenchyma is *not* involved), of viral origin in the majority of cases; however, *Mycoplasma pneumoniae, Chlamydia pneumoniae,* and *Bordetella pertussis* may also cause disease

Differential Dx

- Sinusitis
- Bronchitis
- Viral upper respiratory infection
- Pneumonia
- Influenza
- Pertussis
- Allergic rhinitis
- Pharyngitis
- Meningitis
- Temporal arteritis

Presentation

- Viral URI: Fever, headache, nasal congestion, conjunctivitis, post-nasal drip (may lead to cough), and clear nasal discharge
- Sinusitis: Fever, malaise, headache (corresponds to the involved sinus), nasal congestion, purulent nasal discharge, sinus tenderness to palpation, increased sinus pain when leaning forward, and tooth pain (due to maxillary sinus infection)
- Bronchitis: Malaise, cough, purulent sputum, wheezing; fever may be present

Diagnosis

- Viral URI is a clinical diagnosis
  - Viral cultures are rarely needed nor useful (results do not alter therapy)
  - Chest X-ray may be required to exclude pneumonia
- Sinusitis is usually diagnosed clinically; imaging is optional
  - CT of the sinuses is the gold standard for diagnosis (visualizes thickened sinus tissue and air fluid levels) and may reveal complications of sinusitis (e.g., abscess formation, cavernous sinus thrombosis, subdural empyema)
  - Plain films may also show fluid in the sinuses but are notoriously insensitive
  - Nasopharyngeal or sinus cultures are rarely useful
- Bronchitis is typically diagnosed clinically
  - Chest X-ray to rule out pneumonia is indicated if the lung exam is abnormal, if the patient is immunocompromised, or if there are systemic symptoms (e.g., tachycardia, fever)
  - Blood or sputum culture is rarely helpful

Treatment

- Supportive treatment for viral URIs
  - Over the counter antitussives, antipyretics, analgesics, and decongestants
  - Rest, good nutrition, and increased fluid intake
- Sinusitis
  - Oral antibiotics (amoxicillin, amoxicillin/clavulanate, cefuroxime, or fluoroquinolones) for at least 10 days
  - Decongestants for symptomatic relief
- Acute bronchitis
  - Supportive treatment is generally sufficient for acute bronchitis as most cases are viral
  - Antibiotics (azithromycin, erythromycin) are not recommended except in cases of persistent symptoms, COPD, or immunocompromise
  - Over the counter antitussives and decongestants
  - Rest, good nutrition, and increased fluid intake
  - Inhaled β-agonists (e.g., albuterol) may decrease cough if there is a bronchospastic component

Disposition

- Most patients may be discharged
- Systemically ill or immunocompromised patients should be admitted
- Patients should be advised on good hand-washing techniques to avoid spread of the illness to family or co-workers
- The routine use of antibiotics in the treatment of apparent viral URIs should be avoided, since truly treatable infections occur infrequently

101. Influenza

Etiology & Pathophysiology

- Single-stranded RNA viruses of the orthomyxovirus family; types A and B cause human disease
- Strains change yearly and are designated based on site of origin, year of isolation, and antigen subtype
- Outbreaks occur primarily in the winter months
- Person-to-person transmission via respiratory droplets
- Influenza A is responsible for most cases; type B is often the cause of epidemics
- >100,000 hospitalizations and 20,000 deaths each year in the US
- Complications of influenza include respiratory failure/ARDS, viral pneumonitis (high mortality, often progresses to ARDS), secondary bacterial pneumonia, rhabdomyolysis, myocarditis, myositis, pericarditis, Guillain-Barré syndrome, and encephalitis

Differential Dx

- Common cold
- Pneumonia
- Streptococcal pharyngitis
- Other viral syndromes
- Primary HIV infection

Presentation

- Incubation period of 2 days
- Abrupt onset of fever/chills, headache, malaise, myalgias, sore throat, cough, eye pain, and sensitivity to light
- Elderly may present atypically (e.g., fever, malaise, congestion, and change in mental status)
- Physical exam may show tender, enlarged cervical lymph nodes
- Respiratory distress with crackles and tachypnea in associated pneumonia/pneumonitis
- Deterioration of the patient after 2–4 days of illness indicates likely secondary bacterial pneumonia

Diagnosis

- ELISA rapid antigen test via nose/throat swabs is often used in the ED for screening (sensitivity 50–70%; specificity >90%)
- Viral antigens may be detected in tissue culture or nasopharyngeal swabs (50–80% sensitive)
- Viral cultures of nasal swabs may also be sent
- In severely ill patients, monitor pulse oximetry and arterial blood gases for hypoxemia (often suggests secondary pneumonia)
- Chest X-ray may show interstitial infiltrates (consistent with viral pneumonitis) or lobar infiltrates (consistent with secondary bacterial pneumonia, most commonly due to *S. pneumoniae* or *S. aureus*)

Treatment

- Uncomplicated influenza may be treated symptomatically with antipyretics, analgesics, and decongestants
- Maintain oxygenation
- Antiviral treatment is indicated for high-risk patients (immunodeficiency, old age, co-morbid diseases), patients with severe symptoms, or to shorten illness duration; however, there is no proven efficacy of antiviral treatment if symptoms have been present for >48 hours
    - Amantadine or rimantadine are only used for influenza A infection; may decrease the duration of illness by 50% if given within 48 hours of symptom onset
    - Neuroaminidase inhibitors (e.g., zanamivir, oseltamivir) prevent viral invasion of cells and decrease viral release from infected cells; active against both influenza A and B; may decrease symptoms by 1–1.5 days if given within 48 hours of onset; may be administered prophylactically to prevent influenza in exposed patients
- Prophylactic vaccination of high-risk patients is the best method to prevent infection and transmission of disease

Disposition

- Most people recover from the acute illness within one week; however, significant morbidity and mortality may occur
- Patients with underlying cardiac, pulmonary, metabolic, renal, or immunosuppressive diseases have increased risk of mortality
- Yearly prophylactic vaccination should be given in high-risk individuals and health care workers
- Amantadine, rimantadine, and neuraminidase inhibitors may also be effective for prophylaxis (may be indicated in unvaccinated high-risk patients, some vaccinated high-risk patients, immunodeficient patients, long-term care residents, and staff/household exposures)

102. Sexually Transmitted Diseases

Etiology & Pathophysiology

- Spread via contact with mucous membranes or non-intact skin
- Varying incubation periods from days to months
- Syphilis: Caused by the spirochete *Treponema pallidum;* may cause chronic systemic complications if untreated
- Genital herpes: Caused by herpes simplex virus types 1 or 2; primary infection or latent reactivation of virus (occurs in >80% of patients) may occur
- Chancroid: Caused by the gram-negative bacillus, *Haemophilus ducreyi*
- Genital warts: Caused by the human papillomaviruses
- Lymphogranuloma venereum (uncommon in the US): Due to infection with specific serotypes of *Chlamydia trachomatis*
- *N. gonorrhoeae* or *C. trachomatis* may cause localized cervicitis, urethritis, or pelvic inflammatory disease (see associated entry)
- Refer to "Vulvovaginitis" entry for trichomonas and bacterial vaginosis

Differential Dx

- Urinary tract infection
- Gonorrhea
- Chlamydia
- Bacterial vaginosis
- Trichomonas
- Syphilis
- Chancroid
- Lymphogranuloma venereum
- Genital warts
- Granuloma inguinale
- Genital herpes
- Perineal abscess
- Bartholin's gland abscess
- HIV

Presentation

- Syphilis
    - 1°: Painless genital chancre
    - 2°: Fever, lethargy, rash on palms or soles, adenopathy
    - 3°: Dementia, aortitis, tabes dorsalis, meningitis
- Genital herpes: Painful vesicles on an erythematous base, adenopathy
- Chancroid: Initial tender pustule that ulcerates, painful adenopathy
- Genital warts: Cauliflower-like growths over the genitalia
- LV: Initial vesicle is painful with draining, coalescing lymph nodes
- GC/chlamydia cervicitis: Vaginal discharge, dysuria, absence of abdominal pain

Diagnosis

- Majority of STDs are diagnosed clinically based on lesion morphology
- Pregnancy test in all patients (positive tests influences management and antibiotic choices)
- All patients with STDs require pelvic exams to rule out the presence of PID (i.e., cervical motion, adnexal, and abdominal tenderness) and intravaginal lesions
- Syphilis: Diagnosed by VDRL, RPR, or treponemal antibody tests (most specific)—may be negative in the initial 1–2 wks
- Genital herpes: Tzank smear shows multinucleated giant cells
- Chancroid: Gram stain of fluid draining from lymph nodes will show gram-negative bacilli but culture is often negative
- LV: Culture of lymph node fluid may be diagnostic
- GC/chlamydia: Cervical cultures are diagnostic but therapy should not be delayed while awaiting culture
- Consider HIV testing in all patients

Treatment

- Syphilis: Single dose IM penicillin (oral doxycycline in penicillin allergy)
- Genital herpes: Oral acyclovir, famciclovir, or valacyclovir for 7–10 days (recurrent episodes are treated with a 5-day course of acyclovir or valacyclovir; may require chronic antiviral suppression)
- Chancroid: Single dose of azithromycin or IM ceftriaxone, or a 3-day course of ciprofloxacin
- Genital warts: Outpatient treatment with cryotherapy or topical podophyllin
- LV: Oral doxycycline or erythromycin
- GC/chlamydia cervicitis or urethritis: Use two antibiotics to treat for both GC and chlamydia as they often occur concurrently
    - Single dose ceftriaxone IM, cefixime, ciprofloxacin, or oflaxacin plus either azithromycin 1 g single dose, or a course of erythromycin, doxycycline, or ofloxacin
    - 2 g single dose azithromycin is FDA approved for use but is not recommended due to significant GI upset

Disposition

- Have a low threshold for treatment (even with only suspected disease)
- The diagnosis of a STD should prompt screening for HIV infection, syphilis, and more common infections such as gonorrhea and chlamydia
- Inpatient therapy is reserved for immunosuppressed patients or severe pain
- Partners of affected patients should be treated
- Safe sex should be encouraged
- Most STDs require mandatory reporting to the Health Department

103. HIV Infection and AIDS

Etiology & Pathophysiology

- HIV is an RNA retrovirus that attacks CD4+ cells (e.g., T_h cells)
- AIDS is defined as a T_h count <200 or any AIDS-defining infection
- Viral transmission via mucous membrane contact with body fluids
- Up to 900,000 Americans may be infected with HIV
- Risk factors for infection include IV drug use, intercourse, and contact with blood or body fluids (occupational risk after a hollow bore needle stick is <1%)
- CD4 count provides a clue to the expected complications (e.g., CD4 <200 predisposes to PCP, mycobacteria, CMV, and fungal infection)
- Complications of HIV infection
  - Infections: Bacterial infection, mycobacteria, CMV, HSV
  - Dermatologic: Kaposi's sarcoma, HSV, zoster, other rashes
  - CNS: Cryptococcus, toxoplasma, lymphoma, dementia, psychosis
  - Lung: PCP, TB, CMV, fungal infection
  - GI: Candidiasis, bacterial enteritis, viral enteritis

Differential Dx

- Bacterial infections, TB, HSV, zoster can occur at any time
- CD4 200–500: Bacterial pneumonia, thrush, anemia, ITP, lymphoma
- CD4 <200: PCP, miliary TB, lymphoma, histoplasmosis, coccidiomycosis, dementia
- CD4 <100: Disseminated herpes, pharyngeal candida, toxoplasmosis, cryptococcus
- CD4 <50: CNS lymphoma, disseminated CMV, atypical mycobacteria (e.g., MAI)

Presentation

- Primary infection is an acute flu-like illness (e.g., fever, pharyngitis, arthralgias, headache, rash, aseptic meningitis) 2–6 wks after infection
- An asymptomatic stage of viral replication follows over 2–12 years
- As CD4 counts decline, multiple opportunistic infections occur
  - PCP presents with a dry hacking cough, fever, and hypoxia
  - CMV viremia may cause disease of the retina or liver (mononucleosis-like syndrome)
  - Cryptococcus and toxoplasmosis cause meningitis, encephalitis, fever, focal neurologic deficits, and altered mental status

Diagnosis

- HIV screening tests may be negative until 6 wks post-infection
  - ELISA testing is used as initial screening (sensitivity >99%, but false-positives occasionally occur)
  - Patients with positive ELISA should have confirmatory Western blot testing, which is highly specific for HIV
- In known HIV-positive patients, previously measured CD4 counts and viral loads provide a clue to expected complications
- Patients with fever require complete infectious workup, including blood cultures, urinalysis, CXR, and head CT with LP
- Patients with respiratory symptoms require pulse oximetry; CXR (may be normal despite pulmonary infection); sputum gram stain/culture for bacteria, Grocott stain for PCP, and acid-fast stain; and serum LDH (increased in PCP)
- Patients with neurologic symptoms require head CT to rule out focal lesions with increased ICP, followed by LP; consider MRI
- Patients with GI symptoms require LFTs, amylase, lipase, and stool testing for fecal leukocytes, bacterial, and viral pathogens

Treatment

- Antibiotics: Administer empiric broad-spectrum antibiotics to septic or toxic-appearing patients
  - Add IV TMP-SMX or pentamidine if PCP is suspected
  - Place in respiratory isolation and add anti-tubercular agents if suspect TB or atypical mycobacterial infection
- Antifungals: Consider in toxic-appearing patients with known CD4 counts <200
  - Positive fungal stains or positive fungal culture from blood or CSF warrant immediate IV antifungals
  - Systemic or topical therapy for esophageal candidiasis
- Antiparasitics: Administer pyrimethamine with sulfadiazine and folinic acid for cerebral toxoplasmosis
- Antivirals: Begin IV therapy for patients with systemic CMV or VZV
- Systemic steroids
  - Indicated in patients with possible PCP and hypoxia
  - Indicated in the presence of cerebral mass lesions with associated edema

Disposition

- HIV infection is managed on an outpatient basis with the antiretroviral multiple drug "cocktail"
- Admit patients with infections secondary to HIV infection
- Advances in HIV therapy have transformed HIV into a chronic disease
- Complications of antiretroviral medications should also be considered when evaluating patients with HIV (e.g., pancreatitis, urolithiasis, hepatotoxicity)

104. Lyme Disease

Etiology & Pathophysiology

- Tick-borne illness caused by the spirochete *Borrelia burgdorferi*
- Spread by the bite of the *Ixodes* tick; ticks survive on the white-footed mouse and the white-tailed deer
- Reported in 48 US states, most commonly found in the Northeast
- >10,000 cases per year in the US; most in late spring and summer
- Localized infection (Stage 1) affects the skin only; lasts for weeks
- Disseminated infection (Stage 2) is hematogenously spread to affect the skin, CNS, peripheral nerves, myocardium, cardiac conduction tissue, and/or muscles and joints; symptoms last weeks to months, often waxing and waning and changing locations
- Persistent infection (Stage 3) may develop months to years later to cause arthritis, chronic encephalopathy, or acrodermatitis; symptoms may persist for years
- Most patients do not recall the tick bite

Differential Dx

- Viral syndrome
- Cellulitis
- Arthropod bite
- Chronic fatigue syndrome
- Fibromyalgia
- Bell's palsy
- Bacterial meningitis
- Viral encephalitis
- Viral myocarditis
- Inflammatory arthritis (e.g., SLE, rheumatoid)

Presentation

- Stage 1 (erythema migrans): Initial red papule expands to form an annular lesion with central clearing
- Stage 2: Secondary annular skin lesions, migratory arthralgias and myalgias, headache, adenopathy, mild neck stiffness, constitutional symptoms (e.g., fever, chills, fatigue, malaise), neurologic symptoms (e.g., meningitis, encephalitis, cranial neuritis, peripheral neuropathy), cardiac symptoms (e.g., fluctuating AV block, pericarditis, myocarditis)
- Stage 3: Chronic intermittent arthritis, subacute encephalopathy, polyneuropathy, acrodermatitis

Diagnosis

- Clinical symptoms and history are used to place patients into a risk group
  - Begin empiric therapy for patients with high pretest possibility of Lyme disease
  - Administer ELISA and Western blot testing for patients with intermediate pretest probability
  - Testing is not suggested for patients with low pretest probability
- Serologies include IgM and IgG Lyme antibodies
  - May be negative for weeks after infection; however, a positive antibody response is eventually detected in most patients
  - Titers remain positive for years after infection
  - A 2-step diagnostic approach is recommended (similar to HIV testing): Initially screen patients with an ELISA test, then confirm positive or equivocal results with a Western blot
- Culture of *B. burgdorferi* is difficult and rarely indicated

Treatment

- Oral antibiotic therapy is sufficient for patients with skin lesions, joint lesions, or 1° or 2° heart block
  - Oral antibiotic choices include doxycycline (preferred), amoxicillin, cefuroxime, or erythromycin
- IV antibiotic therapy is generally required for 3° heart block and CNS involvement
  - IV antibiotic choices include ceftriaxone, cefotaxime, or penicillin
- Duration of therapy is generally 30 days; patients with cardiac conduction disease should have therapy continued until high-grade conduction blocks resolve
- Systemic steroids are occasionally administered in patients with complete heart block who do not rapidly respond to antibiotic therapy
- A Lyme disease vaccine is available with 50–75% efficacy; consider administration in high-risk individuals who live in endemic areas; may require a yearly booster to maintain titers

Disposition

- Discharge patients who require only oral antibiotics
- Admit patients with neurologic symptoms or high-grade cardiac conduction disease for IV antibiotic administration
- Patients with high-grade heart block should be admitted to a monitored floor
- Stage 2 disease occurs in 10% of untreated patients
- Stage 3 disease occurs in 60% of untreated patients
- Appropriate antibiotic treatment greatly decreases the development of Stage 2 and 3 disease
- Disease may relapse even with appropriate therapy

105. Tick-Borne Illnesses

Etiology & Pathophysiology

- Tick-borne illnesses include Lyme disease (see related entry), Rocky Mountain Spotted Fever (RMSF), tularemia, erlichiosis, babesiosis, ascending tick paralysis, Colorado tick fever, and relapsing fever
- Patients often do not remember the tick bite
- Consider the diagnosis in all patients with febrile illness and contact with animals or the outdoors
- Tularemia: Due to gram-negative *Francisella tularensis;* occurs with handling of rabbits or deer; skin (ulceroglandular) or inhalation (pneumonic) disease may occur
- RMSF: Infection by the intracellular *Rickettsia rickettsii;* causes a potentially fatal vasculitis with characteristic rash
- Ehrlichiosis: Caused by *Ehrlichia chaffeensis,* which infects leukocytes; primarily occurs in early summer and in the south US
- Babesiosis: Due to the intra-erythrocytic protozoan *Babesia microti*

Differential Dx

- Viral syndrome/viral exanthem
- Bacterial infection
- Pneumonia
- Pulmonary or cutaneous anthrax
- Vasculitis
- Meningitis
- Meningococcemia
- Influenza
- Malaria
- Syphilis
- Other zoonoses (e.g., brucellosis, psittacosis, leptospirosis, plague)
- Guillain-Barré syndrome

Presentation

- All present with a febrile, flu-like illness (e.g., fever, N/V, malaise, myalgias, adenopathy, +/− rash)
- Tularemia: Ulceroglandular disease results in fever, ulcers, and tender lymphadenopathy; pulmonary disease causes pneumonia
- RMSF: Characteristic maculopapular rash beginning on extremities (involves palms and soles) and spreads centrally; may have cardiopulmonary failure or CNS symptoms (confusion, encephalitis, coma)
- Ehrlichiosis: Lung symptoms, rash
- Babesiosis: Rigors, dark urine, hepatosplenomegaly, rash

Diagnosis

- ED diagnosis is generally empiric based on clinical suspicion
- CBC, electrolytes, renal function, and liver function
- Tularemia: ELISA is the gold standard for diagnosis; may see leukocytosis, elevated LFTs, or thrombocytopenia
- RMSF: Serologic testing or immunofluorescent staining of skin biopsy specimens is the gold standard for diagnosis; however, may be negative early in the infection
- Ehrlichiosis: Diagnosis is primarily based on clinical presentation; confirmatory serologic testing is available
- Babesiosis: Diagnosed by identification of intra-erythrocytic organisms on Giemsa or thick smear of a peripheral blood specimen; CBC may show hemolytic anemia

Treatment

- Remove tick by applying viscous lidocaine to kill the tick then using forceps to grab the tick by its head (do not crush or burn the tick)
- Tularemia: IM streptomycin or oral tetracycline for 14 days
- RMSF: Doxycycline, tetracycline, or chloramphenicol for 7–14 days
- Ehrlichiosis: Doxycycline, tetracycline, or chloramphenicol for 7–14 days
- Babesiosis: Treatment is reserved for patients who are moderately to severely ill—IV clindamycin and oral quinine for 7–10 days

Disposition

- Tularemia: Admit patients who appear toxic or who have significant co-morbid conditions
- RMSF: Admit all patients; may be fatal if diagnosis is delayed; complications include renal failure, ARDS, myocarditis, meningitis, and DIC
- Ehrlichiosis: Rarely causes severe systemic illness but complications (in 1% of patients) may include DIC, renal failure, myocarditis, or CNS toxicity
- Babesiosis: Largely self-limited but the clinical course may be prolonged (may last as long as a year); rare complications include hemolytic anemia, renal failure, or liver dysfunction

106. Malaria

Etiology & Pathophysiology

- Malaria is the most important parasitic disease of humans (over 250 million annual infections and 2.5 million deaths worldwide)
- Found throughout the tropics, Central and South America, and occasionally in the southern US along the Gulf of Mexico
- Four distinct species of Plasmodium: *P. vivax* (common in Middle East and India), *P. falciparum* (common in Sub-Saharan Africa and Haiti), *P. ovale,* and *P. malariae*
- Usually transmitted by the bite of a female *Anopheles* mosquito; transfusion of infected blood or maternal-fetal transmission may also occur
- Consider the diagnosis in anyone with recent travel or past malaria
- *P. falciparum* is the most serious form, resulting in erythrocyte stiffness that may obstruct circulation in the brain, kidneys, lungs
- Classic relapsing-remitting symptomatology is due to intermittent erythrocyte lysis with release of merozoites into the circulation

Differential Dx

- Typhoid fever
- Dengue fever
- Babesiosis
- Miliary tuberculosis
- Lymphoma
- Meningoencephalitis
- Yellow fever
- Schistosomiasis
- Leishmaniasis

Presentation

- Incubation period of 10 days to 4 weeks before onset of symptoms
- First symptoms include headache, malaise, fatigue, abdominal pain, myalgias, fever, and chills
- As parasitemia develops, the classic recurrent paroxysms of high-grade fever, chills, rigors, nausea, and severe weakness manifest
- Paroxysms generally occur every 2–3 days; between episodes, patients may be asymptomatic
- *P. falciparum* may cause seizures, ARDS, renal failure, coma (often do not have classic paroxysms)
- Tachycardia, tachypnea, fever, and splenomegaly may be present

Diagnosis

- Peripheral smear is diagnostic by demonstrating the asexual form of the parasite with Giemsa-staining
    - The first blood smear is positive in 95% of confirmed cases
    - Smears should be examined every 12 hours for two days before the diagnosis is ruled out
    - *P. falciparum* blood smear often reveals parasitemia, >4%, crescent shape gametocytes, and multiple infected rings in RBCs
- HRP-2 serologic assay has been developed as a highly sensitive and specific diagnostic test that uses fingerstick blood to identify *P. falciparum* infection
- CBC shows hemolysis, decreased RBCs, normochromic/normocytic anemia, and thrombocytopenia
- Hyponatremia and hypoglycemia may be present
- LFTs are often mildly increased

Treatment

- Severe malaria should be managed in the ICU with close observation, fluid resuscitation, and electrolyte monitoring
- Chloroquine-resistant *P. falciparum* is widespread—assume resistance until proven otherwise
    - Adults: Quinine plus either doxycycline for 7 days or single dose pyrimethamine-sulfadoxine; alternatives include mefloquine plus doxycycline, or halofantrine
    - Children: Quinine for 3 days plus single dose pyrimethamine-sulfadoxine on the third day; or use halofantrine
    - IV antibiotics are indicated for *P. falciparum* if it is chloroquine-resistant and complicated
- If chloroquine-sensitive *P. falciparum* is proven or if blood smear is consistent with *P. malariae, P. vivax,* or *P. ovale* infection, treat with chloroquine for 2 days plus primaquine for 14 days
- Recommended prevention regimens vary depending on region; all travelers to endemic areas should begin prophylaxis and use recommended measures, such as mosquito nets and insect sprays

Disposition

- Widespread antibiotic resistance has hampered treatment
- Cure rates exceed 95% for chloroquine-sensitive strains
- *P. vivax* and *P. ovale* may result in recurrent relapses due to persistent parasites in the liver
- Vaccines are currently in clinical trials
- Admit all patients with *P. falciparum*
- Most patients can be managed as outpatients if *P. falciparum* is ruled out
- Pregnant women and infants should be admitted
- Cerebral malaria may result from *P. falciparum* infection with high mortality
- Treatment updates are available at the CDC hotline: (770) 448-7788

107. Parasitic Infections

Etiology & Pathophysiology

- Frequency of parasitic disease has been increasing in the US due to increases in international travel, immunosuppressed patients, and immigrants from endemic areas
- Parasites are divided into three groups: Protozoa, helminths (worms), and ectoparasites (e.g., scabies, pediculosis)
- Amebiasis (*E. histolytica*): Colonic inflammation with GI symptoms
- Giardiasis: Most common GI protozoan infection in US; results in watery, foul-smelling stool
- *Cryptosporidium:* Significant cause of traveler's diarrhea; results in profuse watery diarrhea
- Babesiosis: Systemic infection transmitted by *Ixodes* ticks
- *Enterobius* (pinworm): Causes GI symptoms and anal pruritus
- Trichinosis: A helminth lodges in muscle, brain, lung, GI tract
- Tapeworms (*Taenia sp*): Transmitted by undercooked meat, pork, fish; may spread to brain, heart, or eye (calcified cysts)

Differential Dx

- Viral or bacterial gastroenteritis
- Rickettsial disease
- Protozoa: Malaria, amebiasis, giardiasis, cryptosporidiosis, toxoplasmosis, trichomoniasis, babesiosis Leshmaniasis, *Trypanosoma* (Chagas disease, African sleeping sickness)
- Helminths: Trichinosis, pinworms, tapeworms, larval migrans, ascariasis (roundworms), *Strongyloides,* filariasis, onchocerciasis, schistosomiasis, hookworms

Presentation

- Nonspecific complaints include HA, fever, malaise, abdominal pain
- N/V (amebiasis, tapeworm, *Giardia, Trichinella, Leishmania*)
- Diarrhea (*Giardia,* amebiasis, tapeworm, hookworm, *Schistosoma, Trichinella, Strongyloides*)
- Pneumonia (*Ascaris, Strongyloides, Trichinella*)
- Eye involvement (Taenia, *Trypanosoma*)
- Cardiac involvement (Taenia, Chagas disease, *Trichinella*)
- CNS invovlement (amebiasis, *Toxocara, Trichinella*, tapeworm, *Trypanosoma* (sleeping sickness)

Diagnosis

- Consider workup for parasitic disease in patients with risk factors (e.g., travel history, nursing home, day-care); in patients with consistent symptoms for >10 days; or in patients with unexplained fever, GI symptoms, rash, and/or eosinophilia
- Stool sample with microscopic exam for ova and parasites is the most common test to establish diagnosis; requires at least 3 separate samples on different days
- Stool sample for fecal leukocytes has poor sensitivity/specificity
- Stool ELISA test is available for *Giardia* and *Cryptosporidia*
- Cellophane tape swab of anus for *Enterobius* (pinworm)
- Duodenal aspirate may diagnose *Giardia* or *Cryptosporidia*
- Peripheral blood smear for babesiosis, malaria, and *Trypanosoma*
- CBC may reveal leukocytosis (amebiasis), anemia (babesiosis, leishmaniasis, hookworm), or eosinophilia (helminth infections)
- Elevated LFTs in schistosomiasis (due to ductal obstruction)
- CT scan and MRI may be used to assess for tissue parasites
- Serologic assays are available for most parasitic infections

Treatment

- Amebiasis: Metronidazole × 10 days plus paromomycin × 7 days
- Ascariasis: Albendazole × 1 dose
- Babesiosis: Clindamycin plus quinine × 7 days
- Intestinal tapeworms: Praziquantel × 1 dose
- Cryptosporidium: Supportive care; consider paromomycin
- Cyclosporiasis: TMP-SMZ × 7 days
- Enterobiasis: Mebendazole × 1 dose and repeat in 2 weeks
- Lymphatic filariasis: Ivernectin × 1 dose; add albendazole × 1 dose in children; or use diethylcarbamazine × 12 days
- Liver flukes: Praziquantel × 1 day
- Giardiasis: Metronidazole × 5 days
- Hookworm: Mebendazole × 1 dose
- Isosporiasis: TMP-SMZ DS × 3 weeks
- Schistosomiasis: Praziquantel × 1 day
- Strongyloidiasis: Ivermectin × 2 days
- Trichinellosis: Albendazole × 14 days
- Trichomoniasis: Metronidazole × 1 dose
- Trypanosoma: Nifurimox or benznidazole for Chagas' disease; suramin or others for sleeping sickness

Disposition

- Most patients can be discharged
- Admission criteria include moderate to severe dehydration, hemodynamic instability, ECG changes (especially in Chagas' disease), and inability to take oral medication
- Travelers should be encouraged to seek medical advice prior to visiting endemic areas
- Travelers should take precautions against insect bites, consume only bottled or carbonated water, avoid undercooked meat, and avoid fresh fruits or vegetables unless peeled or cooked

108. Tetanus

Etiology & Pathophysiology

- Wound infection with spores of the anaerobe *Clostridium tetani,* resulting in increased muscle tone and spasms
- Spores are found worldwide in soil and animal feces
- Tetanospasmin toxin produced by organisms in the wound travels retrograde through axons to the CNS (shorter nerves are affected earlier due to shorter transport time)
- In the CNS, the toxin blocks release of inhibitory neurotransmitters, leading to an excitatory state that causes muscle rigidity
- About 40 cases per year in the US
- Immunity is conferred by vaccine; however, booster shots are required (in the US only 27% of persons over 70 have protective antibody levels but 88% of children ages 6 to 11 are immune)
- Disease is widespread in countries without immunization programs
- Symptoms appear 1–14 days after infection

Differential Dx

- Dystonic drug reaction (e.g., phenothiazines, antiemetics, metoclopramide)
- Hypocalcemic tetany
- Botulism
- Rabies
- Meningitis
- Encephalitis
- Strychnine poisoning
- Other causes of trismus (e.g., dental infection, TMJ syndrome)

Presentation

- Trismus (increased masseter tone) is often the first symptom
- Muscle rigidity and spasms
- Dysphagia
- Pain and stiffness in neck, shoulder, and back muscles
- Abdominal muscle rigidity
- Opisthotonus (arched back due to paravertebral muscle spasm)
- Risus sardonicus (grimace due to facial involvement)
- Respiratory muscle involvement (laryngospasm, poor ventilation, cyanosis)
- Autonomic dysfunction in severe cases includes HTN, tachycardia, dysrhythmias, cardiac arrest

Diagnosis

- Diagnosis is based on clinical findings
- Low risk of infection if immunization status is up-to-date
- Wounds should be cultured; however, *C. tetani* is generally not isolated even in confirmed cases
- CBC may show leukocytosis
- CPK levels may be elevated due to rhabdomyolysis that results from severe muscle spasms
- Electrolytes should be ordered to rule out hypocalcemia
- Lumbar puncture is normal in tetanus infection but may be required to rule out other conditions
- Consider a trial of diphenhydramine or benztropine to rule out dystonic reactions
- Other tetanus syndromes include localized tetanus (weakness and spasm limited to muscles near the wound caused by local effect of toxin on nerve endings) and neonatal tetanus (generalized symptoms with poor feeding, spasms, and rigidity, occurring only in infants of unimmunized mothers)

Treatment

- Supportive care, including supplemental O_2 and IV hydration
- Human tetanus immune globulin (antitoxin) should be promptly given to neutralize toxin; however, it does not cross into the CNS, only neutralizes peripheral toxin
- Tetanus toxoid should be administered to all patients
- Debride and clean the wound after giving antitoxin
- IV metronidazole should be administered to eradicate the organism; alternatives include erythromycin or penicillin
- Muscle spasms may be treated with diazepam or lorazepam (may require very high dosages); intubation with therapeutic paralysis may be needed for uncontrolled spasms
- Intubation may be required for airway compromise due to laryngospasm, oversedation, or upper airway muscle spasm
- Autonomic dysfunction can be managed with β-blockers, clonidine, and morphine (an α-blocker must be administered prior to β-blockade as unopposed α receptor stimulation may cause severe hypertension)

Disposition

- Admit suspected cases to the ICU
- Mortality is about 10%, with poorer outcomes in neonates and elderly
- Outcome is also poorer for patients who have a short interval between the onset of symptoms and frank spasms
- Ventilatory support may be needed for weeks
- Disease usually lasts 4–6 weeks, minor muscle spasms may last for months
- Immunization (tetanus toxoid) should be administered to all patients every 5–10 years (as a booster), to all patients who present with possible tetanus (the disease does not cause immunity), and as a series of 3 shots in those not previously immunized
- Also administer tetanus immune globulin in dirty wounds with unknown primary immunization

109. Botulism

Etiology & Pathophysiology

- *Clostridium botulinum* is an anaerobic, spore forming, gram positive bacillus
- Clinical symptoms occur via a neurotoxin that blocks the release of acetylcholine at the pre-synaptic neuromuscular junction (does not involve the CNS)
- Occurs as food botulism (due to ingestion of preformed toxin), wound botulism (due to local *C. botulinum* infection with toxin release), or infant botulism (due to ingestion of bacterial spores that proliferate in the intestine, often from honey—gut flora in adults is generally protective)
- Botulinum toxin is the most potent toxin known to humans (100,000 times more toxic than sarin nerve gas)
- The toxin has been developed as a potential biological warfare agent to be delivered by aerosol or via contamination of the food supply; however, not an ideal bioweapon (no human-human transmission)

Differential Dx

- Myasthenia gravis
- Cholinergic crisis (therapeutic drug overdose)
- Guillain-Barré syndrome
- Guillain-Barré (Fisher variant)
- Lambert-Eaton syndrome
- Paralytic medications
- Brainstem stroke
- Ocular myopathy
- Thyroid disease
- Idiopathic cranial neuropathy
- Tick paralysis
- Organophosphate poisoning
- Amyotrophic lateral sclerosis
- Poliomyelitis

Presentation

- Initial symptoms include bulbar and extraocular muscle weakness, blurry vision, diplopia, miosis, mydriasis, dysphonia, dysphagia
- Symmetric descending paralysis follows, with progressive weakness, respiratory failure, and death
- Absent pupillary light reflex (normal in myasthenia gravis)
- Constipation, N/V, abdominal pain
- Sensation is intact
- Normal mental status
- Absence of fever
- Infantile botulism presents with poor sucking, poor feeding, constipation, and failure to thrive

Diagnosis

- Botulinum toxin assays of the serum and/or stool may be indicated, but are rarely available in a timely fashion
- *C. botulinum* culture should be attempted from suspected food sources, stool, or wounds
- Consider performing an edrophonium (Tensilon) test to rule out myasthenia gravis; however, false positives may occur occur in botulism
- ESR and WBC count are normal
- In cases of suspected inhalation of toxin secondary to a bioweapon attack, ELISA nasal swab may be diagnostic during the initial 24 hours
- Consider a bioweapon attack if multiple patients present with similar symptoms (see *Disaster Medicine* section)
- Inpatient nerve conduction studies show incrementally improving response on repetitive stimulation (as opposed to decreasing response in myasthenia gravis)

Treatment

- Support ventilation and intubate as necessary
- All patients receive antitoxin immune serum to prevent progression and shorten the duration of illness
    - The most common is an equine-derived trivalent antitoxin; however, severe hypersensitivity may occur (e.g., anaphylaxis, serum sickness), so a skin test is required to rule out hypersensitivity
    - Monovalent human-derived antitoxin is available for treatment of infant botulism from the California Department of Health
    - An equine heptavalent antitoxin is available under certain government-sponsored research protocols
- Wounds with suspected botulism should be debrided to decrease bacterial load; administer penicillin to eradicate the bacteria
- Antibiotics have not been proven beneficial in ingested or infant botulism
- Human botulism immune globulin and vaccines are currently experimental

Disposition

- Admit all patients with proven or suspected botulism
- Weakness often lasts weeks to months, perhaps as long as a year
- Generalized weakness has been reported following medical toxin injection (e.g., Botox) for cosmetic purposes, dystonia, and blepharospasm

110. Rabies

Etiology & Pathophysiology

- A rare disease with near 100% mortality
- Due to infection of the CNS by a rhabdovirus transmitted through contact with infected animals
- Infection typically occurs after a bite but there have been case reports of infection following mucous membrane contact, abrasions, inhalation, scratches, or other non-bite exposures
- Rare in humans; less than 50 cases reported in the US since 1980
- Raccoons, skunks, foxes, bats, dogs and cats may all carry the virus
- Rabbits and rodents are not carriers of the virus
- Initial viral replication occurs in myocytes at the site of inoculation; the virus then crosses the motor end plate and ascends through the peripheral nerves to the CNS where it causes encephalitis
- Virus travels at a slow rate; thus lower extremity bites may not manifest in the CNS for months

Differential Dx

- Guillain-Barré syndrome
- Tetanus
- Meningitis
- Encephalitis
- Brain abscess
- Polio
- Tick paralysis

Presentation

- Initial manifestations include fever, headache, sore throat, and pain and paresthesias at the wound site
- CNS symptoms develop 1–2 weeks after the prodrome (later if lower extremity is the site of inoculation)
  - Encephalitic form: Bulbar and peripheral muscle spasms, opisthotonus, agitation, severe hydrophobia (likely an exaggerated airway protective reflex), autonomic instability
  - Paralytic form: Symmetric, ascending flaccid paralysis
- Disease results in coma, apnea, and death, usually 4–7 days after the onset of CNS symptoms

Diagnosis

- Due to the rarity of human rabies, diagnosis and prophylactic treatment is generally made by identifying at-risk patients at the time of inoculation
- Rabies virus antigen and antibody can be detected in many body fluids by fluorescent antibody testing but are generally negative until 1 week after exposure
- Negri bodies (small, intracellular, eosinophilic inclusions that represent sites of active viral replication) are seen on brain biopsy specimens

Treatment

- Prophylaxis is only successful if administered prior to CNS involvement
- Once full-blown rabies has developed, treatment is supportive—few cases of recovery have ever been reported
- Initial wound cleaning and debridement of devitalized wound tissue is warranted to decrease the viral inoculum
- Prophylaxis for high-risk exposures (the decision to give post-exposure prophylaxis depends on the species of animal, the nature of the exposure, and whether the animal is available for necropsy or observation)
  - Human rabies immune globulin should be administered with half the dose injected around the wound site and the other half given intramuscularly at a distant site
  - Human diploid cell vaccine is given intramuscularly on post-exposure days 0, 3, 7, 14 and 28

Disposition

- Patients with clinical rabies should be admitted to the ICU for respiratory and circulatory monitoring/support
- Post-exposure patients can be managed as outpatients, provided they have good follow-up
- The disease is almost universally fatal once CNS symptoms have developed
- Prophylactic therapy may be deferred in bites if the biting animal has received the rabies vaccine or if the animal is acting normally and is available for observation over a 10 day period

111. Rheumatic Fever

Etiology & Pathophysiology

- Caused by an autoimmune reaction to streptococcal antigens, which cross-reacts with body tissues (especially the heart, joints, CNS, and subcutaneous tissues)
- Follows *Streptococcus pyogenes* (group A strep) pharyngitis infection—no other streptococcal infection is associated with rheumatic fever
- Only certain strains of *S. pyogenes* are likely to result in rheumatic fever
- Symptoms of rheumatic fever begin after initial pharyngitis and a latent period of 2–3 weeks
- Outbreaks of rheumatic fever closely follow epidemics of streptococcal pharyngitis
- Most frequently occurs in children ages 4–9, but may occur at any age

Differential Dx

- Kawasaki disease
- Juvenile arthritis
- Septic arthritis
- Endocarditis
- Other causes of arthritis (e.g., rheumatoid arthritis, systemic lupus erythematosis)
- Leukemia
- Vasculitis
- Drug reaction
- Viral cardiomyopathy

Presentation

- Migratory polyarthritis of large joints
- Pancarditis (pericardial, myocardial, and endocardial inflammation): New onset of chest pain, murmur (typically mitral stenosis), rub, tachycardia, or CHF
- Sydenham's chorea: Involuntary, purposeless movements and muscle weakness
- Subcutaneous nodules (small, firm, painless) occur on extensor surfaces (e.g., wrists, elbows, knees)
- Erythema marginatum: Macular rash with central clearing occurring on the trunk and limbs

Diagnosis

- Modified Jones criteria (1992) are used for diagnosis—require evidence of antecedent streptococcal infection plus either two major criteria or one major and two minor criteria
    - Major criteria: Migratory polyarthritis, carditis, chorea, erythema marginatum, subcutaneous nodules
    - Minor criteria: Fever, arthralgia (subjective pain), previous history of rheumatic fever, elevated ESR or CRP, prolonged PR interval
- Evidence of antecedent streptococcal infection is best assessed by antibody titers—anti-streptolysin O (most sensitive), anti-hyaluronidase, or anti-DNAase B (at least one of these is elevated in 95% of rheumatic fever cases)
- Throat culture is positive in only 40% of cases
- Chest X-ray may show cardiomegaly or evidence of CHF
- ECG may show conduction delays due to carditis
- Echocardiography may be used (generally not in the ED) to assess for valvular disease

Treatment

- Treat all patients for group A streptococcal infection (even if cultures are negative)
    - Oral penicillin V for 10 days or IM benzathine penicillin
    - Macrolides are used in penicillin allergic patients
- Secondary prophylaxis is administered to prevent persistent streptococcal colonization or recurrent infection
    - Monthly IM benzathine penicillin or daily oral penicillin or sulfadiazine
    - Continue prophylaxis for at least 5 years (longer in high-risk or exposed patients); continued for life in those who have had recurrences of rheumatic fever or heart valve damage
- High-dose aspirin (4–8 g/day in adults) is effective for fever and arthritis; should be continued until symptoms resolve and acute-phase reactants normalize
- Severe carditis is treated with standard CHF therapy, systemic steroids, and high-dose aspirin; however, treatment will not prevent valvular damage
- Chorea is treated with haloperidol or benzodiazepines

Disposition

- Admit all patients
- Patients should remain in bed until acute-phase reactants normalize
- Family members and close contacts should have screening throat cultures
- Incidence of recurrence has declined to 2–4% with prophylactic therapy
- Adults may present with joint symptoms only
- Preceding pharyngitis may have been asymptomatic
- Acute disease usually resolves within 3 months
- Persistent valvular heart disease (rheumatic heart disease) is the most common complication

112. Osteomyelitis

Etiology & Pathophysiology

- Infection of bone and marrow due to hematogenous spread (90% of cases), direct inoculation (e.g., trauma, surgery), or direct spread from local soft tissue infection (e.g., diabetic foot ulcer)
- High-risk patients include those with diabetes, peripheral vascular disease, and IV drug use
- *S. aureus* causes 50% of cases; other organisms include gram-negatives, *Staphylococcus epidermidis* (especially in prosthetic joints), anaerobes (especially in diabetics), fungi (especially in immunocompromised), *M. tuberculosis* (e.g., Pott's disease of the spine), and *Pasteurella* (in cat or dog bites)
- In adults, osteomyelitis most commonly occurs in the vertebrae
- In children, osteomyelitis usually occurs in the metaphyses of long bones
- An important cause of fever of unknown origin

Differential Dx

- Cellulitis
- Bone infarction
- Soft tissue infection
- Trauma
- Fracture
- Gout
- Septic arthritis
- Degenerative joint disease
- Rheumatoid arthritis
- Metastatic cancer
- Bone tumor (e.g., Ewing's sarcoma)

Presentation

- Common symptoms include localized bone pain (not relieved by rest), tenderness, warmth, swelling, fever, non-healing ulcer
- Systemic symptoms (e.g., fever, chills, malaise, anorexia, nausea/vomiting) may be present
- Infants may be irritable with a red, warm, tender extremity
- Children more commonly have acute systemic infection; often they will refuse to use the limb or will have decreased weight bearing

Diagnosis

- Plain X-rays are often the first test ordered; however, they are rarely positive early in disease (bony changes may not occur for 10–21 days)—may see periosteal elevation, lytic lesions, cortical changes, or frank bony destruction
- ESR elevation is highly sensitive for osteomyelitis; leukocytosis is less sensitive (neither is specific)
- Blood cultures are only positive in 50–60% of cases
- Needle aspirate or open bone biopsy with culture give the best yield (generally performed by orthopedics)
- Culture of drainage material from open tracts is *not* helpful because it is often contaminated with multiple pathogens
- CT scan is used to determine the extent of disease; however, it also is often negative early in the illness
- Bone scan is very sensitive but not specific; usually not rapidly available in the ED
- MRI is very sensitive and more specific than bone scan; may be obtained in the ED or as an inpatient

Treatment

- IV antibiotics for 4–6 weeks followed by oral antibiotics
  - Begin empiric coverage with two drugs until results of cultures and gram stain are available
  - Always include anti-staphylococcal coverage (e.g., cefazolin, nafcillin, clindamycin, vancomycin)
  - Also cover gram-negatives (e.g., 3rd or 4th generation cephalosporin, gentamicin, ciprofloxacin, imipenem)
  - Consider adding anaerobic coverage (e.g., penicillin/anti-penicillinase, clindamycin) in diabetic patients
  - Tailor antibiotics once gram stain, cultures, and sensitivities return
- Surgical drainage/debridement is indicated emergently in open fractures and if symptoms do not improve within the first 48 hours; more likely to be required in diabetic foot infections

Disposition

- Admit all patients for acute workup and initial IV antibiotics
- Consult orthopedics in all cases for further management
- Rule out septic joint involvement in all suspected cases, as this requires urgent surgical debridement
- Complications include pathologic fracture, vertebral collapse with spinal cord compression, bacteremia, and sepsis
- Osteomyelitis often must be diagnosed clinically, even if all ED imaging is negative; if patients have history and physical consistent with osteomyelitis, obtain cultures and begin antibiotics

113. Hand Infections

Etiology & Pathophysiology

- Due to skin violation from biting, puncture, or penetrating trauma
- May cause significant morbidity due to loss of function
- 85% of cases are caused by *S. aureus* and *Streptococcus pyogenes*
- 15% are caused by anaerobes, *Neisseria, Eikinella corrodens* (human bite), *Pasteurella* (cat and dog bites), and *Capnocytophaga cynodegmi* (dog bites)
- Herpes virus, atypical mycobacterium, aspergillus, candida, and sporothrix species may cause hand infection in special circumstances
- Closed fist injury with skin violation is treated as a human bite wound due to its high infection/complication rate
- Deep space infections of the hand may occur at the thenar space, mid-palmar space, ulnar bursa, or radial bursa (the bursa are synovial spaces containing the flexor tendons)—these are emergencies that require immediate IV antibiotics, orthopedic consultation, and incision and drainage

Differential Dx

- Cellulitis
- Paronychia
- Felon
- Bite wound
- Flexor tenosynovitis
- Herpetic whitlow (especially in health care workers)
- Web space infection
- Deep space infection
- Sporothrix schnekii infection (especially in rose gardeners)

Presentation

- Cellulitis: Warmth, superficial erythema, intact ROM
- Paronychia: Erythema, pain, and swelling along the lateral nail fold
- Felon: Distal palmar pulp space erythema, throbbing pain, swelling
- Flexor tenosynovitis: Infection of distal flexor tendon sheaths
- Bite wounds: Teeth marks, puncture wound, or laceration
- Herpetic whitlow: Painful vesicles on finger tip with burning/pruritus
- Web space infection: Pain and swelling upon finger separation
- Deep space infection: Tenderness, fluctuance in palm, palmar pain upon motion of digits

Diagnosis

- Diagnosis is generally based on the clinical presentation
- Kanavel's four signs of tenosynovitis (an orthopedic emergency):
  - Tenderness over the flexor tendon sheath
  - Symmetrical swelling of the finger (sausage digit)
  - Pain with passive extension of finger
  - Finger held in flexion at rest
- Bite wounds have a high risk of infection (80% of cat bites become infected) and can penetrate deeply; therefore, tendon and joint injury must be ruled out by clinical exam and X-rays should be obtained to rule out open fractures or tooth fragments
- Rapidly spreading infection should raise suspicion of *Pasteurella* infection

Treatment

- Outpatient antibiotics: Amoxicillin/clavulanic acid or cephalexin for 7–10 days
- Inpatient IV antibiotics: Penicillin/anti-penicillinase or clindamycin plus ciprofloxacin
- Cellulitis: Generally managed with outpatient antibiotics
- Paronychia: Incision and drainage by elevating paronychium with a scalpel; add antibiotics if cellulitis occurs
- Felon: Incision and drainage with a high lateral incision into the pulp space; splint finger for protection; oral antibiotics
- Flexor tenosynovitis: Consult orthopedics immediately and administer IV antibiotics and analgesia; most patients proceed to surgery for urgent incision and drainage
- Bite wounds: Clean, irrigate, and dress wounds; however, most are not sutured due to risk of infection; oral antibiotics
- Herpetic whitlow: Most resolve without therapy; consider antivirals; do not incise lesions; dress finger to prevent spread to other areas
- Web space infection or deep space infection: Consult orthopedics immediately and administer IV antibiotics; most patients proceed to surgery for urgent incision and drainage

Disposition

- Discharge cases of mild cellulitis, paronychia, felon, and herpetic whitlow with follow-up exam in 24 hours
- Explain to patients and document the significant risk of morbidity if they fail to follow-up
- Admit patients with severe cellulitis, flexor tenosynovitis, web space infections, or deep space infections for IV antibiotics and possible incision and drainage
- Admit diabetic or immunosuppressed patients, those who are systemically ill, or those who have failed oral antibiotics
- Consider treatment for rabies in animal bite wounds
- Check tetanus status

114. Superficial Soft Tissue Infections

Etiology & Pathophysiology

- Cellulitis: Superficial infection of skin and subcutaneous soft tissue, most commonly due to *S. aureus* or *Streptococcus pyogenes;* other organisms (e.g., anaerobes, pseudomonas) may be present in diabetics and immunocompromised hosts
- Lymphangitis: An extension of cellulitis via the lymphatic system with increased risk of systemic infection
- Erysipelas (St. Anthony's Fire): Painful skin infection with associated lymphangitis, due to *S. pyogenes;* common in children
- Impetigo: Skin infection by *S. aureus* or *Streptococcus pyogenes*, commonly seen in humid, warm weather among infants and children
- Ecthyma: Similar to impetigo but also involves subcutaneous tissue
- Abscesses are walled off collections of pus due to infection
- Diabetic infections are typically polymicrobial (aerobic and anaerobic), resistant to cure, and require more intensive workup

Differential Dx

- Folliculitis
- Furuncle/carbuncle
- Necrotizing tissue infections
- Osteomyelitis
- Scalded skin syndrome
- Toxic shock syndrome
- Meningococcemia
- Bullous impetigo
- Viral exanthem
- Varicella
- Candidiasis
- Bite wound (insect or animal)
- Allergic reaction
- DVT

Presentation

- Cellulitis: Redness and warmth of affected skin, localized induration and pain; some have fever, chills, rigors, and systemic illness
- Lymphangitis: Cellulitis with proximal red streaking
- Erysipelas: Bright red erythema, warmth, and burning pain with lymphangitic streaking; may have bullae or fever/chills
- Impetigo: Pruritic pustules and vesicles that coalesce to a "honey-crust," most commonly on the face
- Ecthyma: "Punched out" ulcers with necrosis, crusting, and inflammation
- Abscess: Fluctuant mass

Diagnosis

- Superficial skin infections are diagnosed clinically based on the disease characteristics, location, and patient age
- Blood or wound cultures are rarely helpful but should be considered in immunocompromised, diabetic, or severely ill patients
- Plain X-rays may reveal subcutaneous air in some cases of fasciitis and may show evidence of osteomyelitis; however, the absence of findings does not rule out these deep infections
- Extremity venous Doppler studies may be necessary to rule out DVT
- Head CT is required in periorbital or orbital cellulitis to evaluate for extension of infection to venous sinuses

Treatment

- Warm compresses and pain control
- Antibiotics should cover *Staph aureus* and *Strep pyogenes*
  - Oral antibiotics may include cephalexin, dicloxacillin, clindamycin, or macrolides
  - IV antibiotics for serious infections may include nafcillin, cefazolin, or clindamycin
  - Diabetic patients require extended-spectrum antibiotics to cover aerobes and anaerobes (e.g., penicillin/anti-penicillinase or a combination of ciprofloxacin and clindamycin)
  - Impetigo may be treated with topical mupirocin or an oral agent as above
  - Erysipelas should be treated with IV antibiotics
- Incise and drain all cutaneous abscesses—if there is minimal cellulitis and good drainage was achieved, antibiotics may not be required unless the patient has risk factors for infections (e.g., diabetes)

Disposition

- Admit patients with systemic illness, immunosuppression, co-morbid conditions, history of diabetes, high fever, hand or facial cellulitis, large area of involvement, or who may have necrotizing disease
- Discharge patients with mild disease and no co-morbid conditions with follow-up in 24–48 hours
- Impetigo rarely needs an inpatient stay
- Erysipelas should be treated as an inpatient with parenteral antibiotics
- Risk factors for cutaneous infections include immunosuppression, diabetes, and peripheral vascular disease
- Complications of cutaneous infections include abscess formation, fasciitis, osteomyelitis, bacteremia, and sepsis

115. Necrotizing Soft Tissue Infections

Etiology & Pathophysiology

- Necrotizing fasciitis: A rapidly developing, life-threatening infection of the superficial and deep fascia that spreads along fascial planes, causing thrombosis of nutrient vessels, gangrene, and necrosis
- Myonecrosis: Rapidly spreading infection of muscle tissue, most commonly due to *Clostridia* species
- Gas gangrene: Gas-forming deep tissue infection, usually due to *Clostridia* species
- Fournier's gangrene: Fasciitis of the genitalia and perineum
- Mixed infections are most common, including anaerobes, *S. aureus, Streptococcus* sp, *E. coli, Clostridia* sp, and *Vibrio vulnificus*
- *Vibrio vulnificus* may cause fasciitis after salt water exposure
- Streptococcal toxic shock-like syndrome ("flesh-eating" bacteria) is also an invasive infection of deep tissues (see related entry)
- Risk factors: Age >50, diabetes, immunocompromised, trauma, renal failure, alcoholism, obesity, IV drugs, malnutrition, vascular disease

Differential Dx

- Cellulitis
- Erysipelas
- Impetigo
- Scalded skin syndrome
- Toxic shock syndrome
- Bullous pemphigoid
- Pemphigus vulgaris
- Candidiasis
- Chickenpox
- Viral exanthems

Presentation

- Rapidly progressive
- Skin erythema, edema, and warmth
- Skin necrosis in some cases
- Subcutaneous crepitus
- Skin discoloration (dusky, purple)
- Loss of sensation in affected areas
- Bullae in some
- Pain out of proportion to physical findings
- Watery, foul-smelling discharge
- Shock or multi-organ dysfunction may occur (fever, tachycardia, hypotension)
- May be difficult to differentiate fasciitis from myonecrosis until surgery

Diagnosis

- Fasciitis and myonecrosis are usually clinical diagnoses
- Plain X-ray may show soft tissue gas but is not sensitive (necrotizing infection may be present without gas accumulation)
- MRI or CT scan may show the soft tissue necrosis and emphysema; however, imaging studies should not delay surgical debridement
- Surgical exploration is required for definitive diagnosis
- Culture and gram stain is usually not helpful if done superficially but should be obtained during surgical debridement
- CBC, electrolytes, BUN/creatinine, LFTs, PT/PTT, DIC screen, urinalysis, and blood cultures may be indicated to monitor for organ system involvement

Treatment

- Emergent surgical debridement is the only definitive therapy and may be life-saving
- Treat shock immediately
  - IV fluid resuscitation with isotonic crystalloid (e.g., normal saline or lactated Ringer's solution)
  - Vasopressors (e.g., norepinephrine or dopamine) if fluids are ineffective
- Emergent broad-spectrum empiric IV antibiotics to cover both aerobes and anaerobes
  - Ampicillin/sulbactam, piperacillin/tazobactam, or ticarcillin/clavulanic acid
  - 3rd generation cephalosporin and clindamycin
  - Penicillin, gentamicin, and clindamycin
  - Imipenem or meropenem
- Hyperbaric oxygen may improve outcomes but is controversial and should only be considered after surgical debridement
- Tetanus immunization if required

Disposition

- Admit all patients for surgical debridement and IV antibiotics
- Most will require ICU care
- Rapid surgical debridement is necessary to decrease mortality
- Complications include renal failure, respiratory failure, myocardial depression, ARDS, sepsis, multi-organ system failure, DIC, and death
- Mortality of necrotizing fasciitis is 40%
- Mortality of myonecrosis is >75%; more likely to cause shock and death than fasciitis

116. Scalded Skin and Toxic Shock Syndromes

Etiology & Pathophysiology

- Multi-system diseases caused by toxin-producing strains of staphylococci and streptococci
- Staphylococcal scalded skin syndrome (SSSS) is an exfoliative disease due to toxin secretion by *Staphylococcus aureus*
  - Cause may be localized skin or bacterial infection (e.g., UTI)
  - Most common in immunosuppressed patients and children <5
- Staphylococcal toxic shock syndrome: Bacterial exotoxin causes diffuse vasodilation and increased capillary endothelial permeability (formally associated exclusively with tampon use but now known to occur in men and women)
- Streptococcal toxic shock-like syndrome: Rapidly invasive soft tissue infection ("flesh eating") by group A streptococcus (*Streptococcus pyogenes*) with exotoxin release and deep tissue invasion (myositis and necrotizing fasciitis)

Differential Dx

- Toxic Epidermal Necrolysis or Stevens-Johnson syndrome
- Scarlet fever (rash spares palms and soles)
- Kawasaki disease
- Rocky Mountain spotted fever (centripetal rash)
- "Gas gangrene" due to *Clostridium perfringens*
- Erythema multiforme
- Pemphigus vulgaris
- Bullous pemphigoid
- Viral exanthem
- Meningococcemia

Presentation

- SSSS: Local skin infection followed by fever, skin pain and tenderness, and scarlatinoform rash progressing to vesicles and bullae
- Staphylococcal TSS: Presents with high fever, malaise, hypotension, diffuse erythematous rash (sunburn-like, centrifugal spread, affects palms and soles), vomiting
  - Desquamation after 1–2 weeks
  - Multisystem organ failure
- Streptococcal TSS: Extremity pain out of proportion to exam, fever, evidence of deep tissue infection, mental status changes; acute onset with rapid decompensation and organ failure

Diagnosis

- CBC, electrolytes, BUN/creatinine, LFTs, PT/PTT, DIC screen, CPK, and urinalysis in all patients
- Blood, urine, wound, and nose/throat cultures
- SSSS is a clinical diagnosis of severe bullous skin disease without multi-organ system involvement
- Staphylococcal TSS is diagnosed by the presence of fever, hypotension, diffuse erythematous rash followed by desquamation, and at least 3 of the following: Vomiting or diarrhea, mental status changes, mucous membrane hyperemia, renal failure, CPK elevation, transaminase elevation, and thrombocytopenia
- Streptococcal TSS is diagnosed by streptococcal soft tissue infection (proven on culture), hypotension, and multisystem organ failure (e.g., renal failure, necrotizing fasciitis or myositis, acute respiratory distress syndrome, cardiac dysfunction, liver inflammation, or coagulopathy)

Treatment

- Remove sources of infection (e.g., tampons, nasal packing)
- Treat shock as necessary
  - Fluid resuscitation with intravenous crystalloid solutions (normal saline or lactated Ringer's)
  - Vasopressors for severe hypotension unresponsive to fluid boluses (e.g., norepinephrine, dopamine)
  - Arterial blood pressure monitoring and invasive monitoring via a Swan-Ganz catheter may be necessary
- Emergently administer IV antibiotics
  - Nafcillin, oxacillin, or clindamycin
  - Strep TSS may also be treated with IV penicillin G plus clindamycin
  - Vancomycin if resistant staphylococcus is suspected
- Incise and drain abscesses
- Surgical consultation for emergent wound debridement in Streptococcal TSS is required and may be life-saving since the bacteria invades deep tissues
- Treat electrolyte abnormalities as appropriate
- Treat coagulopathies with fresh frozen plasma

Disposition

- Admit all patients to an ICU
- Most children with SSSS recover in 2 weeks with treatment
- Staph TSS mortality is 10% even with therapy
- Strep TSS mortality is as high as 80%, depending on the degree of tissue invasion
- Stevens-Johnson syndrome is a similar disorder most commonly due to a drug reaction and causes severe, diffuse bullous skin disease with the epidermis shedding in sheets, exposing dermal layers

INFECTIOUS DISEASE EMERGENCIES

117. Occupational Needlestick Exposures

Etiology & Pathophysiology

- Post-exposure prophylaxis (PEP) is often required following occupational exposures to blood and body fluids
  - Potential transmission may occur with exposure to blood, tissue, and bodily fluids (e.g., CSF, synovial, pleural, peritoneal, pericardial, amniotic)
  - Very low risk of transmission: Feces, saliva, sputum, sweat, tears, urine, vomitus; not infectious unless they contain blood
  - No risk of transmission: Semen and vaginal secretions
- Viruses of concern: Hepatitis B (HBV), hepatitis C (HCV), HIV
- Testing of blood for hepatitis and HIV requires consent of both the source and the exposed individual
- Federal/state reporting requirements for occupational exposures exist
- The CDC intermittently publishes updated guidelines
- National clinicians post-exposure prophylaxis hotline: (888) 448-4911 (24-hour service)

Differential Dx

- Percutaneous exposure
  - Needlestick
  - Cut by sharp object
- Contact with mucous membrane
- Contact with non-intact skin (contact with intact skin is not considered an exposure and does not require PEP)

Presentation

- Evaluate the exposure risk based on body fluid involved, route and severity of the exposure, and the infectious status of the source
- Intact skin: No PEP needed
- Mucous membrane or non-intact skin: Note small volume versus large volume exposure to guide prophylaxis decisions
- Percutaneous exposures
  - Less severe: Solid needle, superficial scratch
  - More severe: Hollow needle, deep puncture, blood on the device, needle used for arterial or venous blood draw

Diagnosis

- Baseline blood work is required in both the exposed and source individuals
  - Exposed: ALT, HepBsAg, HepBsAb, anti-HCV antibody, anti-HIV antibody
  - Source: ALT, HepBsAg, anti-HCV, rapid HIV test (ELISA), anti-HepB core Ab
- HBV: Need for PEP depends primarily on the immune status of the exposed (see below)
- HCV: No PEP exists; test for baseline infection in source and exposed; follow up anti-HCV and ALT in exposed at 4–6 months if the source was HCV positive
- HIV PEP
  - Source HIV negative: No therapy
  - Source HIV positive: Less severe exposures require 2 drugs; more severe exposures require 3 drugs
  - Source unknown HIV: Consider empiric 2 drug PEP
  - Unknown source: PEP based on local HIV patterns

Treatment

- Use standard precautions in all patient contacts
- Wash site thoroughly with soap and water
- Tetanus toxoid if not up-to-date
- HBV: PEP depends on vaccination status of the exposed
  - Unvaccinated: HBV immune globulin plus HBV vaccine
  - Previously vaccinated, known responder to vaccine: No treatment
  - Previously vaccinated, known non-responder: Administer HBV immune globulin and revaccinate
  - Previously vaccinated, unknown response: Test exposed worker for anti-HBsAb and treat if non-responder
- HCV: There are no effective post-exposure therapies
- HIV: Start PEP ASAP
  - Duration of 4 weeks if source is HIV-positive; otherwise continue until HIV status of source is confirmed negative
  - Multiple 2 and 3 drug therapies are available [e.g., zidovudine plus lamivudine +/− (nelfinavir or indinavir)]
  - Consider possible local resistance to anti-HIV drugs
  - Side effects of PEP drugs (in 50%) include N/V, malaise, headache, anorexia, kidney stones, hepatitis

Disposition

- Give PEP ASAP after exposure
- HBV prophylaxis is effective up to 1 week post-exposure but earlier is better
- Risk of transmission
  - HBV: Transmission greatly increased if source is HBVe antigen positive (6% to 30% without treatment)
  - HCV: <2% risk of transmission in percutaneous exposures: rare after mucous membrane exposures
  - HIV: 0.3% after percutaneous exposure; 0.09% after mucous membrane
- PEP decreases the risk of HBV and HIV transmission by >75%
- All patients must follow up with occupational health and must be counseled with regards to risks
- Expert consult is indicated for delayed reporting, unknown source, pregnancy in exposed, source with resistant HIV

Rheumatologic and Allergic Emergencies

TOM MALINICH, MD
ADEMOLA O. ADEWALE, MD

118. Anaphylaxis

Etiology & Pathophysiology

- Allergic reactions vary from mild symptoms to overt anaphylaxis
- Anaphylaxis is a severe, systemic, immune-mediated allergic reaction resulting in urticarial rash, respiratory distress due to upper and/or lower airway obstruction, and vascular collapse due to vasodilation
- Most commonly a Type I Hypersensitivity reaction (IgE-mediated)
- Common causes include drugs (e.g., insulin, penicillin, streptokinase, antiserum), stings and venoms, foods (e.g., nuts, seafood, milk), environmental exposures (e.g., pollen, dust mites, animal dander), latex, and transfusions
- Generally occurs within seconds to minutes after an exposure to an antigen; however, response may be delayed in some cases
- Anaphylactoid reactions (e.g., due to IV dye) result in non immune-mediated mast cell degranulation with similar symptoms as anaphylaxis

Differential Dx

- Simple allergic reaction
- Vasovagal reaction/syncope
- Seizure
- Angioedema
- Epiglottitis
- Asthma exacerbation
- Airway foreign body/obstruction
- Pneumothorax/PE
- MI/arrhythmias
- Septic shock
- Carcinoid syndrome
- Systemic mastocytosis
- Pheochromocytoma

Presentation

- Early symptoms
  - Nasal congestion, hoarseness
  - Dyspnea, wheezing, cough
  - Skin flushing, severe pruritus, urticaria
  - Chest pain/tightness
  - Lightheadedness
  - Nausea/vomiting, abdominal cramping
  - Feeling of impending doom
- Late symptoms
  - Airway obstruction, stridor, angioedema, tongue/pharynx swelling
  - Altered mental status, seizure
  - Hypotension, tachycardia, dysrhythmias

Diagnosis

- Anaphylaxis is a clinical diagnosis; history and physical is helpful in identify inciting agents
- Diagnostic workup concentrates on excluding other diagnoses
  - ECG if a cardiac etiology is suspected
  - CXR to rule out pneumothorax; anaphylaxis may cause hyperinflation
  - ABG to evaluate respiratory status
  - CBC, glucose, electrolytes, BUN/creatinine, and urinalysis
  - Blood cultures if septic shock is considered
- Allergy testing may be done in outpatient follow-up

Treatment

- Establish IV access, high-flow O_2, cardiac monitoring, pulse oximetry
- Assess airway early as swelling can rapidly cause airway compromise
  - Endotracheal intubation if possible; however, swelling may prohibit intubation
  - Surgical airway (jet insufflation or cricothyrotomy) may be necessary
- Rapidly administer IV fluids (2–4 L of NSS or LR)
- Epinephrine decreases airway edema, restores vascular tone
  - IV epinephrine for severe bronchospasm, respiratory arrest, refractory shock, or upper airway obstruction
  - Subcutaneous administration for less severe symptoms
- Antihistamines (IV diphenhydramine plus an H2 blocker) will prevent further mast cell degranulation
- Systemic corticosteroids in all cases
- Albuterol nebulizers to treat bronchospasm
- Dopamine or norepinephrine may be used to maintain vascular tone in patients with persistent hypotension

Disposition

- May be fatal due to respiratory failure or hemodynamic collapse (even mild allergic reactions can progress to anaphylaxis and death)
- Symptoms may recur in 4–8 hours due to a second phase of mediator release
- Mild reactions should be observed for 4–6 hours and discharged if symptoms rapidly resolve
  - Avoid further allergen exposures
  - Continue steroids, H2 blocker, and diphenhydramine for 3 days
  - Consider prescription for pre-filled syringe kits (e.g., Epi-pen)
  - Outpatient follow-up in 1–2 days
- Admit patients with moderate-severe reactions to a monitored bed—ICU admission is warranted if intubated, in respiratory distress, or BP instability

119. Urticaria/Angioedema

Etiology & Pathophysiology

- An allergic reaction with vasodilation and increased vascular permeability, resulting in cutaneous wheals and tissue swelling
  - Urticaria affects superficial cutaneous tissues (dermis) only
  - Angioedema affects dermis and deeper tissues, usually face/neck
- Commonly due to IgE-mediated Type I hypersensitivity reactions with mast cell release of histamine and other mediators; also may be due to activation of complement, arachidonic acid, or kinin systems
- Causes of urticaria include foods, drugs (e.g., aspirin, NSAIDs, morphine, contrast), stings, sunlight, temperature extremes, or physical contact with foods, drugs, plants, or chemicals
- Causes of angioedema include C1 esterase inhibitor deficiency (hereditary or acquired), vasculitis, infections (e.g., hepatitis B), diabetes, thyroid disorders, autoimmune diseases
  - ACE-inhibitors may cause a bradykinin-mediated angioedema that is poorly responsive to therapy and may require intubation

Differential Dx

- Abscess/infection
- Anaphylaxis
- Collagen vascular disease
- Contact dermatitis
- Drug reaction
- Food allergies
- Insect bite
- Systemic lupus erythematosis
- Transfusion reactions
- Vasculitis
- Viral exanthem
- Hypothyroidism
- Urticarial vasculitis

Presentation

- Urticaria: Generalized, erythematous, pruritic wheals that blanch with pressure
- Angioedema: Deep diffuse swelling, most commonly of the head, neck, and upper airway; extremities, genitalia, mucous membranes, and eyelids may also be affected
- Airway edema may be seen on physical exam
- Abdominal pain, nausea, vomiting
- Wheezing or hypotension signal the presence of anaphylaxis

Diagnosis

- Clinical diagnosis
- Family history may provide evidence of hereditary disorders
- C1 esterase inhibitor and complement levels (C2 and C4) may be drawn for specialist follow-up—C2 and C4 are elevated in these diseases; C1 esterase inhibitor is decreased
- CBC, ESR, ANA, TSH, LFTs, and rheumatoid factor may be useful to determine the etiology of chronic cases or to rule out other disease processes
- Skin testing, serum IgE levels, and skin biopsy may be done as an outpatient if the diagnosis is unclear

Treatment

- Allergen avoidance and pulse oximetry
- Cold compresses for comfort
- Subcutaneous epinephrine for severe cases
- IV or oral antihistamines (e.g., diphenhydramine, hydroxyzine)
- H2 blockers may be beneficial as adjuvant therapy
- Systemic steroids are used for significant symptoms or if antihistamines fail to control symptoms
- Continue therapy for several days-to-weeks
- C1 esterase inhibitor concentrate or fresh frozen plasma may be administered if patient has a known deficiency and presents with moderate-to-severe symptoms
- The above measures have not been proven effective for ACE-inhibitor-induced angioedema; supportive care (including intubation) and discontinuation of drug is the primary therapy
- Be prepared to intubate sooner rather than later in cases of angioedema as airway compromise may rapidly ensue

Disposition

- Admission is warranted if symptoms of anaphylaxis are present (e.g., wheezing, respiratory distress, hypotension) or if there is any concern of potential airway compromise
- Patients who are discharged should continue antihistamine and steroid therapy for at least 3 days, avoid allergen if possible, and arrange follow-up with PCP, dermatologist, or allergist
- Acute urticaria lasts less than 6 weeks; chronic urticaria may persist for years (75% of cases are idiopathic)

120. Acute Monoarticular Arthritis

Etiology & Pathophysiology

- Non-inflammatory arthritides include osteoarthritis, trauma, soft-tissue injury, and viral infection
- Septic arthritis occurs due to bacterial infections
  - Disseminated gonococcal infection (DGI) is the most common cause of acute monoarticular arthritis in adults <45
  - Non-gonococcal bacterial arthritis (e.g., *S. aureus*, streptococci, gram negatives, Lyme disease, TB) is the most destructive type of acute monoarthritis; risk factors include diabetes, IV drug use, immunosuppression, rheumatoid arthritis, prosthetic joints
- Crystal deposition diseases occur due to precipitation of crystals in joints, resulting in inflammation, arthritis, and tissue injury
  - Gout: Uric acid crystals precipitate; acute attacks are often triggered by trauma, stress, surgery, illness, alcohol, diuretics, diet
  - Pseudogout: Precipitation of calcium pyrophosphate crystals

Differential Dx

- Traumatic injury
- Osteoarthritis
- Septic joint
- Gout/pseudogout
- Lyme disease
- Hemarthrosis (e.g., due to trauma, coagulopathy)
- Malignancy
- Rheumatoid arthritis
- Spondyloarthropathy
- Systemic lupus erythematosus
- Soft tissue injury (e.g., bursitis, tendonitis)

Presentation

- Warm, swollen, inflamed, painful joint suggests inflammation or infection
- Septic arthritis may result in systemic symptoms (e.g., fever, chills, malaise); often involves knee, hip, or shoulder
- Disseminated gonorrhea: Migrating arthritis (e.g., knee, wrist, ankle), vesiculopustular lesion on fingers, tenosynovitis, urethral discharge
- Gout: 1st MTP joint (podagra), intertarsal joints, ankle, knee, wrist are most commonly involved; fever may be present; palpable tophi develop as crystals deposit in subcutaneous tissues

Diagnosis

- Joint aspiration and analysis is performed in most patients
  - WBC >50,000 suggests an infectious etiology
  - WBC <50,000 suggests inflammatory/autoimmune etiology
  - WBC <2000 suggests a non-inflammatory etiology
  - Gram stain and culture is positive in only 75% of septic joints
  - Crystal analysis may show urate crystals in gout (needle-shaped, negatively birefringent) or calcium pyrophosphate crystals in pseudogout (rod-shaped, positively birefringent)
- Laboratory studies are rarely useful (serum WBC and ESR may be elevated by any cause of inflammation and may be normal in infections; uric acid may be low, normal, or high in acute gout)
- Cervical/urethral cultures if gonorrhea is suspected
- Consider testing for syphilis, Lyme, and HIV
- X-rays may show fracture, tumor, effusion, or osteomyelitis
  - Osteoarthritis: Joint space narrowing, osteophyte formation
  - Gout: Punched-out lytic areas with overhanging bony edges
  - Psuedogout: Chondrocalcinosis

Treatment

- Osteoarthritis: Acetaminophen, NSAIDs, and/or narcotics
- Hemorrhagic joint: Aspirate joint, ice, elevate, pain control; correct coagulopathies
- Septic arthritis requires empiric IV antibiotics to cover *S. aureus* and *N. gonorrhoeae*
  - Nafcillin plus either a 3rd generation cephalosporin or ciprofloxacin
  - Tailor antibiotics based on gram stain and/or culture
  - Prosthetic joint: Vancomycin plus gram negative coverage (e.g., ciprofloxacin, gentamicin, or cefipime)
  - Arthrotomy and open drainage may be necessary (especially for septic shoulder and hip)
- Crystal-induced arthritis
  - Ice, indomethacin and other NSAIDs, and colchicine
  - Corticosteroids (intrarticular/oral/IM/IV) are used in severe disease or in patients with contraindications to NSAIDs; however, be sure joint infection is not present
  - Avoid hypouricemic treatment (e.g., allopurinol) or diuretics during acute attacks

Disposition

- Admit patients with intractable pain, septic arthritis (for IV antibiotic administration), or coagulopathies with joint hemorrhage
- Most other cases of acute monoarthritis can be safely discharged home with early outpatient follow-up
- Do not assume that a patient with a history of a chronic process (e.g., gout) is having an exacerbation—must rule out septic joint if any clinical suspicion exists
- Failure to recognize a septic joint will lead to joint destruction and possible systemic sepsis and death

121. Polyarticular Arthritis

Etiology & Pathophysiology

- May be due to inflammatory, non-inflammatory, or infectious causes
  - Inflammatory arthritis is due to systemic autoimmune diseases (may have extra-articular symptoms), including rheumatoid arthritis, systemic lupus erythematosis, Reiter's syndrome, psoriatic arthritis, and gout
  - Non-inflammatory osteoarthritis (degenerative joint disease) is due to deterioration of articular surfaces and reactive new bone formation; involves large joints and the DIP joints of hand
  - Septic polyarthritis: Gonorrhea, Lyme disease, and other bacteria
  - Post-infectious/reactive arthritis may follow viral illnesses, streptococcal pharyngitis (acute rheumatic fever), serum sickness
- May be symmetric (e.g., rheumatoid arthritis, lupus) or asymmetric (e.g., gonococcal, Lyme, Reiter's, gout)
- Most cases have insidious onset; however, gout and septic arthritis present acutely

Differential Dx

- Systemic rheumatic disease (rheumatoid arthritis, lupus, Reiter's syndrome)
- Osteoarthritis
- Gout
- Septic arthritis
- Viral arthralgias
- Rheumatic fever
- Serum sickness
- Bursitis or tendonitis
- Fibromyalgia
- Soft tissue abnormalities
- Neuropathic pain
- Metabolic bone disease

Presentation

- Morning stiffness (>1 hour in RA)
- Warm, red, swollen, painful joints
- Constitutional symptoms (e.g., fever, chills, night sweats, malaise)
- RA: Symmetric joint involvement, including PIP and MCP
- RF: Migratory polyarthritis; specific major/minor criteria
- Psoriatic arthritis: DIP joint involvement, nail pitting, skin rash
- Reiter's syndrome: Conjunctivitis, urethritis, asymmetric arthritis
- Gonorrhea: Rash, diffuse joint involvement, tenosynovitis of wrist
- Lyme disease: Rash (erythema migrans), migratory arthritis, cardiac or neurologic sequelae

Diagnosis

- X-rays of involved joints
- ESR and WBC may be elevated in inflammatory arthritis
- Serologies may indicate pathology (e.g., RF, ANA)
- Synovial fluid analysis must be performed in all cases of suspected septic arthritis
- Acute rheumatic fever is diagnosed by evidence of antecedent streptococcal infection (positive culture or strep antibodies) plus clinical criteria (2 major and 1 minor or 2 minor and 1 major)
  - Major criteria (polyarthritis, carditis, chorea, erythema marginatum, subcutaneous nodules)
  - Minor (fever, arthralgia, elevated ESR, prolonged PR interval, past history of rheumatic fever)

Treatment

- Osteoarthritis: Analgesia and anti-inflammatory medications (acetaminophen is the preferred initial treatment, then NSAIDs, then narcotics); intra-articular steroids
- Inflammatory arthritis
  - NSAIDs are initial treatment; narcotics may be required
  - Intra-articular steroids are less useful for polyarthritis
  - Systemic steroids may be helpful in some diseases (e.g., polyarticular gout, autoimmune diseases)
  - Anti-rheumatic or cytotoxic drugs (e.g., methotrexate) may be useful in rheumatoid arthritis and SLE, after consultation with a rheumatologist
- Rheumatic fever: Penicillin and high-dose aspirin first line; systemic steroids for cardiac involvement
- Lyme disease: Doxycycline

Disposition

- Most polyarticular arthritic pain can be managed as an outpatient with appropriate follow-up arrangements
- Admission for patients with severe disability, multisystem involvement, intractable pain, inability to ambulate, septic arthritis, and rheumatic fever
- The majority of cases are chronic progressive diseases; prompt anti-inflammatory therapy is necessary to prevent articular degeneration and resulting morbidity

122. Rheumatoid Arthritis

Etiology & Pathophysiology

- A chronic autoimmune disease of joints and other organ systems
- Autoantibodies and immune complexes are deposited in affected organs, resulting in synovial proliferation with pannus formation, cartilage destruction, bony erosion, and eventual joint deformity
- Occurs in 1% of the population; most common in middle-aged adults
- Females and Native Americans have a higher prevalence
- Exact etiology is unknown; genetic predisposition exists (HLA-DR4)
- Complications occur in virtually all organ systems

Differential Dx

- Polyarticular arthritis (>4 joints): Rheumatoid arthritis, osteoarthritis, systemic lupus erythematosis, viral (e.g., HIV) arthritis
- Pauciarticular (2–4 joints): Gonococcal arthritis, Lyme disease, gout/pseudogout, Reiter's syndrome, rheumatic fever, psoriatic arthritis, osteoarthritis
- Monoarticular (1 joint): Trauma, septic joint, Lyme disease, tumor, osteoarthritis, gout/pseudogout

Presentation

- Symmetric polyarthritis, most commonly of small joints in hands and feet (especially PIP and MCP)
- Early morning stiffness >1 hour
- Joint deformities may be present (e.g., ulnar deviation, swan neck deformity, boutonniere deformity)
- Constitutional symptoms: Fatigue, malaise, fever, weakness
- Extra-articular involvement may include cardiac (e.g., pericarditis, myocarditis), dermatologic (e.g., subcutaneous nodules, vasculitis), pulmonary (e.g., interstitial disease, pulmonary nodules, BOOP), ocular (e.g., keratoconjunctivitis), anemia, and C-spine subluxation

Diagnosis

- At least four criteria must be met for diagnosis
  - Morning stiffness for >1 hour
  - Involvement of 3 or more joints
  - Involvement of the wrist, PIP, or MCP joints
  - Symmetric arthritis
  - Rheumatoid nodules
  - Elevated rheumatoid factor (elevated in >75% of patients)
  - Hand X-rays showing bony erosions or decalcification
- CBC may reveal a normochromic/normocytic anemia
- ESR is elevated in >90% of patients but is nonspecific
- CXR in patients with pulmonary symptoms may reveal pulmonary nodules or interstitial disease
- X-rays of involved joints may show erosions or decalcification
- Synovial fluid analysis may be consistent with rheumatoid (i.e., WBC 2000–50,000; >50–75% PMNs; low glucose) and may also rule out other causes of arthritis or infection

Treatment

- Attention to airway, breathing, and circulation in critically ill patients
- Goal of therapy is to prevent inflammation and its resulting damage to joints/organs
- Non-medical therapies include education, physical and occupational therapy, exercise, joint rest, heat/cold modalities, weight loss, and splints if needed
- NSAIDs are first line pharmacologic interventions; if one fails, another may be effective; consider cyclooxygenase-2 (COX-2) inhibitors
- Systemic steroids are used if NSAIDs fail
- Intra-articular steroids may be useful for acute attacks; however, infection of the involved joint must first be ruled out and repeated injections are contraindicated
- Disease modifying anti-rheumatic drugs and/or immunosuppressives may be administered in concert with a rheumatologist, including TNF-α receptor antibodies (e.g., Infliximab), methotrexate, hydroxychloroquine, gold salts, sulfasalazine, azathioprine, penicillamine, and minocycline

Disposition

- The disease follows a chronic course with acute exacerbations
- Criteria for admission include acute complications of RA (e.g., eye involvement, pericarditis, lung disease), unclear diagnosis, sepsis, pain control, and need for social support
- Discharge patients with mild acute exacerbations who have good pain control
- Follow-up with regular doctor or rheumatologist
- Consider cervical spine subluxation as a complication in any trauma patient with RA
- Patients with RA are at significantly increased risk of infection due to steroid use and side effects of systemic drugs—consider infection in any acutely ill patient

123. Systemic Lupus Erythematosis

Etiology & Pathophysiology

- Lupus is a connective tissue disease of unknown etiology characterized by B-cell hyperactivity, activation of complement, and T-cell defects
- Tissue damage occurs via inflammation, vasculitis, and direct damage due to deposition of immune complexes
- Females (9:1) and African-Americans are more frequently affected
- Peak age of onset 15–25 years
- Exacerbations are often preceded by infection, sunlight, trauma, medications, stress, or pregnancy
- Drug-induced lupus (e.g., hydralazine, isoniazid, and procainamide) has similar symptoms

Differential Dx

- Adrenal insufficiency
- Rheumatoid arthritis
- Dermatomyositis
- Polymyositis
- Cardiac disease
- Epilepsy
- Multiple sclerosis
- Sepsis
- Renal disease
- Shock
- Rheumatic fever

Presentation

- Fatigue, fever, malaise
- Symmetric arthritis, myalgias
- Malar (butterfly) or discoid rash
- Photosensitivity
- Headache, seizures, stroke, or psychosis
- Signs of peri-, endo-, myocarditis
- Pleural effusions, pleuritis
- Ulcers, peritonitis
- Hemolytic anemia, TTP, ITP

Diagnosis

- Diagnosis requires 4 of 11 diagnostic criteria: Butterfly rash, discoid rash, photosensitivity, painless oral ulcers, arthritis in >2 joints, serositis (pleural or pericardial inflammation), renal disease (proteinuria >0.5 g/day), seizures, hematologic disorder (e.g., anemia, thrombocytopenia, leucopenia), positive ANA, or positive anti-dsDNA/anti-Sm
- Antinuclear antibodies (ANA) are very sensitive (>95%) for SLE but have poor specificity (may be falsely elevated in the elderly or secondary to certain drugs and other connective tissue diseases)
- Double-stranded DNA (dsDNA) and anti-Smith (anti-Sm) antibodies are less sensitive but much more specific for SLE
- CBC may show thrombocytopenia or decreased RBCs
- Renal function should be checked to rule out nephritis

Treatment

- Avoid sun exposure
- NSAIDs for arthralgias, myalgias, fever, and serositis
- Severe disease (e.g., pericarditis, myocarditis, nephritis, cerebritis, hematologic abnormalities) should be treated with systemic steroids
- Antimalarial drugs (e.g., hydroxychloroquine, chloroquine) and cytotoxic agents (e.g., cyclophosphamide, azathioprine, methotrexate) are used by rheumatology in severe or unresponsive cases or for steroid sparing effects

Disposition

- Admit patients with nephritis or renal failure, CNS involvement, severe lung involvement, pericarditis, pregnancy, severe anemia, or thrombocytopenia
- Infections are the #1 cause of death in these patients (due to decreased immune function from the disease itself and from immunosuppressive medications)

124. Temporal Arteritis

Etiology & Pathophysiology

- An inflammatory vasculitis of medium to large size arteries (also known as giant cell arteritis)
- Generally affects arteries derived from the aortic arch and carotids, most commonly the temporal artery
- The classic picture of temporal arteritis is an elderly patient complaining of a new onset of headache (often unilateral) and/or visual loss
- Etiology is unclear; may be due to deposition of immune complexes in arteries, leading to inflammation
- Retinal artery occlusion may occur, resulting in loss of vision
- Significantly increased risk of thoracic aortic aneurysm; somewhat increased risk of abdominal aortic aneurysm, stroke, and MI
- Closely related to polymyalgia rheumatica (PMR)
  - 50–90% of patients with temporal arteritis have PMR
  - 33% of patients with PMR have temporal arteritis

Differential Dx

- Migraine headache
- Tension headache
- Dental ailments
- Lyme disease
- Otologic disease
- Polyarteritis nodosa
- Retinal vascular accident
- Sinusitis
- SLE
- Takayasu's arteritis
- Thrombosis of artery
- Trigeminal neuralgia
- Wegener's granulomatosis

Presentation

- Headache is the most common symptom (85%); often unilateral but may be diffuse
- Jaw/tongue claudication (65%)
- Tender temporal arteries (70%)
- Visual loss/visual changes (40%) (e.g., diplopia, scotoma, amaurosis fugax); may develop rapidly and lead to irreversible blindness
- Weakness and myalgias
- Fever/weight loss
- Skin color change in scalp/forehead
- Polymyalgia rheumatica presents with proximal (girdle) muscle weakness, stiffness, pain, synovitis

Diagnosis

- Diagnosis via clinical presentation, lab studies, and biopsy
- The presence of 3 of 5 established diagnostic criteria have better than 90% sensitivity and specificity for temporal arteritis:
  - Age >50
  - New localized headache
  - Temporal artery tenderness, node, or decreased pulse
  - Erythrocyte sedimentation rate (ESR)>50 mm/hour
  - Biopsy of temporal artery showing necrotizing arteritis or multi-nucleated giant cells
- Temporal artery biopsy is *not* 100% sensitive because vessel involvement may be segmental; therefore, a negative biopsy does not rule out the disease
- Elevated C-reactive protein (>2.45 mg/dL), normocytic anemia, leukocytosis, and increased PT may be present
- LFTs (especially alkaline phosphatase) are often elevated
- Ultrasound of temporal artery may show decreased blood flow

Treatment

- Systemic steroids are the mainstay of treatment and should be started immediately to prevent blindness, even if there is only a strong suspicion of the disease
  - IV (methylprednisolone) or oral (prednisone)
  - IV therapy may be more helpful in resolving vision changes; however, this has not been definitively proven
  - Steroids may be continued for months to years, depending on symptoms, side effects, ESR, and repeat biopsies
- NSAIDs and aspirin for pain
- Other drugs with limited data or under investigation may be prescribed in consultation with rheumatology (e.g., methotrexate, deflazacort, cyclophosphamide, azathioprine, dapsone, cyclosporine)

Disposition

- Most patients are admitted (especially those with visual loss or aneurysms)
- Rheumatology consult is imperative, especially for outpatient management
- Patients with mild symptoms may be discharged with steroid therapy and close follow-up
- Biopsy of temporal artery should be done within 1–2 days if possible
- Blindness is irreversible; however, proper therapy can prevent visual loss in the other eye

125. Dermatomyositis/Polymyositis

Etiology & Pathophysiology

- Polymyositis is an autoimmune-mediated inflammation of skeletal muscle due that usually progresses over weeks to months
- Dermatomyositis is a similar disease that also presents with characteristic skin involvement
- Most common acquired cause of muscle weakness
- Possible associations with viral infections, connective tissue diseases, and malignancy
- Cardiac muscle/conduction tissue may become involved

Differential Dx

- Collagen vascular diseases (e.g., scleroderma, Sjogren, SLE)
- Myopathies (e.g., drugs, infection, Cushing's disease, hypothyroidism)
- Myasthenia gravis
- Motor neuron disease (e.g., ALS)
- Sarcoidosis or amyloidosis
- Polymyalgia rheumatica
- Electrolyte abnormalities
- Inclusion body myositis
- Nervous system disorders

Presentation

- Muscle weakness
  - Bilateral and symmetrical
  - Proximal (e.g., difficulty climbing stairs, lifting arms, combing hair)
  - Respiratory muscle weakness
  - Dysphagia
  - Ocular muscles are spared
- Heliotropic rash on upper eyelid and knuckles is characteristic of dermatomyositis
- Fever, malaise
- Dysrhythmias, myocarditis

Diagnosis

- Definitive diagnosis is established by abnormal muscle biopsy
- In the ED, myositis is diagnosed by muscle weakness plus lab abnormalities
- Dermatomyositis may be diagnosed by the characteristic rash even without muscle findings
- CPK, aldolase, myoglobulin, creatinine, SGOT, SGPT, and LDH are often elevated secondary to muscle involvement
- ECG may show arrhythmias or signs of myocarditis
- ESR and ANA are often elevated
- Renal function and U/A may reveal signs of rhabdomyolysis

Treatment

- Systemic steroids are the first line therapy
- Cytotoxic agents (e.g., azathioprine, methotrexate, fludarabine, cyclosporine, tacrolimus, cyclophosphamide) may be used in concert with rheumatology in severe disease, unresponsiveness to steroids, and relapses
- Multi-drug regimens are often necessary
- Some patients respond temporarily to IVIG

Disposition

- Admit patients with lung involvement, CHF, myocarditis, dysrhythmias, or significant weakness
- Discharge on steroids if no pulmonary or cardiac involvement
- Complications may include cardiac conduction defects, arrhythmias, dilated cardiomyopathy, interstitial lung disease, joint contractures, subcutaneous calcifications, and an increased risk of neoplasia

Dermatologic Emergencies

KEVIN MACE, MD

126. Eczema and Contact Dermatitis

Etiology & Pathophysiology

- Eczema: Epidermal inflammation with pruritus and indistinct borders
- Nonspecific eczema is most common and is of unclear etiology
  - Types include nummular eczema (oval patches and vesicles), dyshidrotic eczema (vesicles on palms, digits, and soles), autosensitization (generalized rash following a localized dermatitis, due to hypersensitivity to an offending substance), and xerotic eczema (dry fissured skin, common in winter)
- Contact dermatitis is eczema due to contact with a specific source
  - Irritants cause a direct toxic effect on skin (e.g., soaps, detergents, chemicals, diaper dermatitis)
  - Allergic insults cause an immune-mediated reaction (e.g., plants, metal, chemicals, nickel, rubber)
- Atopic dermatitis: Chronic eczema associated with family or patient history of atopy (asthma, allergic rhinitis); common in children
- Seborrheic dermatitis: Chronic eczema of hairy areas (e.g., scalp)

Differential Dx

- Dermatophyte (fungus)
- Insect bite
- Cellulitis
- Impetigo
- Erysipelas
- Herpes zoster
- Drug rash
- Pediculosis (lice)
- Scabies
- Pellagra
- Psoriasis
- Neurodermatitis
- Photosensitivity reaction
- Thermal or radiation burn

Presentation

- Pruritus: *If it doesn't itch, it's not eczema*
- Nummular eczema is a localized lesion that may appear anywhere
- Dishidrotic occurs on palms and soles
- Autosensitization is a diffuse rash
- Contact dermatitis occurs in areas of exposure; symptoms may develop up to 7 days after exposure; history of exposure to irritant or allergen (e.g., detergent, plants such as poison ivy/oak, chemicals, neomycin, turpentine, mercury, nickel on belts or earrings)
- Atopic: Distinctive location on the face, scalp, neck, flexor surfaces (e.g., elbow, knee), and perineum
- Seborrheic: Found on the scalp, face, eyebrows, anterior chest, axilla, groin

Diagnosis

- Diagnosis based on location and appearance of lesions
- Eczema: Appearance depends on the age of the rash
  - Acute: Erythema, vesiculation (fluid filled blisters)
  - Subacute: Xerosis (dry skin), juicy papules, fissuring
  - Chronic: Lichenification (epidermal thickening)
- Contact dermatitis: Well-demarcated plaques and vesicles in exposed areas; may have weeping/crusting
- Rhus contact dermatitis (poison ivy/oak): Streaks of papules on exposed skin
- Atopic dermatitis: Localized erythema, dry skin, facial erythema and perioral pallor, increased palmar markings
- Seborrheic dermatitis: Greasy, scaling patches/plaques
- Consider obtaining gram stain/culture for bacteria, KOH prep for fungus, and/or Tzanck prep for HSV in unclear cases
- Outpatient studies: Biopsy and patch testing (allergen is placed in skin to diagnose allergic contact dermatitis)

Treatment

- Provide symptomatic relief for all patients
  - Oatmeal or cornstarch baths decrease inflammation
  - Moisturizing creams or ointments (emollients)
  - Antihistamines to decrease pruritus; newer non-sedating antihistamines are less effective
- Steroids for nonspecific eczema and contact dermatitis
  - Generally, continue therapy for 2–3 weeks to prevent rebound recurrence of lesions
  - Topical steroids are used in localized disease; available in variable strengths; side effects include skin atrophy with long-term use and hypopigmentation (moderate- and high-potency steroids are contraindicated on the face)
  - Oral steroids are used for severe generalized rash
  - Intralesional injection may be useful in thickened plaques
- Contact dermatitis: Avoid exposures; use protective clothing
- Atopic dermatitis: Treat conservatively with antihistamines, hydration, and emollients; topical steroids are not indicated unless conservative treatment fails
- Seborrheic dermatitis: Anti-seborrheic shampoos with zinc pyrithione, selenium, or ketoconazole

Disposition

- Nonspecific eczema follows a variable course and may recur, but usually responds to therapy
- Irritant contact dermatitis: Course and duration depend upon the concentration of agent causing the reaction and not upon previous exposures; remains localized; resolves in 1–2 weeks if the irritant is removed
- Allergic contact dermatitis: Course depends upon patient sensitivity and not the concentration of the agent; may become generalized; resolves in 1–2 weeks in most cases
- Atopic dermatitis follows a chronic course with intermittent flares; usually spontaneously remits in childhood, but may last for decades
- Seborrheic dermatitis is a chronic condition that responds well to therapy

127. Maculopapular Lesions

Etiology & Pathophysiology

- Macules are small, flat, discolored areas of skin
- Papules are small, raised areas that are <1 cm in diameter (raised lesions >1 cm are called plaques)
- Psoriasis: Inflammatory hyperproliferation of epidermal cells with hyper-keratosis; unclear etiology; increased by stress, during winter months, and by certain drugs (e.g., lithium, β-blockers)
- Guttate psoriasis: Acute, diffuse psoriasis; often due to strep infection
- Lichen planus: Epidermal inflammation; may be idiopathic or caused by drugs (e.g., diuretics, phenothiazines, antimalarials) or hepatitis
- Lichen simplex chronicus: Intensely pruritic rash
- Pityriasis rosea: Exanthem-type eruption in 10–35 year olds; likely due to herpes virus 7; increased incidence in spring and fall
- Discoid lupus: Scaling rash in SLE patients

Differential Dx

- Viral exanthem
- Eczema
- Seborrheic dermatitits
- Drug reaction/eruption
- Disseminated gonococcus
- Kawasaki syndrome
- Meningococcemia
- Fungal infection
- SLE
- Secondary syphilis
- Toxic shock syndrome
- Erythema multiforme
- Rocky Mountain spotted fever
- Cutaneous T-cell lymphoma

Presentation

- Psoriasis causes variably pruritic, slow-growing plaques that occur on the extensor surfaces (i.e., elbows, knees), gluteal cleft, and scalp but spare the palms, soles, and face; nail pitting may occur
- Lichen planus lesions may involve skin, mucosa, palms, and soles
- Lichen simplex chronicus occurs over the ankles, shins, dorsal feet, and genital areas
- Pityriasis rosea involves the trunk, proximal arms, and legs but spares the palms and soles
- Discoid lupus occurs in sun-exposed areas

Diagnosis

- Clinical diagnosis based on location and appearance of the rash
- Psoriasis: Sharply demarcated erythematous plaques and papules with a silvery scale
- Lichen planus: Pruritic, purple, polygonal papules with lacy white markings (Wickham's striae)
- Lichen simplex chronicus: Well-demarcated, intensely pruritic plaques with erythema and hyperpigmentation but minimal scale; chronic changes with lichenification may occur
- Pityriasis rosea: Red-brown oval and round plaques in a "Christmas tree" distribution on the torso (i.e., follows the lines of skin folds); a herald patch is present in 80%
- Discoid lupus: Purple-red plaques with white scale
- Secondary syphilis: Diffuse red-brown papules and plaques that involve the palms and soles

Treatment

- Psoriasis
  - Avoid excess drying of skin
  - Localized disease may be treated with topical steroids, coal tar ointment/baths, or calcitriol
  - Widespread disease should be treated as an outpatient with ultraviolet-A light plus psoralens (PUVA), UV-B light plus either coal tar or anthralin, or retinoids
  - NSAIDs are used for psoriatic arthritis
  - Methotrexate or cyclosporine are also used in widespread skin disease and for psoriatic arthritis
- Lichen planus: Topical steroids and antihistamines
- Lichen simplex chronicus: High-potency topical steroids and anti-histamines
- Pityriasis rosea: Medium potency topical steroids and antihistamines; in some refractory cases, ultraviolet light is used
- Discoid lupus: Topical steroids and sunscreen; some require more intensive anti-rheumatic therapy
- Systemic steriods may be required for diffuse rashes

Disposition

- Psoriasis is a chronic, recurrent disease that waxes and wanes; usually improves in summer due to the effects of sunlight
- Psoriatic arthritis occurs in 5% of psoriasis patients, resulting in progressive damage of the IP joints, knees, hips, spine, and ankles
- Lichen planus usually remits after 1–2 years, but is chronic in some cases; recurrence is uncommon
- Lichen simplex chronicus is a chronic disease that responds slowly to treatment
- Pityriasis rosea usually remits in 6–12 weeks; arrange outpatient biopsy if the rash lasts for a longer period of time
- Discoid lupus follows a chronic course but responds well to therapy

128. Bullous Lesions

Etiology & Pathophysiology

- Bullae are large blisters that occur between the epidermis and sub-epidermal structures
- Pemphigus vulgaris (PV): Formation of intra-epidermal blisters due to an autoimmune process that results in a loss of epidermal cell-to-cell adhesion (acantholysis); caused by immunoglobulin deposits; generally occurs in 50–60 year olds
- Bullous pemphigoid (BP): Autoimmune-mediated, sub-epidermal bullae caused by reaction of autoantibodies with basal keratinocytes; generally occurs in 50–60 year olds
- Dermatitis herpetiformis (DH): Subepidermal blistering due to IgA deposits; associated with gluten enteropathy; occurs in young adults
- Porphyria cutanea tarda (PCT): Abnormal heme synthesis due to absent enzymes leads to porphyrin accumulation and bullae formation; may be familial or sporadic

Differential Dx

- Burn
- Eczematous dermatitis
- Dyshidrotic eczema
- Contact dermatitis
- Herpes infection (HSV, zoster, or varicella)
- Cicatricial pemphigoid
- Erythema multiforme
- Stomatitis
- Toxic epidermal necrolysis
- Stevens-Johnson syndrome
- Bullous impetigo
- PCT: SLE, Sjogren's, sarcoid, secondary syphilis

Presentation

- PV: Blisters occur on the skin and ulcers occur on mucous membranes (may involve pharynx, larynx, esophagus, vagina, penis, or anus); oral lesions often begin months before skin involvement
- BP: Pruritic blisters and eczema occur on the extremities, flexor surfaces, axillae, groin, and lower abdomen; the oral mucosa is involved in 1/3 of cases
- DH: Highly pruritic and grouped vesicles and papules found on the elbows, knees, buttocks, shoulders, and low back
- PCT: Painful blisters and vesicles on the hands

Diagnosis

- Definitive diagnosis by biopsy; in the ED, bullous lesions may be distinguished by location, age group of the patient, and characteristics of the lesions on physical exam
- Nikolsky's sign: Lateral pressure on a bulla causes intra-epidermal shearing with extension of the bulla; positive in diseases that affect intra-epidermal adhesion
- Pemphigus vulgaris: Blisters are flaccid and fragile; erosions often occur after blisters rupture; positive Nikolsky's sign
- Bullous pemphigoid: Blisters are tense and intact; erosions may or may not occur; negative Nikolsky's sign
- Dermatitis herpetiformis: Grouped clusters of vesicles and papules
- Porphyria cutanea tarda: Small blisters and vesicles; 24-hour urine reveals uroporphyrin and coproporphyrin in urine; urine is dark brown and may fluoresce under a Wood's lamp

Treatment

- Secondary bacterial infections must be treated in all cases
- Pemphigus vulgaris: Steroids are the mainstay of therapy (IV in severe cases); severe or generalized disease may require immuno-suppressives (e.g., cyclophosphamide, azathioprine, methotrexate); plasmapheresis for cases unresponsive to other therapy
- Bullous pemphigoid: Oral steroids until the lesions resolve; add immunosuppressives (azathioprine or cyclophosphamide) in severe or resistant cases
- Dermaitts herpetiformis: A gluten-free diet is usually curative; dapsone or sulfapyridine may be used to clear the disease; however, lesions may recur once therapy is stopped
- Porphyria cutanea tarda: Phlebotomy may be used; also consider antimalarials

Disposition

- Pemphigus vulgaris is a severe life-threatening disease with 90% mortality if untreated (10% with treatment)
- Course of pemphigus vulgaris is variable—complete remission occurs in some patients but others suffer indefinitely; sepsis may occur from secondary infection
- Pemphigus vulgaris patients should be admitted in severe cases; will require dermatologic follow-up if discharged
- Bullous pemphigoid has an excellent prognosis; subsides after a few years, even if untreated
- Dermatitis herpetiformis: Medications and diet will improve symptoms but disease may recur if they are stopped

129. Vesicular Lesions (Herpes Viruses)

Etiology & Pathophysiology

- Vesicle: A small, discrete fluid-containing bubble on the skin
- Herpes simplex virus (HSV) affects the epidermis and mucosa; HSV-1 generally causes oral infection, HSV-2 causes genital infection
  - Primary herpes infection is followed by a latent phase where the virus resides in neural ganglia; patient remains infected for life
  - Recurrent infection may occur in the area of the primary lesion
  - Transmission via close contact of a person with active lesions; 90% transmission rate if a sex partner has active lesions
  - Immunocompromised patients can develop systemic infection
- Varicella zoster virus (VZV) is a herpes virus that causes chicken pox; highly contagious, respiratory spread; acute infection lasts about 2 weeks, the patient is infectious until vesicles become crusted; latency occurs after primary infection but may reactivate as shingles
- Herpes zoster causes shingles due to reactivation of Varicella; occurs with advancing age, cancer, stress, immunosuppression

Differential Dx

- Eczema
- Pemphigus foliaceus
- Paraneoplastic pemphigus
- Cicatricial pemphigoid
- Pemphigus vulgaris
- Bullous pemphigoid
- Aphthous stomatitis
- Bullous impetigo
- Erythema multiforme
- Hand-foot-mouth disease
- Herpangina
- Stevens-Johnson syndrome
- Dermatitis herpetiformis
- Porphyria cutanea tarda

Presentation

- HSV primary disease is often asymptomatic or may present with vesicles, pain, and burning (i.e., gingivostomatitis or vulvovaginitis) in a dermatomal distribution
- Recurrent HSV outbreaks usually have a prodrome of burning/itching for 1–2 days prior to appearance of lesions in a dermatomal distribution
- Chicken pox presents with a severely pruritic systemic rash, fever, malaise, and chills
- Shingles occurs in a dermatomal distribution after a prodrome of radicular pain, tingling, and itching; Ramsay-Hunt syndrome results in lesions on the TM and cornea

Diagnosis

- HSV: Peri-oral or peri-genital grouped vesicles with an erythematous base that develop into pustules, which may rupture, weep, and form a crust
  - Primary infection has multiple crops of vesicles
  - Secondary infection has fewer crops of vesicles;
  - "Herpetic whitlow" is infection of fingers by HSV
- Chicken pox: Systemic rash; vesicles on an erythematous base ("dew-drops on a rose petal") progress to pustules, crusts, and scar; lesions will be at varying stages of development
- Shingles: Clinical diagnosis by groups of vesicles in a dermatomal distribution
- Tzanck smear: Unroof lesion using a scalpel; staining of vesicular fluid with Wright's or Giemsa stain reveals multinucleated giant cells; only 60% sensitive
- Consider gram stain, culture, or KOH prep of lesions in unclear cases to confirm diagnosis

Treatment

- HSV: Avoid contact with persons who have vesicles present
  - Oral lesions: Penciclovir 1% cream for 4–7 days decreases viral shedding and time to healing; use in the prodromal stage may prevent the recurrence
  - Primary genital lesions: Oral antiviral (e.g., acyclovir, famciclovir, valacyclovir) for 10 days
  - Recurrent genital lesions: Oral antiviral for 5 days (must treat within 2 days of onset for benefit)
  - Chronic suppression: Oral antiviral (e.g., acyclovir bid, famciclovir bid, or valacyclovir qd)
  - Immunocompromised patients or severe systemic disease: IV acyclovir
- Chicken pox: Immunization (Varivax) is 80% effective at preventing disease; symptomatic treatment includes lotions, antihistamines, oatmeal baths, and antipyretics; IV acyclovir in immunosuppressed patients
- Shingles: Oral antiviral; prednisone is controversial; must start therapy within 3 days of rash for best results; IV acyclovir for patients with eye or nose involvement; narcotics and amitriptyline for post-herpetic neuralgia

Disposition

- HSV: Primary disease has 1 week incubation and lasts 3 weeks
  - Active viral shedding begins even before recurrent lesions appear (i.e., infected patient may be infectious even in the absence of lesions)
  - Recurrence may occur from stress, fever, sunlight, menses
  - Complications: Chronic ulceration, generalized mucocutaneous spread, systemic infection
- Chicken pox: Self-limited in healthy children; bacterial superinfection, pneumonia, or encephalitis may develop; maternal varicella may result in maternal-fetal spread
- Shingles: Rash persists for 2–3 weeks; post-herpetic neuralgia may cause severe neuropathic pain lasting months

130. Lacerations

Etiology & Pathophysiology

- Account for up to 10% of ED visits
- Wound healing is a process that requires weeks to months; full return to pre-injury tissue strength is achieved at 150 days
- Goal of repair is to achieve cosmesis and prevent wound infection
- Primary closure: Closure at time of initial evaluation using suture, adhesive, or staples
- Secondary closure: Wound is not closed but is allowed to heal gradually by granulation tissue; used for wounds with a high risk of infection (e.g., puncture wounds, >8 hours since injury)
- Tertiary closure (delayed primary closure): Wound is packed without closing; closure follows a week later if the wound is not infected; used for large wounds with high infection risk
- Risk factors for infection include poor vascular supply (e.g., wound to hands or feet), moist skin folds, foreign body, co-morbid medical illness (e.g., diabetes), steroid use, elderly, crush wounds

Differential Dx

- Lacerations
- Crush wound
- Bite wound (human, cat, dog)
- Puncture wound
- High-pressure injection injury
- Foreign body
- Nailbed injury
- Tendon injury
- Amputation
- Open fracture/joint space
- Needle stick injury

Presentation

- Note the following wound characteristics:
  - Time since wound occurred
  - Length of wound
  - Depth of wound (tissue layers– subcutaneous, fascia, muscle)
  - Shape of wound
  - Location and tension
  - Risk of foreign body or gross contamination
  - Distal neurovascular symptoms
  - Tendon function
  - Handedness
  - Keloid or scar formation from previous wounds
  - Tetanus status

Diagnosis

- Anesthetize the area with an injectable or topical agent
- Hemostasis either locally or with a blood pressure cuff
- Explore the wound for foreign bodies (significantly increase the risk of infection); X-rays may be used to evaluate metal, stone, and most glass; CT may be required for wood or plastic
- Debride devitalized, dead, or contaminated tissue to allow for healthy wound edges
- Irrigate the area with adequate volume (>500 cc) and pressure (sufficient pressure to dislodge bacteria is generated by a syringe and 18 gauge angiocatheter)
- Closure: Slightly evert wound edges and match skin layers; use a deep layer of sutures if the fascia is penetrated or there is high tension on the wound
- Wound care: Cover with antibiotic ointment and a dressing for 48 hours (change dressing daily); follow up in 24–72 hours for re-check; advise on long term care to minimize scar (e.g., avoid sunlight, use suntan lotion for 1 year, use vitamin E or aloe)

Treatment

- Tetanus toxoid should be administered if the last booster was >10 years ago or if >5 years ago and wound is contaminated
- Pain control with NSAIDs, acetaminophen and/or narcotics
- Close the wounds using
  - Sutures: Absorbable (polyglactin, chromic gut, plain gut) or non-absorbable (nylon, polypropylene, silk, polyester)
  - Staples: In areas where scars will not be seen (e.g., scalp)
  - Adhesives (cyanoacrylate glue): In wounds <5 cm in length with minimal tension (cosmesis equal to sutures)
  - Tape (steri-strips): For small wounds with little tension
- Antibiotics are not routinely used; indicated in bites, plantar punctures, intra-oral lacerations, or contaminated wounds
  - Dicloxacillin or cephalexin (staph and strep coverage)
  - Amoxicillin/clavulanic acid for bite wounds
- Injectable anesthetics may be used to achieve local or regional nerve block (e.g., digits, face, teeth); epinephrine is often added to cause vasoconstriction in order to decrease bleeding and prolong anesthetic presence/effectiveness (not used on digits, ears, nose, penis as ischemia may ensue)

Disposition

- Consultation is required for some eyelid wounds, open fracture or joint, extensive facial wounds, involvement of tendons, nerves, or major vessel, loss of significant skin surface area
- Bite wounds/closed-fist injuries require antibiotics and frequent follow-up; be wary of retained tooth fragments
- Closed-fist injuries often involve the MCP joint space
- Puncture wounds should be opened as needed to inspect for foreign bodies; high infection rate
- High-pressure injection (e.g., paint gun, air gun) may result in significant deep tissue involvement; often requires surgical exploration
- Despite proper care and management 3–5% of wounds will become infected; warn patients of signs of infection

Ophthalmologic Emergencies

MARY DAVIS, DO
JEFFREY M. CATERINO, MD

131. The Red Eye

Etiology & Pathophysiology

- Common causes include glaucoma, infection, trauma (see entries)
- Keratitis: Inflammation of the cornea due to herpes simplex, herpes zoster, bacteria, UV light, contact lenses, or dry eye syndrome
- Anterior uveitis: Inflammation of iris and ciliary body; most often idiopathic but may be due to trauma, infection (e.g., TB, syphilis, herpes, Lyme), sarcoid, IBD, SLE, RA, Sjogren's, or Reiter's
- Scleritis: Inflammation of the sclera; may be the initial symptom of connective tissue disease (e.g., SLE, RA, Wegener's, vasculitis, sarcoid) or infection (e.g., syphilis, TB, Lyme, zoster)
- Episcleritis: Benign, idiopathic inflammation near the sclera
- Keratoconjunctivitis sicca (KS): Benign cause of dry, red eyes; may be due to drugs (e.g., antihistamines, anticholinergics), Sjogren's syndrome, or sarcoidosis
- Subconjunctival hemorrhage: Benign rupture of small vessels due to underlying coagulopathy, trauma, coughing, or eye rubbing

Differential Dx

- Entropion or ectropion
- Infection (conjunctivitis, blepharitis, dacrocystitis, endophthalmitis, orbital cellulitis)
- Allergic conjunctivitis
- Keratoconjunctivitis sicca
- Keratitis
- Anterior uveitis (iritis)
- Scleritis/episcleritis
- Subconjunctival hemorrhage
- Acute closed angle glaucoma
- Corneal perforation
- Trauma (foreign body, corneal abrasion, globe injury)

Presentation

- Pain, pruritus, discharge, sensation of foreign body, and photophobia are often present
- Keratitis: Pain, redness, tearing, decreased vision
- Uveitis: Pain, perilimbal injection
- Scleritis: Unilateral severe pain, decreased vision, and injection; no discharge
- Episcleritis: Mild pain, localized redness
- Subconjunctival hemorrhage: Painless localized hemorrhage
- Infectious conjunctivitis: Watery, purulent discharge with injection
- Allergic conjunctivitis: Watery discharge with injection

Diagnosis

- Ocular exam with topical anesthetic may identify hallmarks of uveitis (i.e., constricted, minimally reactive pupil and pain with accommodation) or glaucoma (i.e., hazy cornea and dilated, non-reactive pupil)
- Slit lamp exam with fluorescein stain
  - May demonstrate foreign body or corneal abrasion
  - May show anterior chamber reaction/inflammation due to uveitis, keratitis, scleritis, corneal ulcer, gonococcal or bacterial infection
- Consider tonometry if suspect increased intraocular pressure
- Culture of discharge if suspect keratitis or bacterial infection
- Consider CT of orbits if foreign body is suspected
- Consider PT/PTT and platelet count to evaluate coagulopathic causes of subconjunctival hemorrhage
- Additional workup may be warranted for recurrent or bilateral uveitis and scleritis (e.g., ESR, ANA, PPD, VDRL, CXR for sarcoid and TB, toxoplasma and CMV titers)

Treatment

- Provide appropriate oral analgesics as needed
- Keratitis
  - Topical broad-spectrum antibiotics (quinolone or aminoglycoside)
  - Antivirals (topical and/or oral) if HSV is suspected
  - Cycloplegics for pain control if iritis is present
- Uveitis/iritis
  - Cycloplegics decrease pain by preventing ciliary muscle spasm
  - Topical steroids may be used to decrease inflammation as long as infection has been definitively ruled out after consulting with ophthalmology
- Scleritis: Topical/systemic steroids are administered in absence of infection after consulting with ophthalmology
- Episcleritis: Topical vasoconstrictors or anti-inflammatory medications (e.g., NSAIDs, steroids)
- Keratoconjunctivitis sicca: Discontinue offending medications and treat with artificial tears and eye lubricants
- Subconjunctival hemorrhage: No therapy required

Disposition

- Consult ophthalmology and consider admission for patients with unclear diagnosis, diminished vision, uveitis, scleritis, keratitis, acute closed angle glaucoma, bacterial infection, corneal ulcer, endophthalmitis, or perforation/globe injury
- Discharge patients with clear diagnosis, intact vision, and good follow-up
- Non-herpetic keratitis usually resolves in 2–3 days; however, herpes keratitis is vision threatening
- Uveitis: Complications include cataract, glaucoma, and pupillary dysfunction
- Episcleritis is usually self-limiting
- Scleritis should resolve with treatment, but may recur

132. Acute Vision Loss

Etiology & Pathophysiology

- Differentiate rapid, acute vision loss from slow, chronic degeneration (e.g., commonly due to cataract or proliferative diabetic retinopathy)
- Retinal detachment: Vision loss due to trauma or proliferative retinopathy
- Vitreous hemorrhage: Loss of vision due to bleeding within the globe secondary to coagulopathy, proliferative retinopathy, or trauma
- Central retinal artery occlusion (CRAO): Sudden, painless loss of vision caused by embolism, atherosclerosis, or temporal arteritis
- Central retinal vein occlusion (CRVO): Subacute, painless venous thrombosis or occlusion; associated with diabetes or HTN
- Temporal arteritis: Vasculitis of medium-sized arteries (especially the carotids) that affects patients > age 50
- Optic neuritis: Rapid, painful loss of vision due to optic nerve injury
    - Most common non-traumatic cause of vision loss in patients <50
    - Due to MS, virus, connective tissue disease, sarcoid, TB

Differential Dx

- Glaucoma
- CVA
- TIA (amaurosis fugax)
- Intracranial mass lesion
- Cerebral aneurysm
- Migraine
- Cavernous sinus thrombosis
- Malingering
- Uveitis
- Methanol ingestion

Presentation

- Retinal detachment: Painless; flashing lights, floaters, and curtain or shadow over the visual field; grayish area on the retina
- Vitreous hemorrhage: Painless; floaters or cobwebs; hemorrhage
- CRAO: Painless; pale retina with cherry red spot
- CRVO: Painless; swollen optic disc, retinal hemorrhages, cotton wool spots
- Temporal arteritis: Severe headache and tenderness over the temporal area, fever, malaise
- Optic neuritis: Painful; usually unilateral; afferent pupillary defect; normal fundoscopy

Diagnosis

- Fundoscopic exam is *mandatory* (cycloplegics facilitate exam)
- Tonometry to measure eye pressures
- Test visual acuity alone and while looking through a pinhole
    - Pinhole improves vision in lens, vitreous, or corneal pathology
    - Vision is unimproved in retinal, vascular, or CNS pathology
- Swinging flashlight test for afferent pupillary defect
    - Marcus-Gunn pupil: The pupil inappropriately dilates to direct light but has an appropriate consensual response (i.e., constricts when the light is shined in the other eye)
    - Present in optic nerve injury (optic neuritis), temporal arteritis
- Visual field testing
    - Retinal detachment may have partial or complete field loss
    - CNS lesions have characteristic visual field loss patterns
    - Optic neuritis results in central loss with peripheral sparing
- Head CT may show vitreous hemorrhage and retinal detachment
- Temporal arteritis: Elevated ESR; temporal biopsy is diagnostic

Treatment

- CVA requires workup and therapy for acute stroke
- Intracranial mass lesions may require surgical decompression
- Central retinal artery occlusion: There are no proven ED therapies; however, attempts are made to move the clot peripherally to improve blood flow
    - Ocular massage may dislodge the clot
    - Topical β-blocker and IV acetazolamide will decrease intraocular pressure to allow clot mobility
    - Anterior chamber centesis may also decrease IOP (generally performed by ophthalmology)
    - CO_2 re-breathing dilates cranial arterioles
- Central retinal vein occlusion may require photocoagulation
- Temporal arteritis: Immediate high-dose systemic steroids must be administered to prevent permanent vision loss, even if the diagnosis is not yet confirmed by biopsy
- Retinal detachment: Surgical repair by banding or laser
- Optic neuritis: Often treated conservatively with analgesia and ophthalmology follow-up; may require systemic steroids

Disposition

- Emergent ophthalmology consultation is *required* in all cases of acute vision loss
- Many patients will require admission or urgent surgical intervention (e.g., retinal detachment)
- May discharge if diagnosis is clear and visual loss is minimal or has resolved
- Retinal detachment is often successfully repaired
- CRAO is a true emergency with a poor prognosis; irreversible damage begins to occur within 60 minutes
- Temporal arteritis has good prognosis if steroid therapy begins before vision loss occurs
- Optic neuritis improves within 6 weeks in 95% of cases

133. Eye Infections

Etiology & Pathophysiology

- Conjunctivitis is the most common eye infection
  - Viral: The most common cause of red eye (especially adenovirus); easily transmissible and may become epidemic
  - Bacterial: Staph, strep, H flu; pseudomonas in contact lens users
  - Gonorrhea: Very aggressive; may spread to deep structures
  - Neonatal: Herpes, gonorrhea, and chlamydia are common
- Bacterial keratitis/corneal ulcer: Rapidly progressive infection of the cornea, conjunctiva, and anterior chamber with corneal ulceration and uveitis; usually occurs following corneal abrasion
- Herpes infections: Usually due to reactivation of latent virus (HSV or zoster); may affect skin, conjunctiva, and cornea; vision-threatening
- Suspect fungal cause in immunosuppressed or persistent infections
- Endophthalmitis: Serious, vision-threatening fungal or bacterial infection of the intraocular cavity caused by trauma or surgery; associated with diabetes mellitus and immunosuppression

Differential Dx

- Traumatic eye injury (e.g., corneal abrasion)
- Conjunctivitis
- Bacterial keratitis/corneal ulcer
- Viral conjunctivitis
- HSV keratitis
- Allergic conjunctivitis
- Fungal conjunctivitis
- Acute anterior uveitis (iritis)
- Corneal abrasion
- Ultraviolet keratitis
- Blepharitis (eyelid inflammation)
- Orbital cellulitis
- Periorbital cellulitis

Presentation

- Conjunctivitis: Diffuse redness, edema, watery (viral) or purulent (bacterial) discharge, morning crusting; normal visual acuity
- Gonococcus: Extremely copious discharge, scleral hemorrhage
- Chlamydia: Mucous discharge; swollen bulbar conjunctiva follicles
- Herpes: Pain, blurry vision, tearing, decreased corneal sensation, photophobia, redness, vesicles on skin or nose (Hutchinson's sign)
- Bacterial keratitis: Pain, discharge, injection, pain with consensual or direct light reflex, photophobia
- Endophthalmitis: Pain, decreased vision, headache, redness

Diagnosis

- History and physical exam, including sexual history
- Visual acuity
- Tonometry exam to measure eye pressures
- Slit lamp exam with fluorescein stain may be diagnostic
  - No corneal dye uptake or anterior chamber reaction in simple conjunctivitis
  - Localized dye uptake in corneal abrasions
  - Punctate corneal dye uptake in keratitis
  - Dendritic-shaped uptake indicates HSV or zoster
  - May show anterior chamber reaction/inflammation in keratitis, corneal ulcer, gonorrhea, herpes
  - Corneal ulcer has a hazy or white appearance
- Culture and gram stain of exudate if suspect gonorrhea, bacterial keratitis, or corneal ulcer; in neonates; and in non-resolving infections (also consider fungal cultures)

Treatment

- Conjunctivitis: Supportive therapy with cool compresses and ocular decongestant drops (e.g., Naphcon-A)
  - Viral: No treatment is required; empiric topical antibiotics are often used but there is no evidence of benefit
  - Bacterial: Topical antibiotics for 5 days; antipseudomonal antibiotic drops (e.g., aminoglycoside, quinolone) for contact lens users
  - Gonorrhea: Systemic antibiotics (e.g., ceftriaxione and doxycycline in adults, penicillin in neonates)
  - Chlamydia: Systemic antibiotics (e.g., azithromycin or doxycycline in adults, erythromycin in neonates)
  - Neonates: Treat for chlamydia and gonorrhea (e.g., topical erythromycin and IV ceftriaxone)
- Herpes virus: Topical or systemic antivirals for HSV; systemic antivirals for zoster; avoid steroids due to risk of corneal perforation
- Bacterial keratitis/corneal ulcer: Alternate topical quinolone and aminoglycoside drops every 15 minutes
- Endophthalmitis: Systemic and/or intraorbital antibiotics

Disposition

- Conjunctivitis can be very contagious for up to 7 days; use gloves when examining the patient
- Emergent ophthalmology consult and likely admission for bacterial keratitis, suspected gonorrhea, corneal ulcer, herpes infections, and endophthalmitis
- Discharge patients with uncomplicated conjunctivitis
- Contact lens users must not wear lenses until symptoms resolve
- Never place a patch in contact lens users due to risk of pseudomonas infection and perforation
- Complications of eye infections may include vision loss, glaucoma, or corneal scarring

134. Glaucoma

Etiology & Pathophysiology

- Due to elevated intraocular pressure (IOP)—either acute or chronic—that results in corneal edema, optic nerve damage, and blindness if not corrected
- Aqueous humor (AH) is normally produced by the ciliary body in the posterior chamber, circulates to the anterior chamber, and is reabsorbed by the trabecular meshwork
- Open angle glaucoma is a chronic disease of inadequate trabecular reabsorption of aqueous humor—may be asymptomatic until significant optic nerve damage has occurred
- Closed angle glaucoma is caused by a narrowed anterior chamber that prevents aqueous humor from reaching the trabecular meshwork
  - Acute angle closure glaucoma is a medical emergency with a rapid increase in IOP and severe symptoms; precipitated by pupillary dilatation (e.g., dim light, stress, fatigue); some medical illness and medications increase the risk of disease (secondary glaucoma)

Differential Dx

- Red eye (e.g., infection, uveitis, allergy, abrasion, trauma)
- Headache (e.g., migraine, cluster, tension, temporal arteritis)
- GI causes of nausea/vomiting
- Vision loss (e.g., vascular occlusion, retinal injury)
- Secondary glaucoma: Diabetes, endocrine disease, trauma, or drugs (e.g., steroids, atropine, antidepressants, anxiolytics, sympathomimetics, antihistamines, mydriatics)

Presentation

- Open angle glaucoma is asymptomatic except for gradual vision loss
- Acute angle closure glaucoma
  - Severe eye pain
  - Eye redness
  - Headache
  - Blurry vision
  - Halos around lights
  - Nausea/vomiting, abdominal pain
  - Ocular exam: Globe is firm to palpation, cloudy cornea, minimally reactive pupil
- Chronic angle closure may present only with vague eye pain

Diagnosis

- Check visual acuity and visual field exam
- Tonometry measures intraocular pressure (normal 10–21 mmHg)
  - Acute angle closure presents with elevated pressures
  - Chronic glaucoma may be present even if pressure is normal
  - Asymptomatic, chronically elevated pressure does not necessarily indicate glaucoma (i.e., glaucoma cannot be diagnosed unless optic nerve damage is present)
- Pupils are fixed and mildly dilated in acute angle closure glaucoma but are normally reactive in chronic angle closure
- Cornea has a cloudy appearance in acute angle closure glaucoma
- Flashlight test is positive in angle closure glaucoma
  - Hold light at the temporal limbus and shine medially
  - If the nasal half of the iris is shadowed, the angle is narrowed and glaucoma is likely (80% sensitive)
- Fundoscopy will show cupping of the optic nerve or optic disc in open angle glaucoma

Treatment

- Treatment is aimed at decreasing aqueous humor production and increasing outflow
- Topical β-blockers (e.g., timolol, betoxolol) decrease AH production and increase outflow; systemic side effects may occur due to nasolacrimal absorption (e.g., bradycardia, bronchospasm)
- Topical α-agonists (e.g., apraclonidine, brimonidine) decrease AH production; side effects may include dry mucous membranes and mild hypotension
- Carbonic anhydrase inhibitors (topical, oral, or IV) also decrease AH production
- IV mannitol increases serum osmolality, which shifts fluid out of the eye to decrease IOP
- Topical pilocarpine is a cholinergic agonist that improves AH outflow by constricting the pupil and ciliary body; however, it is ineffective if IOP is greater than 40 mmHg
- Topical prostaglandin analogues (e.g., latanoprost) also increase AH outflow
- Marijuana has been shown to decrease IOP; however, side effects and legal issues limit its use

Disposition

- All patients with acute angle closure glaucoma require emergent ophthalmology consultation and admission
- Patients with chronic glaucoma may be discharged with ophthalmology follow-up
- Risk factors for open angle glaucoma include advanced age, African-American, family history, diabetes mellitus, severe myopia, and steroid use
- Risk factors for closed angle glaucoma include Asian descent, family history, hyperopia, past uveitis, medications
- Frequently re-check IOP
- Elderly patients may present atypically (e.g., they may complain only of abdominal pain)

135. Trauma to the Anterior Eye

Etiology & Pathophysiology

- The anterior segment of the eye includes the cornea, anterior sclera, conjunctiva, iris, lens, and the anterior chamber
- Corneal epithelial injury ("corneal abrasion"): Superficial injury caused by minor trauma (e.g., scratch), foreign body, contact lens use, or UV light
- UV keratitis: Radiation burn due to tanning booths, welding, altitude
- Posttraumatic corneal ulcer: Due to bacterial or fungal infection
- Corneal or scleral laceration/rupture: Deep injuries that can extend into the anterior chamber or globe
- Traumatic iritis: Inflammation of the iris due to blunt trauma
- Iris/ciliary body injury: Blunt trauma can cause transient miosis or mydriasis, or may cause iridodialysis (avulsion of the iris)
- Hyphema: Blood in the anterior chamber, usually originating from the iris or ciliary body; causes include trauma, coagulopathy, and leukemia

Differential Dx

- Posterior segment injury
- Corneal injury (abrasion, laceration, foreign body, posttraumatic ulcer)
- Ultraviolet keratitis
- Conjunctival laceration
- Cornea/sclera perforation
- Hyphema
- Iris/ciliary body injury
- Traumatic iritis (iridocyclitis)
- Iridodialysis
- Posttraumatic glaucoma
- Lens subluxation/dislocation
- Chemical injury (acid, alkali, airbag, skin glue)

Presentation

- General symptoms include pain, redness, sensation of foreign body, photophobia, tearing, conjunctival injection, blepharospasm
- Corneal perforation: Teardrop pupil (due to prolapsed iris), hyphema
- Corneal ulcer: Cloudy white/gray
- Iridodialysis: Double pupil
- Lens dislocation: Monocular diplopia, quivering/displaced lens
- Iritis: Perilimbal injection, pain upon accommodation or consensual light reflex
- Scleral laceration: Bloody chemosis (conjunctival hemorrhage/swelling)
- Hyphema: Anterior chamber RBCs

Diagnosis

- Ocular exam with topical anesthetic (note: prolonged anesthetic use may cause delayed healing, further damage due to lack of corneal sensation, or toxic chemical keratitis)
- Tonometry to measure intraocular pressure and rule out posttraumatic glaucoma (contraindicated if suspect scleral /corneal laceration or globe penetration)
- Evert lid to identify foreign bodies
- Slit lamp exam will show foreign bodies and lacerations, and allow examination of anterior chamber for cell and flare (inflammation, iritis, infection, hyphema) and RBCs (hyphema)
- Fluorescein stain
  - Corneal abrasions fluoresce
  - "Ice rink sign": Multiple linear abrasions suggest FB under lid
  - Seidel test: Streaming of fluorescein indicates aqueous humor leakage due to a full-thickness corneal or scleral injury
- Consider CT to rule out intraocular foreign body and to examine for posterior eye and orbital injuries

Treatment

- Corneal epithelial injury/UV keratitis
  - Provide analgesia with acetaminophen, topical NSAIDs (e.g., ketorolac), and short-acting cycloplegics
  - Topical antibiotics are frequently prescribed; however, there is no definitive evidence that they improve outcome
  - Contact lens wearers require anti-pseudomonal coverage (e.g., aminoglycoside or a quinolone)
  - Eye patch may be worn for comfort; no benefit in healing
- Chemical injury: Immediately irrigate until eye pH is normal then administer antibiotics, analgesics, and cycloplegics
- Foreign body: Remove with a stream of sterile saline, cotton tip applicator, eye spud, or 25-gauge needle; deep foreign bodies should be removed by ophthalmology
- Corneal ulcer: Frequent topical or systemic antibiotics
- Corneal/scleral laceration: Metal eye shield, tetanus shot, IV antibiotics, antiemetics, and analgesics; may require surgery
- Traumatic iritis: Cycloplegics; consider steroids
- Hyphema: Analgesics, antiemetics, eye shield, head elevation, and eye rest (no reading or TV)

Disposition

- Must rule out posterior segment and orbital injuries
- Admission and ophthalmology evaluation for serious injuries
  - Decreased visual acuity
  - Large amount of visual axis involved
  - Multiple foreign bodies
  - Hyphema
  - Posttraumatic corneal ulcer
  - Corneal or scleral laceration or perforation
  - Chemical injury
  - Any iris or ciliary body injury
  - Lens dislocation/subluxation
  - Posttraumatic glaucoma
- Reevaluate all eye injuries in 24 hours
- Return to ED immediately if decreased vision or increased pain

136. Trauma to the Posterior Eye and Globe

Etiology & Pathophysiology

- Posterior eye structures include the vitreous body, retina, choroids, posterior sclera, and optic nerve
- Any posterior eye injury may result in permanent loss of vision
- Vitreous cavity hemorrhage: Bleeding due to vitreous body detachment or injury to the iris, ciliary body, retina, or choroid
- Retinal injury: Includes breakage and detachment of the retina
- Intraocular foreign body: Suspect in any injury with a high velocity projectile (e.g., grinding, sanding); may be painless
- Open globe injury: Full thickness injury caused by blunt trauma (resulting in a rapid increase in IOP) or penetrating trauma
- Retrobulbar hemorrhage (orbital compartment syndrome): Bleeding behind the globe resulting in increased intraorbital pressure
- Posttraumatic endophthalmitis: Infection of posterior eye structures
- Eyelid trauma: Suspect globe injury in full thickness injury, puncture wounds, or if prolapsed fat is present

Differential Dx

- Anterior eye segment injury
- Optic nerve injury
- Globe luxation (globe lies external to orbit)
- Orbital fracture
- Adnexal injury
- Eyelid laceration
- Shaken baby syndrome (retinal hemorrhages)

Presentation

- Vitreous hemorrhage: Hazy or decreased vision, floaters/cobwebs, afferent papillary defect; blood in the posterior chamber
- Retinal injury: Painless, floaters or flashes of light, curtain/shadow over visual field
- Foreign body: Symptoms of open globe injury may be present
- Globe injury/rupture: Pain, redness, swelling, enophthalmos, normal or decreased vision, subconjunctival hemorrhage, hyphema, irregular pupil, shallow anterior chamber
- Retrobulbar hemorrhage: Proptosis, pain, elevated IOP, decreased extraocular movement, vision loss

Diagnosis

- Fundoscopic exam: Examine for blood; retinal injury may result in a boat- or flame-shaped hemorrhage or a hazy gray retina
- Extraocular movement abnormalities suggest intraorbital injury
- Tonometry is contraindicated if open globe injury, globe rupture, or intraocular foreign body is suspected
- Seidel's test for open globe injury or intraocular foreign body is positive if a fluorescein-stained stream of aqueous humor is present
- Orbital CT is diagnostic for most posterior eye injuries (e.g., vitreous hemorrhage, retinal injury, intraocular foreign bodies, orbital fracture, and retrobulbar hemorrhage)
- MRI may be more effective to visualize intraocular foreign bodies but is contraindicated if metal foreign body is suspected
- Facial plain films or CT are helpful in suspected orbital fractures

Treatment

- Vitreous hemorrhage: Bed rest with head elevated and analgesia; avoid NSAIDs and ASA due to platelet inhibition
- Retinal injury: Treatment by ophthalmology with laser or scleral buckling; treat within 24 hours if possible
- Intraocular foreign body: Eye shield, antiemetics, broad-spectrum systemic antibiotics, and possible surgical removal
- Open globe injury: Prevent episodes of elevated intraocular pressure, which may cause further extrusion of contents; eye shield, pain control, antiemetics, sedation, IV antibiotics, surgical repair
- Retrobulbar hemorrhage: Emergent therapy with topical β-blockers and carbonic anhydrase inhibitors to decrease IOP; emergent decompression may be required
- Eyelid injury/laceration
  - Partial thickness injury may be repaired in ED
  - Ophthalmology must repair full thickness lacerations; injuries with involvement of the lid margin, lacrimal duct, or levator apparatus; and injuries with orbital penetration
- Posttraumatic endophthalmitis: Broad-spectrum systemic, topical and intraocular antibiotics

Disposition

- Maintain a high degree of suspicion for posterior injury in eye trauma and consult ophthalmology in unclear cases
- Emergent ophthalmology consult for all posterior eye pathology
- Most patients require admission for further therapy, surgical intervention, and/or systemic antibiotics
- Prognosis depends on presenting visual acuity, mechanism and extent of injury, presence of retained foreign body, and presence of lens defect

ENT
Emergencies

SERVE WAHAN, MD, DMD
JEFFREY M. CATERINO, MD

137. Ear Pain

Etiology & Pathophysiology

- Otitis media: Infection of the middle ear, commonly due to *Streptococcus pneumoniae, H. influenzae,* or *Moraxella catarrhalis;* most often in infants and children
- Acute otitis externa (swimmer's ear): Infection of the external auditory canal, usually by *Pseudomonas aeruginosa* or *S. aureus*
- Malignant otitis externa: Infection of the external canal by *Pseudomonas,* which spreads to the structures of the ear, skull, parotid gland, cranial nerves, carotid vessels, meninges, and/or TMJ; most common in elderly, diabetics, or immunosuppressed patients
- Bullous myringitis: Infection and formation of bullae in the auditory canal and tympanic membrane (TM)
- Traumatic hematoma of the external ear cartilage may cause deformity or necrosis if not properly treated
- TM perforation may occur due to trauma, pressure, or loud noises

Differential Dx

- Otitis media
- Acute otitis externa
- Malignant otitis externa
- Bullous myringitis
- Tympanic membrane perforation
- Barotrauma
- Cerumen impaction
- Foreign body
- Frostbite

Presentation

- Otitis media: Ear pain; red, bulging, or retracted TM with or without fluid buildup; poor movement of TM on pneumatic otoscopy; may have fever or hearing loss
- Otitis externa: Pain, erythema, tenderness, crusting, and drainage of the external canal; hearing loss
- Malignant otitis externa: Otitis externa symptoms plus trismus, parotitis, cranial nerve findings, meningitis, or neck pain
- Bullous myringitis: Visible bullae, severe pain, and hearing loss
- Hematoma: Pain and swelling
- TM perforation: Pain and possible discharge

Diagnosis

- Diagnosis by visual inspection and palpation of the ear structures
- The entire tympanic membrane must be visualized for the exam to be adequate
- Malignant otitis externa requires head CT to define the degree of tissue invasion
- ESR will be markedly elevated in malignant otitis externa

Treatment

- Otitis media requires oral antibiotics for 10–14 days
  - Children: High-dose amoxicillin, amoxicillin/clavulanic acid, cefprozil, cefuroxime, cefpodoxime, a macrolide, TMP-SMX, or single dose IM ceftriaxone
  - Adults: Amoxicillin, amoxicillin/clavulanic acid, cefuroxime, or a quinolone
- Otitis externa requires pain control, cleaning with hydrogen peroxide, and topical antimicrobials for 10 days
  - Consider ear wick if a large amount of edema is present
  - If perforation occurs, apply Cortisporin otic suspension (solution is middle ear toxic) or Floxin otic
- Malignant otitis externa requires double-coverage of *Pseudomonas* with IV antibiotics: Antipseudomonal penicillin/penicillinase inhibitor, aminoglycoside, cefipime or ceftazadine, and/or a quinolone
- Bullous myringitis is treated with azithromycin, analgesics, anti-inflammatory medications, and warm compresses
- Drain traumatic hematomas and apply a pressure dressing
- TM perforation requires only topical antibiotics if contamination is suspected

Disposition

- Discharge patients with acute otitis externa or otitis media
- Malignant otitis externa is a life-threatening emergency that requires urgent ENT consultation and admission for IV antibiotics
- Hematoma requires follow-up in 24–48 hours
- Uncomplicated TM perforation does not result in hearing loss; presence of hearing loss should prompt a search for more serious etiologies
- Majority of TM perforations will heal; may be discharged with ENT follow-up
- Complications of otitis media include mastoiditis, dural abscess, meningitis, lateral sinus thrombosis, and cholesteatoma

138. Epistaxis

Etiology & Pathophysiology

- Differentiate anterior nasal bleeding from posterior nasal bleeding
- Anterior epistaxis (90% of nosebleeds) is generally a benign process that quickly resolves with ED therapy
  - Most commonly originates in Kiesselbach's plexus of vessels in the anterior nasal septum
- Posterior epistaxis is a much more serious bleed that originates in the large posterior nasal vessels and is more difficult to control—may result in significant blood loss, hypotension, or airway compromise
- Cases of epistaxis occur more frequently during the dry winter months, in dry heat, or with abrupt temperature changes

Differential Dx

- Dry nasal mucosa
- Trauma
- Infection
- Allergic rhinitis
- Hypertension
- Anticoagulant therapy or other coagulopathy
- Cocaine use
- Hereditary telangiectasia
- Juvenile nasopharyngeal angiofibroma
- Foreign body
- Tumor

Presentation

- Anterior epistaxis
  - Unilateral bleeding
  - Minimal or no blood in the posterior pharynx
  - Dried clots
  - Visible bleeding site
- Posterior epistaxis
  - Bilateral bleeding
  - Blood or clots in the oropharynx
  - No visible anterior lesions
  - Fails to resolve with anterior packing

Diagnosis

- Visualize interior of the nose with a head lamp and nasal forceps
- CBC and PT/PTT may be ordered in cases of anterior epistaxis if a coagulopathy is suspected
- CBC, blood type and screen, and PT/PTT in significant cases of posterior epistaxis
- Consider CT of the head and facial bones if epistaxis is the result of trauma

Treatment

- Anterior epistaxis
  - Maintain direct pressure for a minimum of 10 minutes
  - Intranasal vasoconstrictors (e.g., phenylephrine)
  - Anesthetize the mucosa with liquid or viscous lidocaine
  - Silver nitrate cautery may be attempted if the site of bleeding is identified—avoid cauterizing large areas as it may result in future bleeding or septal perforation
  - Nasal packing should be attempted if cautery fails—a nasal sponge is coated with antibiotic ointment, inserted into the nose, and expands as blood is absorbed
  - Antibiotics covering *Staphylococcus* should be given after packing to prevent toxic shock syndrome
  - Consult ENT if packing fails to control hemorrhage
  - Consider antihypertensives in patients with severe HTN
- Posterior epistaxis
  - Vasoconstrictors and anesthetics may be attempted
  - Nasal packing with balloon tamponade is usually required
  - Intubation may be necessary in severe cases
  - Definitive care may require embolization or ligation

Disposition

- Discharge patients with controlled anterior epistaxis with PCP or ENT follow-up in 2–3 days
- Patients with anterior packing must follow up with ENT in 2–3 days for removal
- ENT consult and admission for all patients with posterior epistaxis or poorly controlled anterior epistaxis
- Encourage discharged patients to frequently use normal saline nose drops and avoid aspirin and NSAIDs, nose blowing, bending over, and straining
- Complications of posterior packing include sinusitis, otitis media, airway obstruction, cardiac arrhythmia or arrest, necrosis of the nasal mucosa, and hypoxia

139. Neck Emergencies

Etiology & Pathophysiology

- Pharyngitis: Superficial infection of the pharynx and tonsils, usually of viral etiology (80%); the most common bacterial cause is group A β-hemolytic *Streptococcus;* may progress to deep tissue infection
- Peritonsillar abscess: Spreading of bacterial tonsillitis to deeper tissue with abscess formation; rare in patients <12 years old
- Retropharyngeal abscess: Deep space infection of the retropharyngeal space due to extension of nearby infection (e.g., local neck/pharynx infection, croup, otitis media, dental infection) or trauma from a foreign body or medical procedure (e.g., endoscopy); almost all cases occur in children <6 years old
- Submandibular abscess (Ludwig's angina): Deep space infection of the submandibular spaces, often secondary to dental disease
- Epiglottitis: Bacterial infection of the epiglottis
- Most common causes of deep space infections are *Streptococcus, Staphylococcus, H. influenzae,* and anaerobes (often polymicrobial)

Differential Dx

- Pharyngitis
- Tonsillitis
- Peritonsillar abscess
- Epiglottitis
- Diphtheria
- Viral croup
- Retropharyngeal abscess
- Infectious mononucleosis
- Allergic reaction
- Foreign body
- Mumps
- Botulism
- Tetanus
- Tumor

Presentation

- Sore throat, dysphagia, fever
- Pharyngitis: Erythema, adenopathy; may have purulent discharge
- Peritonsillar abscess: Hoarseness, toxic appearance, trismus, muffled "hot potato" voice
- Retropharyngeal abscess: Toxic appearance, preceding infection or trauma with gradual symptom onset, no trismus, decreased neck movement; may have torticollis
- Submandibular abscess: Toxic appearance, jaw and neck pain/swelling, drooling and/or voice change
- Epiglottitis: Copious secretions and drooling (worse when supine)

Diagnosis

- Rapid strep testing or cultures may be indicated if streptococcal pharyngitis is suspected (see associated entry)
- Physical exam may suggest the diagnosis
  - Peritonsillar abscess: Swollen fluctuant tonsillar mass, uvula deviates away from the abscess, palatal erythema/edema
  - Retropharyngeal abscess: Retropharyngeal bulging/fluctuance
  - Submandibular abscess: Local induration and tenderness, elevated tongue, dental caries
  - Epiglottitis: Pain with palpation/movement of larynx/trachea
- Neck CT is the imaging study of choice to identify neck infections and involvement of other structures
- Lateral X-rays of the neck are inferior to CT but may be used in patients with an unstable airway who are unable to undergo CT
  - Submandibular abscess: Edema of submandibular soft tissue
  - Retropharyngeal abscess: Prevertebral soft tissue widening or retropharyngeal air
  - Epiglottitis: Thumb-shaped epiglottis, soft tissue swelling

Treatment

- Deep space infections (i.e., peritonsillar, retropharyngeal, or submandibular abscess) and epiglottitis can rapidly cause airway occlusion—emergent intubation may be required (surgical airway if necessary)
- Pharyngitis: Treat with penicillin or amoxicillin and consider steroids to decrease swelling
- Peritonsillar abscess: Needle aspiration and drainage plus oral antibiotics (penicillin/anti-penicillinase or clindamycin)
- Submandibular and retropharyngeal abscesses: IV antibiotics (penicillin plus metronidazole, penicillin/anti-penicillinase, clindamycin, or cefoxitin); surgical drainage may be required in refractory cases
- Epiglottitis: All children require immediate ENT consultation for intubation in the operating room; stable adults may be observed in the ICU; administer IV antibiotics (cefotaxime, ceftriaxone, or ampicillin-sulbactam) and steroids (to decrease airway edema)

Disposition

- Discharge patients with simple pharyngitis
- Consult ENT for all neck abscesses
- Admit patients with peritonsillar abscess if there is any concern of airway compromise, if they appear toxic, and young patients
- ICU admission for all patients with epiglottitis and retropharyngeal or submandibular abscesses
- Peritonsillar abscess may extend to deeper neck tissues, mediastinum, or carotid vessels
- Submandibular and retropharyngeal abscesses may result in airway obstruction, aspiration, or extension of abscess into airway, carotid blood vessels, spinal canal, mediastinum, or pericardium

140. Dental Emergencies

Etiology & Pathophysiology

- Dental caries: Bacteria penetrate through the enamel to the dentin and pulp
- Periradicular periodontitis/periapical abscess: Severe tooth pain due to pulp and root inflammation (very common ED presentation)
- Post-extraction alveolar osteitis ("dry socket" syndrome): Exposure and inflammation of the alveolar bone, occurring 2–3 days after tooth extraction
- Dental fractures: Classified as Ellis I (enamel only), Ellis II (enamel and dentin), or Ellis III (enamel, dentin, and pulp)
- Injuries to tooth supporting structures are classified as concussion (pain without mobility of the tooth), subluxation (pain and mobility of the tooth), and luxation (partial avulsion of the tooth from the alveolar bone; may be associated with alveolar fracture)
- Avulsion: Total removal of the tooth from the alveolus (tooth socket)—reimplantation is most successful if done within 1 hour

Differential Dx

- Myocardial infarction
- Tooth eruption (secondary teeth, "wisdom" teeth)
- Gingivitis/periodontitis
- Periodontal abscess
- Facial cellulitis
- Orbital cellulitis
- Submandibular abscess
- Acute necrotizing ulcerative gingivitis ("trench mouth")
- Trigeminal neuralgia
- Oral candidiasis

Presentation

- Dental caries: Tooth pain, pain with percussion, temperature sensitivity
- Periradicular periodontitis: Constant severe pain, caries, and tenderness to percussion; may have a fluctuant abscess
- Post-extraction osteitis: Severe pain following tooth extraction
- Ellis I fracture: Chipped enamel
- Ellis II: Chipped tooth with visible dentin (creamy yellow color), temperature sensitivity
- Ellis III: Chipped tooth, visible pulp (pink), bleeding from pulp
- Luxation: Abnormal tooth position
- Avulsion: Absence of tooth

Diagnosis

- Teeth are systematically numbered 1–32—percuss each tooth to identify which tooth is associated with pain
- Minimal diagnostic studies are necessary
- Obtain a chest X-ray of patients with avulsion to rule out aspiration of tooth (if tooth is not in their possession)
- Jaw X-rays to look for retained root fragment in cases of dry socket syndrome
- Panoramic X-ray (Panorex) may show bony erosion around affected teeth or a fracture of alveolar bone

Treatment

- Pain relief with ice, NSAIDs or narcotics, and/or dental nerve block is generally the most useful ED treatment
- Dental caries/periapical disease: Provide adequate pain relief, incise and drain abscesses, and treat infection with penicillin VK or clindamycin (pain and inflammation will decrease after 24–48 hours)
- Post-extraction osteitis: Irrigate with saline and pack with eugenol (oil of cloves) gauze to decrease pain
- Ellis I: No ED treatment, except filing down of sharp edges
- Ellis II: Cover dentin with dental cement to protect the pulp and provide pain relief
- Ellis III: A dental emergency requiring emergent dental consult; eugenol (oil of cloves) and dressing for pain relief
- Concussion/subluxation: Pain control only
- Luxation: Replace tooth in original position and splint to the neighboring teeth; dental consult is often necessary
- Avulsion: Rinse tooth and replace in socket ASAP (do not re-implant primary teeth); stabilize by splinting to adjacent teeth—transport avulsed tooth in saliva, Hank's solution, saline, or milk to preserve tooth until re-implantation

Disposition

- All dental cases should have dental follow-up with an appropriate specialist
- Conditions that require dental visit within 24 hours include painful lesions, luxations, and avulsions
- Emergent ED dental consults are indicated for Ellis III fractures, some Ellis II fractures, luxations (especially if alveolar bone fracture is present), and avulsions
- Complications of caries and periapical periodontitis include facial or orbital cellulitis and submandibular abscess
- Complications of traumatic dental injury include pulpal necrosis and tooth or root resorption

Toxicology

CHRISTOPHER R. CARPENTER, MD

141. General Approach to the Poisoned Patient

Etiology & Pathophysiology

- 3 million poisonings annually in the US, which account for nearly 10% of all ED visits; however, only 20% of poison exposures present to a health care facility for treatment
- 85% of poison exposures are unintentional; 90% occur at home; 40% occur in children under 3 years old
- A single substance is implicated in nearly 90% of poison exposures
- Drug overdose is the second leading cause of cardiac arrest in patients under 40
- Recognition of toxidromes (easily identifiable clusters of clinical signs and symptoms) facilitates the diagnosis and guides therapy—refer to the presentation section for common toxidromes
- Toxidromes and some associated agents include cholinergic (e.g., insecticides), anticholinergic (e.g., atropine, scopolamine), opioid (e.g., morphine, heroin), sympathomimetic (e.g., amphetamines, cocaine), serotonin syndrome (e.g., SSRIs, other antidepressants)

Differential Dx

- Accidental ingestion
- Acute delirium
- Adverse drug reaction
- Date rape
- Homicide attempt
- Hypoglycemia
- Hypothermia
- Hypoxia
- Intracranial hemorrhage
- Metabolic encephalopathy
- Sepsis
- Trauma

Presentation

- Cholinergic (*DUMBELS*): Diarrhea/diaphoresis, urination, miosis/muscle fasciculations, bradycardia/bronchospasm, emesis, lacrimation, salivation/seizure
- Anticholinergic: Dry skin, urinary retention, decreased bowel sounds, delirium, tachycardia, dilated pupils, seizures, dysrhythmias
- Sympathomimetics: Tachycardia, hypertension, dilated pupils, delusions, psychosis, seizures, dysrhythmia; difficult to differentiate from anticholinergics
- Opioids: Respiratory depression, coma, constricted pupils

Diagnosis

- Obtain history from paramedics, family, friends, pharmacist, and/or primary care physician, if possible
- Obtain all medication bottles from scene and clothing
- Measure vital signs, note respirations, and evaluate for trauma
- Note any unusual odors, which may give clues to the exposure
- Do not rely on the drug screen—labs do not routinely test for many substances, the initial drug level may be below the detection threshold, and the identified drugs may not be responsible for the clinical findings
- Initial workup includes pulse oximetry, glucose, electrolytes, urinalysis, urine pregnancy test, and acetaminophen, salicylate, and blood alcohol levels
- Quantitative blood levels for those drugs whose treatment is based on the level
- Consider head CT, CXR, and ECG
- Consider empiric treatment in lieu of definitive diagnosis in known or strongly suspected overdoses

Treatment

- Airway/breathing: Intubate as needed
- Circulatory support as necessary
  - If hypotensive with sinus tachycardia, treat with IV fluids
  - If hypotensive with wide-complex tachycardia, treat with bicarbonate (suspect Na^+ channel blocker overdose, e.g., TCA)
  - If hypotensive with bradycardia, treat with IV fluids, atropine, glucagon, and catecholamines
- Consider dextrose, oxygen, thiamine, naloxone, flumazenil
- Consider empiric treatment in known or suspected overdoses
  - In general, ipecac and other forms of induced emesis and gastric lavage are *not* indicated in the ED
  - Activated charcoal is the treatment of choice for most toxic ingestions; utility is limited with hydrocarbons and metals; it is recommended that activated charcoal not be given in non-toxic or minimally toxic exposures
  - Hemodialysis may be indicated for lithium, methanol, ethylene glycol, or aspirin
  - Treat seizures with benzodiazepines or barbiturates

Disposition

- Treat the patient not the poison!
- 60% of poison exposures are treated and released
- 10% are admitted to an ICU
- If patient is stable in the ED, determine if a non-toxic exposure has occurred—
  - Toxin definitely identified
  - Exposure unintentional
  - Patient asymptomatic during period of observation corresponding to the expected period of toxin peak effect
- Non-toxic exposures may often be discharged
- Otherwise, admit to hospital as appropriate for expected toxic side effects
- Psychiatry consultation for suicide attempts

142. Pediatric Toxic Ingestions

Etiology & Pathophysiology

- 4 million pediatric poisonings occur annually (75% are unreported)
- 50% of all exposures reported to poison centers in the US are children <6 years old (96% are essentially asymptomatic; 0.002% prove fatal)
- Most commonly ingested toxins correlate with household availability (cosmetics > cleaning products > analgesics > plants > non-prescription medications)
- The most lethal exposures are cocaine, anticonvulsants, antidepressants, and iron supplements
- Typical household products contain many toxic compounds
  - Ethanol (e.g., mouthwash, perfumes, cold medicine)
  - Isopropanol (e.g., rubbing alcohol)
  - Ethylene glycol (e.g., antifreeze)
  - Methanol (e.g., windshield washer fluid)
  - Methacrylic acid, toluidine, and acetonitrile (e.g., nail products)

Differential Dx

- Child abuse
- Dehydration
- Hypoglycemia
- Encephalitis
- Meningitis
- Sepsis
- Foreign body aspiration
- Intracranial bleed/mass
- Metabolic encephalopathy
- New onset diabetes mellitus
- Occult trauma
- Seizure disorder
- Toxic shock syndrome
- Viral gastroenteritis

Presentation

- Physical exam should concentrate on identification of specific toxidromes (refer to "General Approach to the Poisoned Patient")
- General symptoms include nausea/vomiting, confusion, obtundation, ataxia, urinary retention, and seizures
- Other symptoms of caustic ingestions may include
  - Pain/odynophagia
  - Oral burns
  - Stridor, drooling
  - Hoarseness
  - Tachypnea
  - Evidence of mediastinitis or peritonitis

Diagnosis

- In most cases, the ingestion is known or suspected based on known household exposures (e.g., chemicals, medications) and diagnostic testing can be directed accordingly
- All children with altered level of consciousness should have serum glucose monitored for hypoglycemia
- Quantitative serum levels should be obtained as indicated for acetaminophen, carboxyhemoglobin, ethanol, ethylene glycol, iron, methanol, methemoglobin ingestions, salicylates, phenytoin, digoxin, phenobarbital, theophylline, and valproic acid ingestion
- Other diagnostic tests may include ECG, urine crystal analysis, and radiographs of the abdomen (to reveal heavy metals or iron)
- A number of ingestions are rapidly fatal to a 10 kg toddler even if given just one swallow (e.g., camphor, chloroquine, imipramine, quinine, theophylline, chlorpromazine, nifedipine) while many others may initially be asymptomatic, requiring prolonged observation

Treatment

- Airway, breathing, and circulation
- GI decontamination is not required for every toxic ingestion but should be administered on an individual basis based on the potential toxin(s) ingested
  - Activated charcoal is the only intervention generally required (administer via NG tube if >20 minutes since ingestion)
- Ipecac, gastric lavage, and cathartics do not improve outcomes compared with charcoal alone and are associated with many adverse side effects—they should not be used in pediatric ingestions
- Treat hypoglycemia as necessary
  - > age 2: 3 cc/kg of D_{50} plus $D_{10}W$ for 1 day
  - < age 2: 2.5 cc/kg D_{10} plus $D_{10}W$ for 1 day

Disposition

- Admit any child with abnormal ECG, altered consciousness, airway compromise, acid-base abnormality, or caustic injury to an ICU
- Admit hypoglycemic children for 24-hour dextrose infusion
- Children with caustic ingestions require immediate GI or surgical consultation with endoscopic evaluation within the first 4 hours
- Asymptomatic children with no evidence of oropharyngeal burns and who are playful and eating/drinking 6 hours after a suspected caustic ingestion probably have no significant caustic injury and can safely be discharged home from the ED
- Ensuring parent education and ability to contact poison control can prevent recurrence and adverse outcomes

143. Acetaminophen Overdose

Etiology & Pathophysiology

- Acetaminophen (APAP) overdoses result in more hospitalizations than any other overdose; causes 10% of ingestion fatalities
- Acute overdose (ingestion within a 4-hour period) and chronic usage are both toxic to the liver
- Hepatic metabolism of APAP results in production of N-acetyl-p-benzo-quinonimine, a potent oxidizing agent that damages hepatocytes
- Risk of hepatotoxicity and need for treatment is determined by a nomo-gram that is based on serum APAP levels at 4–24 hours and time since ingestion
- Chronic alcohol use increases the risk of liver toxicity (even at therapeutic doses of APAP); whereas acute alcohol intoxication is somewhat hepato-protective

Differential Dx

- Other toxic ingestions
- Peptic ulcer disease
- Viral hepatitis
- Alcoholic liver disease
- Wilson's disease
- Biliary colic
- Carbon tetrachloride
- Gastroenteritis
- Metabolic encephalopathy
- Mushrooms (Amanita)
- Other hepatotoxic drugs (e.g., methotrexate, amiodarone, methyldopa, statins)
- Reye's syndrome
- Sepsis

Presentation

- Pre-injury period (the initial 24 hours after ingestion) is generally asymptomatic; nausea, vomiting, or malaise may occur
- Initial liver injury (12–36 hours) results in RUQ and epigastric dis-comfort
- Maximum liver injury (2–4 days post-ingestion) may result in symp-toms of fulminant hepatic failure and renal failure
- Recovery period may take weeks to months

Diagnosis

- Measure APAP concentration
  - Toxicity in acute ingestions is predicted by APAP concentration at a given time post-ingestion, as determined by the Rumack-Matthew nomogram
  - Toxicity in chronic ingestion is predicted by both APAP concen-tration and LFT abnormalities
- AST/ALT, chemistry panel, and prothrombin time should be obtained in many cases of acute overdose and all cases of chronic ingestions
- Check aspirin level due to possible concurrent ingestion
- Consider a urine drug screen for other co-ingestants

Treatment

- Activated charcoal should be administrated immediately, unless contraindicated
- Oral N-acetylcysteine (NAC) is administered as a 140 mg/kg loading dose followed by seventeen additional doses of 70 mg/kg every four hours (initiate within 8 hours of overdose for optimal results)
  - IV NAC may be needed in cases of intractable vomiting not controlled with anti-emetics
- Supportive care of liver dysfunction with vitamin K and fresh frozen plasma as indicated

Disposition

- If APAP concentration in acute inges-tions is above the nomogram treatment line, a course of NAC should be admin-istered with inpatient observation and psychiatry evaluation as appropriate
- In chronic ingestions, no treatment is required if the APAP concentration and LFTs are within normal limits
- Poor prognostic signs include acidosis, coagulopathy, elevated creatinine, and encephalopathy
- Hepatic failure may cause death due to hemorrhage (lack of clotting factors), sepsis, cerebral edema, or multiorgan failure

144. Aspirin Overdose

Etiology & Pathophysiology

- Commonly ingested agent in suicide attempts among adolescents and adults
- Also seen as an accidental chronic overdose in the elderly secondary to treatment of chronic disease states
- Overdose initially produces respiratory alkalosis due to stimulation of CNS respiratory drive; however, prolonged elevation of serum aspirin level ultimately depresses the respiratory drive and causes metabolic acidosis (due to inhibition of the Kreb's cycle)
- Salicylate half-life can approach 30 hours in toxic ingestions
- Pediatric exposures may occur from salicylate-containing ointments and breast milk

Differential Dx

- ARDS
- Acute renal failure
- CHF
- CVA
- Dehydration
- Hyperthermia
- Meniere's disease
- Seizure disorder
- Subdural hematoma
- Viral syndrome
- Asthma
- Delirium

Presentation

- Nausea and vomiting are the most common symptoms
- Tinnitus and hearing loss (both are reversible) may occur
- Hyperventilation and hyperthermia may occur
- Irritability may progress to stupor and coma
- Chronic ingestions may present only with tinnitus and/or CNS effects (e.g., confusion, agitation, paranoia, impaired memory)
- Less common effects include non-oliguric renal failure, non-cardiogenic pulmonary edema, and cerebral edema

Diagnosis

- Ingestions >300 mg/kg are potentially toxic; >500 mg/kg are potentially lethal
- Measure serum salicylate concentration 6 hours after ingestion and re-check every 4 hours until levels begin to decline
- Evaluation following significant ingestions should include arterial blood gas, CBC, electrolytes, prothrombin time, and chest and abdominal films
  - Respiratory alkalosis initially occurs, progressing to combined respiratory alkalosis and anion-gap metabolic acidosis, and finally a combined respiratory and metabolic acidosis
  - May have hyper- or hypoglycemia
  - May have hypokalemia
  - Closely monitor arterial pH
- When assessing severity of exposure, do not rely solely on blood concentration; be sure to assess age, co-morbidities, dose ingested, type of pill ingested (e.g., sustained release), acid-base status, and clinical appearance

Treatment

- Administer activated charcoal if no contraindications are present
- Monitor fluid status carefully—administer IV fluids with added sodium bicarbonate and glucose to maintain urine pH >7.5 (caution: overhydration may predispose to pulmonary and cerebral edema)
  - Urinary alkalinization with IV sodium bicarbonate infusion enhances renal elimination of salicylates and potassium
- Replete potassium
- Consider hemodialysis if patient fails to respond to the above measures or if pulmonary edema, seizures, worsening acid-base disorders, renal or hepatic failure, or coma occurs
- In pregnant patients with salicylate intoxication, consider immediate delivery due to heightened fetal sensitivity to salicylates

Disposition

- Admit any patient with acid-base disorders or cases of infant salicylism
- ICU admission in patients with evidence of pulmonary or cerebral edema or a need for hemodialysis
- Admit to psychiatry or discharge home once salicylate concentration is <25 mg/dL and symptoms have resolved
- Mortality of chronic salicylate toxicity is 25% (versus just 1% for acute ingestions)

145. SSRI and MAOI Overdoses

Etiology & Pathophysiology

- Selective Serotonin Reuptake Inhibitors (SSRIs) are generally less toxic than cyclic antidepressants
- Serotonin is present in the CNS, where it regulates mood, circadian rhythms, and temperature, and in GI enterochromaffin cells
- SSRI overdose may cause direct symptoms or serotonin syndrome
- Serotonin syndrome (SS) results when a serotonergic agent is added to an established medication regimen or when an SSRI is increased
  - SS is an idiosyncratic reaction, usually not associated with ingestion of large amounts of drug, and associated with behavioral/cognitive, autonomic, and neuromuscular symptoms
  - A number of medications can precipitate SS, including codeine, cocaine, meperidine, MAOIs, TCAs, and newer antidepressants
- MAO inhibitors (MAOIs) prevent metabolism of biogenic amines
- MAOI toxicity results from overdose or new diet/drug interactions
  - Tyramine containing foods can precipitate symptoms

Differential Dx

- Sedative-hypnotic withdrawal
- Neuroleptic malignant syndrome
- Opioid withdrawal
- Salicylate overdose
- Seizure
- Sepsis
- Sympathomimetic overdose
- Thyrotoxicosis

Presentation

- Many SSRI overdoses are asymptomatic
- 20% of SSRI overdose patients will develop drowsiness or sinus tachycardia with tremors, hypertension, and GI upset
- Diagnosis of SS requires three of the following: Agitation, ataxia, diaphoresis, diarrhea, hyperreflexia, hyperthermia, mental status changes, myoclonus, shivering, or tremors
- Signs/symptoms of MAOI overdose usually occur within 12 hours, including HA, tachycardia, agitation, mydriasis, muscular rigidity, hyperthermia, or coma

Diagnosis

- SSRI overdose requires a complete history (including a thorough review of medications and recent dose changes or additions) and vigilant observation of subtle signs/symptoms
- Lab tests and drug levels do not assist in establishing the diagnosis
- Serotonin syndrome is a clinical diagnosis
- Workup might include salicylate and acetaminophen levels, CBC, urinalysis, thyroid studies, and CPK
- MAOI use is the most helpful clue to toxicity
- MAOI drug and enzyme levels are not clinically useful
- Foods that commonly precipitate the tyramine reaction include cheese, aged meats, fava beans, avocados, sauerkraut, chocolate, bananas, ginseng, and undistilled alcoholic beverages

Treatment

- ABCs and supportive care are most important for both SSRI and MAOI overdoses
- Activated charcoal is useful to decrease absorption of either substance
- SSRI overdose is treated with supportive care
- SSRI-induced ventricular dysrhythmias are treated with lidocaine
- SSRI-induced seizures are treated with benzodiazepines, phenobarbital, or propofol
- Serotonin syndrome: Discontinue causative medications and provide supportive care; cyproheptadine (an anti-serotonergic agent) may be effective in severe cases
- MAOI malignant hypertension is treated with nitroprusside or phentolamine

Disposition

- Patients with asymptomatic SSRI overdose may be discharged home after 6 hours of cardiac monitoring
- Admit all patients with serotonin syndrome or symptomatic SSRI ingestion
- All patients with MAOI overdose of >1 mg/kg, suspected serotonin syndrome, or MAOI interactions should be admitted for 24-hour cardiac monitoring
- MAOI overdose complications can include hypoxia, renal failure, rhabdomyolysis, hemolysis, metabolic acidosis, DIC, asystole, seizures, death

146. Tricyclic Antidepressant Overdose

Etiology & Pathophysiology

- Antidepressants cause 20% of poisoning deaths
- Toxicity may occur in certain susceptible patients even at therapeutic doses (e.g., in slow metabolizers or those with pre-existing illness)
- Tricyclics act as non-selective sodium channel and receptor blockers
  - Fast sodium channel blockade causes a prolonged QRS complex
  - α_1-receptor antagonism causes hypotension and mydriasis
  - Serotonin and norepinephrine reuptake inhibition causes sympatho-mimetic effects, such as agitation, confusion, seizure
  - Blockage of potassium efflux prolongs the QT interval
  - Antihistamine effect causes CNS sedation and may cause coma
  - Antimuscarinic effects include CNS depression, ileus, and dry skin
  - Anti-GABA effects disinhibit the CNS and cause seizures
- Drug kinetics are characterized by rapid absorption, large volumes of distribution, high protein binding, and hepatic metabolism

Differential Dx

- Anticholinergic overdose
- Antidysrhythmic (Type Ia, Ic)
- Hallucinogen abuse
- Intracranial hemorrhage
- Meningitis
- Metabolic encephalopathy
- Neuroleptic malignant syndrome
- Psychosis
- Seizure
- Sepsis
- Sympathomimetic abuse
- Thyroid storm

Presentation

- Consider overdose in patients with altered level of consciousness, tachycardia, prolonged QRS, or right deviation of the terminal QRS
- Do not be falsely reassured by an initial lack of symptoms—25% of patients are intact immediately prior to seizure and death
- Deterioration usually occurs within 60 minutes of ED presentation
- Signs/symptoms may include mental status changes (from confusion to coma), seizures, dry mucous membranes, tachycardia, hypotension, dysrhythmias, hyperthermia, ileus, myoclonus, and urinary retention

Diagnosis

- Clinical suspicion, history from EMS, family, or friends, or a suicide note are most useful in establishing the diagnosis
- Urine and serum drug levels are not clinically useful in the overdose setting
- Workup should include cardiac monitoring, pulse oximetry, ECG, and acetaminophen and salicylate levels
- Additional workup might include CBC, electrolytes, BUN, creatinine, cultures, cardiac enzymes, thyroid function tests, urine drug screen, head CT, and lumbar puncture as appropriate
- ECG often has a characteristic appearance
  - Sinus tachycardia
  - Prolonged PR, QRS, and QT intervals
  - An R wave in a VR >3 mm (signifying rightward deviation of the terminal 40 msec of the QRS axis)
  - Rhythm may degenerate into ventricular arrhythmias (especially if limb-lead QRS is >160 msec)
- Hypotension may occur with or without QRS widening

Treatment

- Remember that deterioration occurs rapidly and often with minimal initial symptoms
- Have a low threshold to intubate patients
- Activated charcoal $+/-$ gastric lavage to decrease absorption
- Hypotension is treated initially with isotonic saline; refractory hypotension should be treated with norepinephrine or dopamine
- IV sodium bicarbonate bolus for any QRS prolongation, refractory hypotension, seizures, or life-threatening dysrhythmias; continue administration until the problem resolves or serum pH is >7.55
- Prolonged seizures should be treated with benzodiazepines, phenobarbital, or propofol; phenytoin is ineffective
- Hyperthermia (rectal temperature >40°C) should be treated with evaporative cooling, nondepolarizing neuromuscular blockade, and mechanical ventilation
- Treat dysrhythmias with sodium bicarbonate and lidocaine (judiciously—may cause seizures); Class IA, IC, and III, β-blockers, and Ca-channel blockers are contraindicated
- Hemodialysis is not useful for removal of TCAs

Disposition

- Discharge after 6 hours of observation if workup is normal and there is no evidence of altered level of consciousness, respiratory depression, hypotension, hypoxemia, dysrhythmias, cardiac conduction blocks, seizures, or ileus
- All other patients should be admitted, preferably to an intensive care unit

147. Benzodiazepine and GHB Overdose

Etiology & Pathophysiology

- Benzodiazepines account for 2/3 of psychotropic medications prescribed worldwide and are the most frequently ingested prescription drugs in suicide attempts; however, they are far less fatal than other sedative-hypnotics (e.g., barbiturates, alcohol)
- Three unique benzodiazepine receptors have been identified in the central and peripheral nervous system; all increase the frequency of $GABA_A$ chloride-channel opening, thereby hyperpolarizing the cell membrane and inhibiting neural transmission
- γ-hydroxybutyrate (GHB) is a non-benzodiazepine sedative-hypnotic that is a metabolite of GABA; it binds weakly to $GABA_B$ receptors and GHB-specific receptors in the reticular activating system
- GHB is a popular euphoric drug of abuse and is commonly used as a date-rape drug (colorless, slightly salty, half-life of ~30 minutes)
- Benzodiazepines and GHB produce tolerance to their effects and life-threatening withdrawal symptoms may occur with abrupt cessation

Differential Dx

- Alcohol intoxication
- Barbiturate intoxication
- Opioid, alcohol, or barbiturate co-ingestion
- Anoxic encephalopathy
- Date rape
- Hypoglycemia
- Intracranial injury
- Meningitis
- Occult head injury
- Polypharmacy abuse
- Sepsis
- Suicide attempt

Presentation

- Slurred speech is the most common sign of benzodiazepine overdose
- CNS depression ranges from drowsiness to coma
- Decreased respiratory tidal volumes are common
- Respiratory rate depression may be seen with large overdoses or when combined with opioids
- Benzodiazepines may also cause nausea, vomiting, and headache
- The hallmark of GHB intoxication is rapid unconsciousness alternating with severe agitation
  - Emesis, bradycardia, and hypothermia may be present
  - Complete resolution within 8 hrs

Diagnosis

- Benzodiazepine overdose is diagnosed by history or response to flumazenil
- Most urine benzodiazepine drug screens recognize only the oxazepam glucuronide metabolite and will not identify many common agents (e.g., midazolam, lorazepam, alprazolam)
- Serum drug concentrations are not readily available in the ED nor do they correlate with clinical severity
- GHB should be suspected by exam significant for the characteristic stimulation-induced combativeness that returns to deep coma upon lack of stimulation
- GHB is not detected on routine urine toxicology screens and is rapidly metabolized

Treatment

- Most benzodiazepine overdoses require only supportive care
- Administer activated charcoal if the airway is secure
- Flumazenil is a nonspecific competitive antagonist of benzodiazepine receptors
  - Half-life (about 1 hour) is shorter than many benzodiazepines, so repeat doses may be necessary
  - Co-ingestions of substances that lower the seizure threshold (e.g., cyclic antidepressants) or prodysrhythmics (e.g., chloral hydrate), head injury, or use of a benzodiazepine to control seizures are all relative contraindications to the use of flumazenil
- Supportive treatment is sufficient for GHB toxicity
  - Naloxone and flumazenil have no effect
  - No role for gastric lavage, whole bowel irrigation, dialysis
  - Neostigmine and physostigmine have been shown to be effective, but are not generally required

Disposition

- Asymptomatic benzodiazepine ingestions may be discharged to psychiatry or home after 6 hours of observation
- GHB ingestions show no delayed toxicity; however, ensure that there are no co-ingestions prior to discharge
- Counsel patient on the dangers of continued GHB use and obtain substance abuse referral as indicated
- Legal authorities should be notified as appropriate for suspected cases of date rape

148. Barbiturate and Chloral Hydrate Overdose

Etiology & Pathophysiology

- Barbiturates and chloral hydrate (CH) enhance the CNS inhibitory effect of GABA at postsynaptic membranes, thereby inhibiting neurotransmission
- Barbiturates were once a popular, readily accessible suicide agent; however, with diminished clinical applications today, they are rarely encountered
- Barbiturates produce tolerance to their effects and can produce a life-threatening withdrawal syndrome similar to delirium tremens upon abrupt cessation
- Barbiturates depress respiratory drive at the brainstem and directly depress the myocardium
- CH is utilized as a sedative-hypnotic in the elderly and for pediatric procedural sedation
- CH increases myocardial sensitivity to catecholamines

Differential Dx

- Alcohol intoxication
- Benzodiazepine intoxication
- GHB intoxication
- CHF
- Environmental (e.g., hypothermia)
- Intracranial hemorrhage
- Occult trauma
- Polysubstance abuse
- Seizure disorder
- Sepsis
- Suicide attempt

Presentation

- Symptoms begin within 1 hour
- Presentation may be confused with alcohol or benzodiazepine intoxication in mild cases
- CNS depression ranges from mild sedation to coma/respiratory arrest
- Other symptoms include slurred speech, ataxia, and drowsiness
- Hypothermia, apnea, and hypotension with cardiovascular collapse may occur in severe cases
- CH may also result in hemorrhagic gastritis and dysrhythmias (Afib, SVT, VT, and torsades de pointes)

Diagnosis

- Serum barbiturate levels >80 μg/mL are potentially fatal; however, serum levels do not accurately reflect CNS concentrations or correlate with clinical severity
- Serum CH levels are unavailable; serum TCE levels may confirm ingestion, but are not readily available and do not guide management or predict outcomes
- Lab testing should include electrolytes, glucose, CBC, and blood cultures
- Additional workup for barbiturate intoxications may include head CT, ECG, and CXR

Treatment

- Airway, breathing, and circulatory support—intubation is often required due to apnea and impaired consciousness
- No specific antidote exists for either drug
- Administer multiple doses of activated charcoal
- Treat hypotension and cardiovascular collapse
  - Rapid infusion of crystalloid to support BP
  - Add inotropic agents and vasopressors (e.g., dopamine or norepinephrine) if fluids are insufficient to maintain BP
  - Be aware of possible pulmonary edema in cases of barbiturate intoxication—early pulmonary artery catheterization may guide fluid resuscitation
- Treat hypoglycemia
- In cases of phenobarbital overdose, alkalinize the urine via bicarbonate infusion to maintain urine pH 7.5–8
- β-blockers are generally used to counteract dysrhythmias

Disposition

- Patients should be observed for 6 hours in the ED for hypotension, respiratory depression, or altered mental status
- All symptomatic patients should be admitted
- Asymptomatic ingestions without other co-ingestions or co-morbid medical problems may be discharged to psychiatry after 6 hours

149. Antipsychotic Overdose

Etiology & Pathophysiology

- Antipsychotics block dopamine and serotonin receptors to alleviate psychotic (e.g., hallucinations in schizophrenic patients) or agitated states
- These are a diverse group of medications that have many applications outside of psychiatry, including antiemetics (e.g., chlorpromazine, prochlorperazine, droperidol) and antihistamines (e.g., hydroxyzine)
- Acute overdoses and chronic side effects may present in the ED
- Side effects are thought to occur either from antagonism/blockade or upregulation of dopamine receptors in the nigrostriatum (movement disorders) or hypothalamus (temperature dysregulation)
- Neuroleptic malignant syndrome is an idiosyncratic life-threatening side effect resulting in hyperthermia and muscular rigidity

Differential Dx

- Acute psychosis
- Anticholinergic syndrome
- Heat stroke
- Meningitis
- Occult head trauma
- Opioid overdose
- Seizure disorder
- Sepsis
- Serotonin syndrome
- Hypoglycemia

Presentation

- Acute overdoses result in sedation, coma, and tachycardia that may mimic opioid intoxication; extrapyramidal symptoms may be present
- Side effects of chronic use
  - Extrapyramidal symptoms, such as akathisia (muscle restlessness), bradykinesia, or dystonic reactions (muscle spasm of head and neck)
  - Tardive dyskinesia (quick, involuntary muscle movements of tongue and face)
  - Neuroleptic malignant syndrome (fever, muscular rigidity, autonomic instability, and altered mental status)

Diagnosis

- Drug levels are not indicated
- Cardiac monitoring for dysrhythmias and prolonged QT syndrome with torsades de pointes
- In patients with neuroleptic malignant syndrome, check electrolytes (metabolic acidosis, hyperkalemia), BUN/creatinine (renal failure), CPK, TSH, glucose, and CBC
- Patients with altered level of consciousness may require pulse oximetry, head CT, lumbar puncture, aspirin and acetaminophen levels, electrolytes, and/or ECG

Treatment

- No specific antidote exists
- Activated charcoal should be given within 2 hours of acute ingestion
- Treat extrapyramidal syndromes and dystonic reactions with anticholinergic medications (e.g., diphenhydramine, benztropine) for 48 hours
- Akathesia may respond to benzodiazepines
- Neuroleptic malignant syndrome requires emergent IV benzodiazepines, hydration, and active cooling
- Dantrolene may be used to facilitate muscle relaxation
- Treat torsades de pointes with IV $MgSO_4$, overdrive pacing, and/or isoproterenol
- Hypotension refractory to fluid administration should be treated with α-agonists
- Some atypical antipsychotic overdoses have responded well to physostigmine

Disposition

- All overdose patients should be observed on a monitor for a minimum of 4 hours post-ingestion
- ICU admission is warranted for severe symptoms, such as airway compromise, neuroleptic malignant syndrome, or coma
- Discharge is acceptable following appropriate psychiatric evaluation for patients with normal mental status, vital signs, and ECG after 4 hours of ED observation
- All other patients should be admitted to a monitored bed for observation
- *Atypical* antipsychotics are a new group of medications with similar effects but fewer side effects (tardive dyskinesia and extrapyramidal symptoms) than classic anti-psychotics

150. Opioid Overdose

Etiology & Pathophysiology

- Opioids include naturally occurring agents (opiates), endogenous peptides (endorphins), and their synthetic equivalents
- Opioid receptors are concentrated in the central and peripheral pain pathways; stimulation of the receptors inhibits adenylate cyclase, activates potassium channels, and/or inhibits calcium channels, thereby modifying CNS pain perception
- Heroin is the most commonly abused opioid—most deaths occur in chronic abusers 1–3 hours after use and involve polysubstance abuse
- 70% of heroin is absorbed into the brain, compared with just 5% of IV morphine; in the brain, heroin is metabolized to morphine

Differential Dx

- Hypoglycemia
- Hypoxemia
- Intracerebral hemorrhage, especially pontine hemorrhage
- Sedative-hypnotic use/abuse (e.g., benzodiazepines, GHB)
- Alcohol intoxication
- Hepatic encephalopathy
- Hypothermia
- Hyponatremia
- Occult head trauma
- Seizure disorder
- Meningitis, encephalitis, sepsis
- Serotonin syndrome
- Suicide attempt

Presentation

- CNS depression and respiratory depression are the classic presenting symptoms
- Miosis
- Bronchospasm and non-cardiogenic pulmonary edema are common in overdoses
- GI effects include nausea, vomiting, and biliary colic
- Other neurologic manifestations may include spongiform leukoencephalopathy and serotonin syndrome
- Seizures may occur if meperidine is used in patients with renal or hepatic insufficiency

Diagnosis

- The classic clinical toxidrome of respiratory depression, miosis, and CNS depression is highly sensitive and relatively specific for the diagnosis of opioid overdose
- Therapeutic response to naloxone is highly suggestive of opioid toxicity (failure to respond to 10 mg of naloxone should prompt evaluation for another cause of altered mental status); however, non-opioids (e.g., ethanol) may also be reversed by naloxone
- Opioids are detected by most urine toxicology screens with the exception of synthetic opioids (e.g., fentanyl, meperidine)
- Respiratory acidosis and hypoxemia on ABG are supportive of the diagnosis; other labs are not helpful
- Consider checking acetaminophen and salicylate levels due to common use of combination products
- Consider abdominal X-rays if packing or stuffing is suspected
- ECG should be evaluated for widened QRS, suggesting propoxyphene toxicity
- CXR may show pulmonary edema

Treatment

- Respiratory depression is the most common immediately life-threatening complication—immediate attention to airway protection and opioid antagonism is essential
    - Naloxone is the most widely used antidote for any intoxication; unfortunately, the duration of action is only 1–2 hours so most opioid overdoses should be observed beyond that period to ensure no further reversal is required
    - Nalmefene has a much longer half-life (8–11 hours) but has the theoretical disadvantage of causing prolonged withdrawal symptoms if administered to a chronic addict
- Activated charcoal may be administered, especially if a co-ingestant (e.g., aspirin, acetaminophen, alcohol) is suspected
- Correct metabolic abnormalities (e.g., hypoglycemia)
- Withdrawal symptoms can be treated with methadone, L-α-acetyl-methadol, or clonidine
- Propoxyphene cardiotoxicity can be treated with sodium bicarbonate

Disposition

- Asymptomatic, untreated patients should be observed 4–6 hours prior to discharge
- Patients treated prior to arrival or in ED should be observed 6–12 hours and discharged if asymptomatic
- Symptomatic patients should be admitted to an ICU
- Drug packers should have whole bowel irrigation and remain until passage of contents is confirmed by radiography
- Appropriate substance abuse counseling should be obtained and documented prior to discharge
- Due to delayed or prolonged toxicity, certain opioid ingestions require admission (e.g., lomotil, methadone, propoxyphene, fentanyl patch)

151. Digitalis Toxicity

Etiology & Pathophysiology

- Digoxin is one of the most commonly prescribed medications in the US, most often for rate control of atrial fibrillation and relief of symptomatic congestive heart failure
- Digitalis occurs naturally in plants, such as foxglove and oleander
- Digitalis is a positive inotrope that blocks the Na^+/K^+ pump and also slows conduction through the atrioventricular node
- At toxic levels, digitalis suppresses SA and AV nodal activity and sensitizes the myocardium to the effects of catecholamines, resulting in both bradydysrhythmias and tachydysrhythmias
- Digitalis toxicity is the most common cause of preventable, iatrogenic cardiac arrest
- Increased risk of toxicity occurs in patients with underlying heart disease, use of multiple cardiovascular medications, renal insufficiency, and electrolyte abnormalities

Differential Dx

- Acute psychosis
- β-blocker overdose
- Ca-channel blocker overdose
- Intrinsic sinus node disease
- CVA
- Depression
- Food poisoning
- Hypoglycemia
- Occult trauma
- Sedative overdose
- Seizure disorder
- Sepsis
- UTI
- Viral gastroenteritis

Presentation

- Most intoxications present with nonspecific complaints, such as headache, fatigue, and confusion
- Nausea/vomiting
- Altered mental status
- Blurred or discolored vision (e.g., yellow-green halos around objects)
- Bradycardia (commonly) or tachycardia (less commonly)

Diagnosis

- Diagnosis is primarily based on clinical suspicion and symptoms
- Digoxin levels are not the sole predictor of intoxication (i.e., patients may have digitalis toxicity despite normal serum levels)
  - Levels are often elevated in acute toxicity, but may be normal in patients who chronically take the medication
  - Levels above 2–6 ng/mL are potentially fatal; however, steady-state serum levels are not achieved until ~6 hours after intake
- Electrolyte abnormalities are common
  - Hyperkalemia is a common effect of acute digitalis toxicity, due to blockade of the Na^+/K^+ pump
  - Some abnormalities (e.g., hypokalemia, hypercalcemia, hypomagnesemia) may predispose the patient to digoxin toxicity by altering membrane potentials
- ECG abnormalities include PVCs (most common), heart block, bradydysrhythmias (sinus, junctional or ventricular rhythms), and ventricular fibrillation

Treatment

- Digoxin-specific Fab fragment antibody that binds digoxin, lowering effective circulating levels
  - Indicated for refractory bradycardias, ventricular arrhythmias, and hyperkalemia >5.5 mEq/L
  - Dosing can be empiric (6 vials for chronic overdoses, 10 vials for acute overdose), based on the amount ingested, or based on the steady-state digoxin level
  - Also administer activated charcoal and magnesium
- Maintain proper potassium balance
  - Chronic ingestions are exacerbated by *hypo*kalemia; therefore, maintain serum potassium near 4 mEq/L
  - Acute ingestions often cause *hyper*kalemia; if potassium is >5 mEq/L, consider empiric digoxin-specific antibody; do not use calcium as it increases ventricular irritability
- Dysrhythmias—Digoxin-specific antibody is the definitive treatment
  - Atropine for symptomatic bradycardias
  - IV magnesium decreases ventricular irritability
  - Transvenous cardiac pacing is ineffective

Disposition

- All suspected cases should be admitted with cardiac monitoring
- Psychiatry evaluation for intentional overdose
- Digoxin specific Fab fragments improve mortality from 25% to <10%
- Although allergic reactions to digoxin-specific antibodies are rare, patients should be monitored for side effects, such as CHF exacerbation, excessive ventricular response to atrial fibrillation, or hypokalemia
- Chronic digoxin poisoning has a higher mortality than acute ingestions

152. β-blockers and Calcium Channel Blockers

Etiology & Pathophysiology

- Widely used for dysrhythmias, hypertension, angina, migraine prophylaxis, glaucoma, and other conditions
- β-blockers competitively inhibit endogenous catecholamines at the β receptor, thereby acting as negative inotropes and chronotropes
  - Toxicity depends to some extent on lipophilic properties and cardioselectivity (e.g., the highly lipophilic and less cardioselective propranolol has higher mortality than other agents)
  - Symptoms may occur even with ophthalmic preparations
- Calcium channel blockers (CCB) prevent calcium influx into muscle cells, resulting in decreased contraction and automaticity
  - 2000 poisonings and 30 deaths annually (mostly due to verapamil)
  - Verapamil and diltiazem are negative inotropes and chronotropes
  - Dihydropyridines (e.g., nifedipine) cause systemic vasodilation with minimal direct cardiac effect

Differential Dx

- Acute myocardial infarction
- Digoxin overdose
- Dysrhythmia
- Hyperkalemia
- Hypothyroid
- Increased vagal tone
- Intracranial hemorrhage
- Oral hypoglycemic overdose
- Occult infection
- Opiate overdose
- Sedative overdose
- Seizure
- Sepsis
- Viral gastroenteritis

Presentation

- Onset of symptoms within 30–60 minutes of ingestion
- β-blockers: Hypotension, bradycardia, obtundation, respiratory depression, seizures, nausea, bronchospasm
- CCB: Hypotension, bradycardia progressing to asystole, pulmonary edema
  - Dihydropyridines generally cause hypotension with tachycardia, but may cause bradycardia at very high doses

Diagnosis

- Clinical diagnosis may be difficult in the absence of known ingestion, especially if non-cardiac symptoms manifest first
- Ingestion should be suspected in patients with unexplained dysrhythmias associated with obtundation and nausea or with hypotension and bradycardia
- Serum levels are neither generally reliable nor readily available
- If ingestion of β-blockers or CCB is known or strongly suspected, treatment should progress immediately to maintain hemodynamic stability
- ECG should be checked in all patients and will generally show bradycardic dysrhythmias (e.g., sinus bradycardia, junctional or ventricular escape rhythms)
- CCBs may also cause hyperkalemia

Treatment

- Activated charcoal administration
- Consider whole bowel irrigation
- β-blockers
  - IV glucagon is first-line therapy as it has both inotropic and chronotropic effects that bypass the β-receptor
  - Atropine for symptomatic bradydysrhythmias
  - Inotropic support with dopamine, norepinephrine, and/or isoproterenol
  - Amrinone, pacing, and intra-aortic balloon pump may be considered for refractory hypotension
  - Hemodialysis may be useful for non-lipophilic drugs (e.g., atenolol, nadolol)
- CCB
  - IV calcium chloride administration
  - Glucagon may be effective as above
  - Atropine, dopamine, norepinephrine as above
  - Insulin and glucose infusion improves contractility
  - Hemodialysis may also be effective in refractory cases

Disposition

- β-blockers
  - Patients who are asymptomatic after 6 hours may be transferred to Psychiatry
  - Sustained-release ingestions should be monitored for 24 hours
  - Patients with hypotension, AV block, or dysrhythmias should be admitted to a monitored floor or ICU
- CCB
  - Patients who are asymptomatic after 6 hours may be transferred to Psychiatry
  - Continuous cardiac monitoring is required if sustained-release preparations were ingested or symptoms are present

153. Sympathomimetic Overdose

Etiology & Pathophysiology

- Cocaine and amphetamine derivatives are common sympathomimetics
- Cocaine remains the most common cause of drug-related death (up to 25% of ED patients with chest pain and 6% of those with enzymatic evidence of myocardial infarction test positive for cocaine)
- 25 million Americans have used cocaine once and 1.5 million are current users
- Cocaine stimulates the release of biogenic amines and inhibits synaptic reuptake, resulting in α- and β-receptor stimulation
- Cocaine also inhibits the movement of sodium across the cell membrane, delaying nerve impulses and prolonging the QRS complex (amphetamines do not inhibit sodium channels)
- Amphetamines, including methamphetamine ("ice" or MDA) and MDMA, enhance the release and block reuptake of catecholamines

Differential Dx

- Acute psychosis
- Anticholinergic overdose
- Delirium tremens
- Heat stroke
- Hypoglycemia
- Hypoxemia
- Ma huang ingestion
- Meningitis
- Neuroleptic malignant syndrome
- Salicylate overdose
- Sedative-hypnotic withdrawal
- Sepsis
- Thyrotoxicosis
- Serotonin syndrome

Presentation

- Toxidrome: Hypertension, tachycardia, mydriasis, diaphoresis, and hyperthermia
- Cardiac effects include chest pain due to myocardial ischemia or aortic dissection and arrhythmias
- CNS effects include hallucinations, seizures, CVA, and intracranial hemorrhage
- Pulmonary effects (in patients who inhale the drug) include barotrauma, pneumonitis, pneumothorax, and bronchospasm
- Syncope may indicate aortic dissection or dysrhythmias
- Rhabdomyolysis with renal failure may occur

Diagnosis

- Clinical recognition of the sympathomimetic toxidrome
- Immediate rectal temperature for malignant hyperthermia
- Glucose and pulse oximetry should be assessed immediately
- Dysrhythmias may include sinus tachycardia, SVT, and wide-complex or ventricular tachycardia
- Serial ECGs and troponin if MI is suspected
- CPK to rule out rhabdomyolysis
- Head CT and lumbar puncture should be done to exclude subarachnoid hemorrhage in severe persistent headache
- Other labs may include DIC panel, electrolytes, cultures, and liver function tests
- Urine drug screens detect cocaine and amphetamine metabolites for several days after last use, so a positive test in the absence of the sympathomimetic toxidrome is probably not clinically useful
- Abdominal radiographs for suspected body packers

Treatment

- Activated charcoal +/− gastric lavage is useful in ingestions to prevent drug absorption
- Aggressively lower core temperatures >106°F to prevent organ failure via ice water immersion, benzodiazepines, and rapid fluid resuscitation
- Hypertension should be treated with benzodiazepines; refractory hypertension may be treated with phentolamine (α-antagonist), nitroglycerin, or nitroprusside
- Never use β-blockers in cocaine abuse (e.g., to treat hypertension, MI, or aortic dissection) as the unopposed α-adrenergic effect will produce paradoxically increased vasoconstriction and hypertension
- Treat chest pain with aspirin, nitroglycerin, and benzodiazepines
- Wide-complex tachycardia should be treated with sodium bicarbonate
- Body packers swallow large quantities of packaged drugs for transport across borders; administer charcoal and whole bowel irrigation; if symptoms of intoxication are present, surgical extraction may be necessary

Disposition

- Patients with mild agitation can be treated with benzodiazepines and discharged with a responsible adult after 6 hours of observation
- Admit agitated, violent, or symptomatic patients
- Patients with chest pain should be admitted if pain is persistent or is associated with ECG changes, elevated cardiac enzymes, or cardiovascular decompensation
- Route of intake may suggest associated complications: Inhaled (barotrauma), snorted (nasal septum perforation), or injected (endocarditis, abscess, DVT)
- Body packers should be admitted to a monitored floor for observation and whole bowel irrigation; radiological confirmation of packet clearance is necessary

154. Cholinergic/Anticholinergic Overdose

Etiology & Pathophysiology

- Cholinergics include organophosphate insecticides, carbamates, and nerve agents used in warfare (e.g., GA, GB, VX)
  - Organophosphates competitively inhibit acetylcholinesterase (AChE), thereby activating nicotinic and muscarinic acetylcholine receptors
  - Carbamates are shorter-acting AChE inhibitors
  - Organophosphate will covalently bind to AChE ("aging"), carbamates will not
  - Early mortality occurs due to bronchorrhea-induced airway compromise; late mortality is due to respiratory muscle fatigue
- Anticholinergics include atropine, scopolamine, glycopyrrolate, benztropine, oxybutynin, antipsychotics, tricyclics, and antihistamines
  - Competitively antagonize the muscarinic effects of acetylcholine

Differential Dx

- Cholinergics
  - Allergic reaction
  - Caustic ingestion
  - Food poisoning
  - Foreign body aspiration
  - Irritable bowel syndrome
  - Seizure disorder
  - Urosepsis
- Anticholinergics
  - Acute psychosis/delirium
  - Carbon monoxide
  - Sympathomimetic abuse
  - Steroid psychosis
  - Thyrotoxicosis
  - Serotonin syndrome

Presentation

- Cholinergic toxidrome
  - DUMBELS: Diarrhea/diaphoresis, urination, miosis/muscle fasciculations, bradycardia/bronchorrhea/ bronchospasm, emesis, lacrimation, salivation/seizure
- Anticholinergics:
  - *"Hot as hades, blind as a bat, dry as a bone, red as a beet, mad as a hatter"*
  - Hot and flushed, dilated pupils, dry mucous membranes, urinary retention, tachycardia, hypoactive bowel sounds, psychosis, seizures

Diagnosis

- Cholinergics
  - Clinical diagnosis based on classic toxidrome findings or known exposure
  - Response to empiric therapy confirms diagnosis
  - RBC cholinesterase activity may be measured
- Anticholinergics
  - Also a clinical diagnosis
  - Specific drug levels are neither readily available nor specific for anticholinergic intoxications
  - ECG may show widened QRS, prolonged QT, SVT, or wide-complex tachycardia

Treatment

- Cholinergics
  - Remove clothes, irrigate skin/membranes, stabilize airway
  - GI decontamination is unnecessary as vomiting and diarrhea are part of the toxidrome
  - IV atropine 5 mg every 5 minutes until bronchorrhea resolves; however, this will only reverse muscarinic effects without affecting nicotinic receptors
  - Early administration of pralidoxime will break apart the organophosphate-acetylcholinesterase complex
  - Long-acting IV/IM benzodiazepines for patients with severe toxicity, agitation, or seizures
- Anticholinergics
  - Ensure adequate volume replacement
  - IV physostigmine blocks acetylcholine metabolism; used for pure anti-cholinergic overdose, but not for drugs with mixed effects (e.g., TCAs); caution in patients with underlying coronary disease, reactive airway disease, or myasthenia gravis
  - Sodium bicarbonate for wide-complex tachycardias
  - Benzodiazepines for agitation or seizures

Disposition

- Cholinergic toxicity generally requires admission
- Anticholinergics
  - Patients with mild symptoms may be discharged home after psychiatric evaluation and/or assessment of child's home safety
  - Patients with moderate to severe symptoms should be observed in a monitored setting
  - Antihistamine overdoses should be observed on monitor for 8 hours because of delayed onset of symptoms

155. Cyanide Poisoning

Etiology & Pathophysiology

- Cyanide (CN) inhibits the final step of oxidative phosphorylation, forcing cells to utilize anaerobic metabolism to produce ATP and resulting in an anion-gap metabolic acidosis
- In cases of CN poisoning, oxygen is not used for cellular respiration; it remains bound to hemoglobin, producing bright red venous blood
- Exposure may occur due to inhalation, ingestion, or percutaneous exposure
- Exposures may occur in fires, the workplace (e.g., metal plating, paper, fertilizer, plastics industries), foods (e.g., apricots, bitter almonds), and in some non-traditional cancer therapies (e.g., Laetrile)
- Elimination of CN occurs via the enzyme *rhodanese,* which converts it to water-soluble thiocyanate
- Concurrent carbon monoxide poisoning may occur in smoke inhalations

Differential Dx

- Hypoxia
- Carbon monoxide poisoning
- Hydrogen sulfide inhalation
- Alcoholic ketoacidosis
- Methanol, ethanol, or ethylene glycol ingestion
- Isoniazid poisoning
- Acute lung injury/ARDS
- Hydrogen sulfide
- Intracranial bleed
- Salicylate overdose
- Seizure disorder
- Sepsis
- Viral syndrome

Presentation

- Affects the CNS, cardiac, and pulmonary systems
- CNS symptoms begin as headache, restlessness, and fatigue; may progress to seizures, loss of consciousness, and coma
- Cardiac symptoms begin as tachycardia and may progress to hypotension, bradycardia, asystole
- Pulmonary symptoms include dyspnea and tachypnea (as a compensatory response to metabolic acidosis)
- Patients are not cyanotic
- Post-mortem findings include a cherry-red retina and retinal hemorrhages

Diagnosis

- All fire victims should be suspected of carbon monoxide and cyanide exposure until proven otherwise
- History is the most important diagnostic factor; supporting labs may include cyanide level, lactate level, and electrolytes for anion gap acidosis
- Serum cyanide level will determine the magnitude of exposure but is generally unavailable for rapid diagnosis in the ED (toxic levels are >0.5 mg/L and fatal levels are >3 mg/L)
- Electrolytes will reveal an anion gap metabolic acidosis (typically anion gap >30)
- Lactate will be elevated
- ABG reveals a normal PaO_2 and metabolic acidosis; spectrophotometric co-oximetry should be checked to discern the presence of carboxyhemoglobin
- Pulse oximetry will be normal

Treatment

- Administer 100% oxygen by a non-rebreather face mask
- Activated charcoal if ingestion is suspected
- Cyanide antidote kit is indicated for symptomatic patients
   - Inhaled amyl nitrite pearls and IV sodium nitrite generate methemoglobin to bind to CN
   - Sodium thiosulfate provides a sulfur moiety to improve *rhodanese* elimination of CN
   - Methemoglobin formed by nitrites may further decrease oxygen-carrying capacity and worsen ischemia—as a result, the antidote kit should only be used in patients with symptoms
- Hyperbaric oxygen is not effective

Disposition

- All patients with symptomatic exposures should be admitted for observation
- Patients with asymptomatic exposures may be monitored for 6–8 hours and released

156. Carbon Monoxide Poisoning

Etiology & Pathophysiology

- Carbon monoxide (CO) is a colorless, odorless gas produced by the incomplete combustion of hydrocarbons
- CO has an affinity for hemoglobin 250-fold greater than oxygen, thereby decreasing oxygen dissociation from hemoglobin in the tissues (via shifting the oxygen-hemoglobin dissociation curve to the left) and decreasing the oxygen carrying capacity of blood
- CO also inhibits the last step of oxidative phosphorylation, forcing cells to undergo anaerobic metabolism to produce ATP
- At high concentrations, CO also binds to myoglobin and inhibits cardiac contractility
- Exposures occur due to fires, gas or oil heaters, engine exhaust, smoking, and industrial occupations
- CO poisoning is the most common cause of fire-related death

Differential Dx

- Cyanide poisoning
- Alcoholic ketoacidosis
- Lactic acidosis
- Acute lung injury/ARDS
- Hydrogen sulfide
- Intracranial bleed
- Salicylate overdose
- Seizure disorder
- Sepsis
- Viral syndrome
- Respiratory infection

Presentation

- Toxicity manifests as vague, non-specific complaints, including headache, nausea, weakness, dizziness, and confusion
- Common signs include lethargy, tachycardia, and tachypnea
- Severe cases may present with syncope, seizure, coma, chest pain, myocardial ischemia, hypotension, or cardiac arrest
- Strongly consider CO poisoning when an entire family/group presents with similar complaints at the same time

Diagnosis

- Suspect carbon monoxide exposure in all fire victims
- Arterial blood gases and pulse oximetry cannot distinguish carboxyhemoglobin (COHb) from oxyhemoglobin—spectrophotometric co-oximetry can be ordered on arterial or venous blood to reliably distinguish the two (pulse oximetry may misidentify COHb as oxyhemoglobin and therefore overestimate oxygen carrying capacity and tissue oxygenation)
- History is the most important diagnostic factor; supporting labs may include cyanide level, elevated lactate level, and electrolytes (reveal anion gap metabolic acidosis)
- Additional workup should include a pregnancy test, CBC, CPK, urinalysis, cardiac enzymes, salicylate level, ECG, and CXR
- Consider using the Carbon Monoxide Neuropsychological Screening Battery to provide a baseline for mental status changes

Treatment

- Remove the patient from the source of carbon monoxide
- Administer supplemental O_2 via a non-rebreathing facemask
- Hyperbaric oxygen therapy should be considered in pregnant patients with COHb >10%, coronary disease with COHb >20%, patients with any cardiac symptoms, and all other patients with COHb >20–40% or severe/deteriorating symptoms
  - Hyperbarics speed resolution of symptoms and decrease rates of delayed sequelae
  - The half-life of COHb is 6 hours on room air, <90 minutes on 100% oxygen at 1 atmosphere, and <30 minutes on 100% oxygen at 3 atmospheres

Disposition

- COHb levels do not correlate with symptom severity
- 10–30% of symptomatic CO exposures develop delayed sequelae of cognitive or personality changes, parkinsonism, or chronic headaches
- Complications of CO exposure include myocardial infarction, brain ischemia, noncardiogenic pulmonary edema, rhabdomyolysis, DIC, and renal failure
- Discharge patients with CO exposure whose symptoms resolve after 4 hours of oxygen therapy
- Admit all patients who have severe or persistent symptoms

157. Ethanol Intoxication

Etiology & Pathophysiology

- Most frequently used/abused drug in the US
- Ethanol is found in the blood of 15–40% of ED patients
- Acts as a CNS depressant by inhibiting neuronal activity
- Metabolism primarily occurs in the liver via alcohol dehydrogenase and acetaldehyde dehydrogenase
- See entry on *Withdrawal Syndromes* for further information
- Alcohol use is a significant risk factor for trauma
- Legal intoxication is generally defined as blood level 80–100 mg/dL
- Metabolized at approximately 30 mg/dL/hour
- One drink (e.g., 12 oz beer, 4 oz wine, 1 shot 80-proof liquor) increases blood alcohol by 20–30 mg/dL
- Complications of chronic use: CNS (e.g., cognitive impairment, cerebellar degeneration, peripheral neuropathy, dementia), GI (e.g., fatty liver, alcohol hepatitis, cirrhosis), cardiomyopathy, malignancy
- Wernicke and Korsakoff's syndromes are due to thiamine deficiency

Differential Dx

- Alcohol withdrawal
- Toxic alcohol ingestion (e.g., methanol, ethylene glycol)
- DKA
- Hypoglycemia
- Illicit drug use
- Traumatic injury
- Seizure disorder
- Metabolic disturbance (e.g., electrolyte abnormality, infection)
- Meningitis
- Encephalitis

Presentation

- Commonly causes slurred speech, disinhibited behavior, poor judgement, decreased coordination, CNS depression, respiratory depression (in severe cases)
- Cardiac arrhythmias or hypotension with reflex tachycardia may occur
- Gastritis, esophagitis, GI bleed, or pancreatitis may occur
- Increased sexual desire, decreased ability to perform
- Wernicke's syndrome: Ataxia, ophthalmoparesis, encephalopathy
- Korsakoff's syndrome: Alcohol-induced amnesia (antegrade greater than retrograde)

Diagnosis

- Complete physical exam is required to assess for the presence of associated traumatic injuries and hypothermia
- Ethanol levels are readily available but are not absolutely required; clinical effects of ethanol depend both on blood level and degree of patient tolerance
- CBC reveals increased MCV and thrombocytopenia
- Electrolyte abnormalities may include hypokalemia, hypomagnesemia, hypocalcemia, and hypophosphatemia
- Alcoholic ketoacidosis (anion gap metabolic acidosis) may occur due to decreased oxidation of fatty acids and poor diet, resulting in increased serum ketones, large anion gap, and either mildly increased or normal serum glucose
- Hypoglycemia is often present due to impaired liver gluconeogenesis
- Consider urine drug screen if co-ingestants are suspected—cocaine is especially common

Treatment

- Observe until clinically sober
- Occasionally, patients require intubation for respiratory depression or airway protection
- Activated charcoal is ineffective; administration is only indicated if a co-ingestant is suspected
- Gastric lavage is rarely required
- Treat dehydration with IV fluids containing dextrose if volume depletion or clinical dehydration is present
- Administer thiamine and folate (prior to glucose administration) to prevent acute Wernicke's encephalopathy
- Treat hypoglycemia with D50 bolus or IV fluids containing glucose

Disposition

- Patients who are clinically intoxicated may be held against their will if they pose a danger to self or others
- Patients may be discharged if they are clinically sober and able to care for themselves—a specific blood ethanol level is not required
- Do not overlook associated injuries (e.g., altered mental status may be due to intracerebral hemorrhage secondary to a fall rather than EtOH intoxication)
- 1–2 drinks per day may have beneficial health effects by decreasing cardiovascular disease rates
- Alcohol intake during pregnancy is rapidly transferred across the placenta and may cause fetal alcohol syndrome
- Provide referrals to patients who are problem drinkers

158. Toxic Alcohols

Etiology & Pathophysiology

- All alcohols are metabolized by the enzymes alcohol dehydrogenase and acetaldehyde dehydrogenase
- Methanol (MetOH) is also known as wood alcohol or wood spirits
  - Found in antifreeze, windshield fluid, inks, glass cleaners, solvents, and paint thinners
  - Metabolized to formic acid (the true toxin); antagonizes cellular respiration causing anion-gap metabolic acidosis, ocular toxicity
- Ethylene glycol
  - Primarily found in antifreeze and engine coolants
  - Metabolized to toxic organic acids
  - Forms characteristic calcium oxalate crystals in the urine
- Isopropanol
  - Found in rubbing alcohol and solvents
  - Metabolized to acetone causing metabolic acidosis
- Ethanol: See related "Ethanol Intoxication" entry

Differential Dx

- MUDPILES mnemonic for an anion gap metabolic acidosis
  - Methanol
  - Uremia
  - DKA
  - Paraldehydes
  - Iron or isoniazid overdose
  - Lactic acidosis
  - Ethanol (alcoholic ketoacidosis) or ethylene glycol
  - Salicylates
- Consider other causes of altered mental status

Presentation

- Methanol toxicity may occur up to 3 days after ingestion
  - Early toxicity mimics ethanol ingestion (N/V, abdominal pain, ataxia, decreased mental status)
  - 50% develop visual changes, from blurred vision to blindness
- Ethylene glycol has 4 stages
  - Neurologic (1–12 hrs): Drunken behavior, CNS depression
  - Cardiopulmonary (12–24 hrs): HTN, tachycardia, pulm edema
  - Nephrotoxic (24–72 hrs): CVA tenderness, renal failure
  - Delayed neurologic sequelae
- Isopropanol: Respiratory and CNS depression, gastritis, coma, death

Diagnosis

- Check glucose, CBC, electrolytes, renal function, and urinalysis
- Toxic alcohols generally cause an elevated anion gap (minimal in ethanol and isopropanol, moderate to severe in ethylene glycol and methanol) and an elevated serum osmolal gap
- Serum levels of each alcohol are available and should be obtained for the suspected ingestant
- Methanol
  - Occupational exposure history may provide the diagnosis
  - Head CT may show characteristic bilateral putaminal lesions
- Ethylene glycol
  - Calcium oxalate crystals in the urine is diagnostic
  - Urine fluorescence with a Wood's lamp, if present, is helpful; however, lack of fluorescence does not rule out poisoning
- Isopropanol
  - Causes only a mild acidosis with ketonemia and ketonuria
  - May have severe hypoglycemia

Treatment

- Profound bicarbonate-resistant metabolic acidosis may occur; therefore, the goals of therapy are to rapidly correct the acidosis and immediately inhibit further production of toxic metabolites
- Both methanol and ethylene glycol are treated with IV ethanol or fometizole to competitively antagonize the dehydrogenase enzyme, hindering further production of toxic metabolites
- Early hemodialysis is the most effective means of removing toxic organic acid metabolites; indications for hemodialysis vary with the toxin ingested
  - Methanol: Any visual impairment, base deficit >15 mmol/L, serum [MetOH] >50 mg/dL, or consumption of >40 mL
  - Ethylene glycol: Refractory acidosis or renal failure
  - Isopropanol: Refractory hypotension or level >400 mg/dL
- Activated charcoal is ineffective and has no role in isolated alcohol ingestion; administer only if a co-ingestion is suspected

Disposition

- 90% of exposures are unintentional
- All toxic alcohol ingestions should be admitted
- If treated early, alcohol poisonings have low mortality; however, failure to initiate prompt therapy can be fatal within 1–2 days
- Methanol: Predictors of mortality include coma, initial pH <7, or seizure on presentation
- Ethylene glycol: Predictors of mortality include coma, low pH, hyperkalemia, and seizures

159. Heavy Metal Poisoning

Etiology & Pathophysiology

- Lead has no known biological functions; it impairs various enzymes by binding to sulfhydryl groups, primarily of the hematopoietic, neurologic, and renal systems
  - 5% of US children have toxic blood lead levels due to exposures to paint, soil, contaminated food storage cans, and herbal remedies
- Iron toxicity depends on elemental iron level ingested (<20 mg/kg no symptoms, 20–60 mg/kg moderate symptoms, >60 mg/kg severe)
  - Once transferrin becomes saturated, free iron circulates in serum, moves into cells, and uncouples oxidative phosphorylation
  - Iron also causes direct damage to the GI tract
- Arsenic is an odorless, tasteless metal that binds sulfhydryl groups, inhibiting glycolysis and replacing phosphorus in ATP-dependent cellular energy production; found in pesticides and high-tech industries
  - Exposures may be occupational or criminal (attempted homicide or as a biological weapon)

Differential Dx

- Acute renal failure
- Bowel obstruction
- Carbon monoxide
- Child abuse
- Cyanide toxicity
- Mercury poisoning
- Gastroenteritis
- Hepatitis
- Homicide attempt
- Peptic ulcer disease
- Sepsis
- Suicide attempt
- Causes of altered mental status

Presentation

- Lead poisoning may present as chronic toxicity (anemia, peripheral neuropathy, abdominal pain, pica, and intellectual impairment) or acute overdose (GI distress, encephalopathy, seizures)
- Iron presents in 5 distinct phases
  - GI toxicity (90 minutes)
  - Incomplete recovery (12–24 hrs)
  - Deterioration with GI bleed and CNS depression (12–48 hrs)
  - Rapid hepatic failure (2–5 days)
  - Bowel scarring and strictures
- Arsenic: Violent vomiting, prolonged gastroenteritis, CNS symptoms, white lines in nails, hypotension, arrhythmias, alopecia

Diagnosis

- Lead: Blood lead level (BLL) is diagnostic
  - Other tests include head CT, CBC (demonstrates anemia +/− basophilic stippling), electrolytes, liver function tests, and urinalysis
  - X-ray of long bones in children may reveal lead lines (increased metaphyseal deposition) in the distal ulna or fibula
- Iron: Blood iron level is diagnostic and correlated with severity
  - CBC and electrolytes may show leukocytosis or hypoglycemia
  - Abdominal X-rays may be helpful to visualize GI iron tablets, but absence does not rule out the diagnosis
- Arsenic: 24-hour urine arsenic level >100 μg/day or spot urine >50 μg/L requires therapy
  - In chronic ingestions, hair or nails should be examined for traces of arsenic
  - May also see anemia with basophilic stippling and an active urinary sediment (e.g., casts, WBCs, RBCs)

Treatment

- All heavy metals are readily removed by hemodialysis
- Lead: Chelation therapy for significant toxicity
  - Parenteral chelators include dimercaprol and calcium disodium ethylenediaminetetraacetic acid (EDTA)
  - Enteral chelators include succimer (a water-soluble dimercaprol analog) or D-penicillamine
  - <20 μg/dL: No chelation therapy required
  - 20–44: Consider outpatient chelation
  - 45–69: Outpatient enteral chelation
  - >69: Inpatient parenteral chelation
- Iron
  - Whole bowel irrigation if tablets are seen on X-ray (activated charcoal, gastric lavage, and induced vomiting are ineffective)
  - Continuous deferoxamine infusion (forms a water-soluble complex with iron, which is then renally excreted)
- Arsenic
  - Dimercaprol, succimer or D-penicillamine chelation
  - Gastric lavage, activated charcoal, or bowel irrigation

Disposition

- Lead
  - All lead levels >10 μg/dL require family evaluation, health department assessment, and blood screening to ensure lead-free environment
  - Admit symptomatic patients or those with lead levels >69 μg/dL
  - CNS damage is often permanent
- Iron
  - Patients with ingestions <20 mg/kg of elemental iron may be discharged if asymptomatic after 6 hours
  - Admit patients with ingestions >20 mg/kg; consider treatment with bowel irrigation and supportive therapy
  - Patients with serum levels >350 μg/dL require chelation therapy
- Arsenic exposures are generally admitted

160. Hydrocarbon Poisoning

Etiology & Pathophysiology

- Hydrocarbons are carbon-based structures, most often petroleum distillates (e.g., gasoline, other fuels, adhesives/glues, paint, varnish, paint/stain/varnish removers, cleaners, and other solvents)
- As a group, these are among the most commonly reported poisonings; generally fall into one of four clinical scenarios—toddler ingestion, adolescent recreational abuse (e.g., glue-sniffing, huffing), accidental dermal/inhalational exposure, or suicide attempt
- 1/3 of toddler exposures result from drinking from a reused beverage container used to store hydrocarbons!
- Because hydrocarbons are used as solvents for many substances (e.g., pesticides), the composition of the ingested substance should be ascertained
- Toxicity is noted primarily in the lungs, cardiovascular system, and CNS

Differential Dx

- Asthma
- Caustic ingestion
- Child abuse
- Congenital heart disease
- Foreign body aspiration
- Pesticide ingestion
- Polysubstance abuse
- Pneumonia
- Suicide attempt
- Other causes of mental status changes (e.g., meningitis)

Presentation

- Respiratory: Hypoxia, pneumonitis with direct alveolar injury, or bronchospasm
- Cardiovascular: Dysrhythmias or sudden death; may enhance myocardial sensitivity to catecholamines
- CNS: Narcotic-like euphoria, tremor, agitation, seizures
  – May result in long-term neurodegeneration with encephalopathy and neuropathy
- Dermal exposures typically cause burning pain, swelling, or blisters

Diagnosis

- Note the characteristic smell of breath in conjunction with presenting complaints
- Paramedics and family members should be encouraged to bring the ingested substance from the scene so that any co-toxicities may be anticipated (e.g., pesticides)
- Laboratory levels of hydrocarbons are not clinically useful
- Chest X-ray may manifest abnormalities within 30 minutes of ingestion (even in the absence of auscultatory findings)
- ABG may show hypoxemia or increased A-a gradient
- ECG may show ventricular dysrhythmias (due to increased catecholamine availability)
- Check CBC, electrolytes, and liver and renal function
- In suspected recreational abuse, a characteristic rash around the mouth and nose ("huffer's rash" or "glue-sniffer's rash") may support the diagnosis; be sure to exclude other common drugs of abuse

Treatment

- Supportive therapy is the key to successful management; recognize potential complications and the potential for a rapid deterioration following asymptomatic presentation
- Generally, do not give charcoal, ipecac, or GI lavage unless another toxic ingestion is suspected (these are generally not effective and increase the risk of hydrocarbon aspiration)
- GI decontamination may be used for specific hydrocarbons
  – Camphor (seizures)
  – Halogenated hydrocarbons (dysrhythmias and hepatotoxicity)
  – Aromatic hydrocarbons (bone marrow suppression)
  – Metals, such as lead and mercury
- Keep patients calm (use sedation if necessary) because of the enhanced myocardial sensitivity to catecholamines
- Arrhythmias are best treated with β-blockers due to the excess of catecholamines
- Wash dermal exposures copiously with soap and water
- No specific antidotes exist for isolated hydrocarbon toxicity

Disposition

- Patients may remain asymptomatic for several hours after exposure; thus, all reported exposures should be observed in the ED for a minimum of six hours
- Patients who are asymptomatic after 6 hours may be discharged following repeat pulmonary auscultation, chest X-ray, pulse oximetry, and/or ABG
- All discharged patients should have appropriate follow-up
- Admit patients with symptomatic cough or dyspnea
- Psychiatry should be consulted for chronic abusers and suicide attempts
- Glue sniffers or huffers are at risk for chronic CNS toxicity

161. Caustic Ingestions

Etiology & Pathophysiology

- Caustic injuries to the esophagus primarily occur in two age groups: Children ages 1–5 (due to accidental ingestions) and young adults ages 15–30 (usually due to larger ingestions as a suicide attempt)
- Injury progresses in three stages
  - Acute inflammation with necrosis and ulcer formation
  - Granulation (days 4–14) with risk of perforation
  - Chronic cicatrization (days 14–90) with stricture formation
- Alkali results in liquefaction necrosis and protein disruption (deep tissue penetration may occur) whereas acids produce coagulation necrosis and eschar formation (limiting tissue damage to superficial)
- Alkali primarily damages the esophagus whereas acids may damage the esophagus or stomach
- Acute complications include airway compromise, pneumonitis, and esophageal or gastric perforation with mediastinitis or peritonitis
- Caustic ingestions increase the risk of esophageal cancer 3000-fold

Differential Dx

- Abdominal catastrophe (e.g., perforation)
- Child abuse
- Electrical burn
- Esophageal cancer
- Esophageal dysmotility
- Fungal/viral esophagitis
- GERD
- Pill esophagitis
- Periodontal infection
- Radiation esophagitis
- Schatzki's ring

Presentation

- Airway edema and perforation of a viscus require emergent management
- Common presenting complaints include oral pain, abdominal pain, vomiting, and drooling
- Stridor, dysphonia, chest pain, respiratory distress, and lip/facial burns are also common
- Hypovolemic shock, fever, and acidosis may be present
- Dermal burns may occur if the substance touched the skin
- Hydrofluoric acid dermal burns uniquely cause severe pain with minimal physical findings

Diagnosis

- The key to diagnosis and treatment is to elicit the exact agent ingested; injury severity is a function of the type of agent, concentration, volume, viscosity, duration of contact, pH, and whether food was present in the stomach
- Labs should include electrolytes, CBC, and PT/PTT
- Obtain ABG to evaluate for systemic acidosis
- Upright chest and abdominal plain films are required to identify perforations (free air in the abdomen or mediastinum) and pleural effusions—evidence of either necessitate immediate surgical exploration for source of perforation
- Endoscopy (safest within the initial 24 hours) should be performed urgently (<6 hours) in any symptomatic or intentional ingestions to determine degree of injury
- Chest and abdominal CT is used in stable patients to identify any questionable perforations, but is not 100% sensitive
- Hydrofluoric acid exposures require cardiac monitoring and serum Ca^{+2} and Mg^{+2} levels

Treatment

- Airway management with endotracheal intubation may be required for severe pharyngeal or oral injuries
- Patients with alkali ingestion who are not vomiting or displaying evidence of perforation can be given 1–2 glasses of water or milk to neutralize the caustic agent within 15 minutes of ingestion
- Copious irrigation of ocular, dermal, and oral lesions
- Do not induce emesis (may increase esophageal or pulmonary injury) or administer activated charcoal (does not bind caustics and may obscure endoscopic evaluation)
- Do not place NG tube in alkali burn due to perforation risk
- Corticosteroids may be considered in circumferential, second-degree alkali burn injuries of the esophagus to decrease stricture formation; not indicated in acid burns
- Antibiotic prophylaxis against oral pathogens if steroids are utilized or perforation has occurred
- Surgery is required emergently in most perforations
- Hydrofluoric acid dermal burns are treated with topical calcium gluconate gel or benzalkonium chloride until pain is relieved; refractory pain requires calcium gluconate injection

Disposition

- All symptomatic patients require ICU admission
- After 4–6 hours of observation, asymptomatic patients require ED endoscopy or outpatient follow-up within 12 hours for re-evaluation
- Psychiatry should be involved for all intentional ingestions
- Parents should be advised not to store caustic substances in spaces accessible to toddlers or in containers usually reserved for beverages
- Acid ingestion has higher mortality than alkali despite more superficial tissue invasion (likely due to systemic absorption of the acid)
- Long-term complications include esophageal stricture formation (especially after alkali burn)

162. Hallucinogen Overdose

Etiology & Pathophysiology

- Hallucinogens are a heterogeneous group of compounds
- LSD-like agents include mescaline, psilocybin, and *Amanita muscaria* mushrooms—these all produce altered thought process and perception of surroundings by interruption of serotonergic (5-HT) signal processing to the cerebral cortex
- 3,4-methylenedioxymethamphetamine (MDMA, "ecstasy") is known as an "enactogen" or "empathogen" due to the enhanced sense of empathy it produces; commonly used by teenagers at raves
  - Alters 5-HT transmission and increases dopamine release
  - Composed of an amphetamine-like moiety and a mescaline-like moiety, resulting in both hallucinogenic euphoria and stimulation
  - Death may occur due to cardiac arrhythmias or intracranial hemorrhage
- PCP (angel dust) is a synthetic dissociative anesthetic that blocks glutamate; clinical effects vary from agitation to sedation

Differential Dx

- LSD-like agents
  - Anticholinergic toxin
  - Delirium tremens
  - Schizophrenia
  - Sympathomimetics
- MDMA/PCP-like agents
  - All the above
  - Tricyclic antidepressant overdose
  - Head trauma
  - Heat stroke/neuroleptic malignant syndrome
  - Meningitis, sepsis
  - Salicylate overdose
  - Thyrotoxicosis

Presentation

- Illusions (abnormal perception of sensory inputs) and/or hallucinations (sensory perceptions without any external stimuli)
- LSD-like agents: Sympathomimetic symptoms (e.g., tachycardia, HTN, flushing, mydriasis); a "bad trip" occurs with acute panic and paranoid delusions, which may foster dangerous/suicidal behavior
- MDMA: Sympathomimetic symptoms, euphoria; may cause hyperthermia, seizures, acute panic, mydriasis, muscle spasm
- PCP: Altered mental status, HTN, rotatory nystagmus, and violent and agitated misbehavior

Diagnosis

- LSD-like agents are readily identified by mass spectrometry of serum, urine, or gastric contents; however, results of these tests are rarely available in the ED
  - Not detected on common urine drug screens
- MDMA is identified by urine drug screens; diagnosis is confirmed by urine chromatography
  - Obtain ECG if arrhythmias are suspected
  - Severe hyponatremia is possible due to SIADH
- PCP is detected by urine drug screens; however, false positives are common with other agents (e.g., dextromethorphan diphenhydramine)
  - May cause hypoglycemia
- Depending on the presentation, additional workup may include a drug screen for additional substances of abuse, acetaminophen and aspirin levels if suicide attempt is suspected, and bacterial cultures to exclude infection

Treatment

- Charcoal may be beneficial if given within 1 hour of ingestion or if co-ingestions are suspected
- LSD-like agents
  - Calm, comfortable environment
  - Benzodiazepines, haloperidol, or droperidol as needed for sedation
- MDMA
  - IV fluids and active cooling—the length of time of hyperthermia correlates directly with adverse outcome
  - Benzodiazepines for seizures or agitation
  - β-blockers, calcium-channel blockers, or procainamide for dysrhythmias
  - Benzodiazepines or β-blockers for HTN
  - Dantrolene for hyperthermia
- PCP
  - Airway management
  - Active cooling
  - Benzodiazepines or phenobarbital for seizures
  - Haloperidol or droperidol for agitation

Disposition

- LSD-like agents
  - Onset 30 minutes; lasts 2–12 hours
  - Admit if symptoms persist >8 hours
  - Complications: Persistent psychosis and/or "flashbacks"
- MDMA
  - Discharge patients if asymptomatic after 4–6 hours
  - Admit patients with persistent thought disorders, dysrhythmias, seizures, or renal failure
  - Complications: Dysrhythmias, HTN with intracerebral hemorrhage, DIC, hyperthermia, seizure, rhabdomyolysis
- PCP
  - Admit agitated or violent patients
  - Discharge if asymptomatic for 6 hrs
  - Complications: Seizures, coma, rhabdomyolysis

163. Botanical Ingestions and Herbal Toxicity

Etiology & Pathophysiology

- Herbal remedies are used by over 30% of the general public
- Most ED herbal toxicities result from product contamination (unintentional), overdoses, and drug interactions
- Botanical ingestions peak in summer and fall, when colorful berries and leaves attract children and mushroom enthusiasts mistake toxic species
- Herbal supplements include ephedra (causes sympathetic hyperactivity), echinacea (used for URIs), ginkgo (used to improve mental status; inhibits platelets), ginseng (used for ulcers, fatigue, and stress), and many others
- 5% of poison center calls involve plant ingestions (usually age <6); however, <5% of plant ingestions produce adverse effects and mortality is less than 1:1,000,000
- Fatal plant ingestions include water hemlock and oleander
- Most mushroom fatalities are from *Amanita phalloides* ingestion

Differential Dx

- Alcohol intoxication
- Caustic ingestion
- Gastroenteritis
- Hallucinogen abuse
- Hepatitis
- Homicide attempt
- Hypersensitivity reactions
- Intracranial hemorrhage
- Seizure
- Suicide attempt

Presentation

- Herbals
  - Ephedra: Tachycardia, tachypnea, hypertension, cardiac ischemia, and diaphoresis
  - Chamomile, echinacea: Anaphylaxis
  - Ginkgo: Bleeding
  - Ginseng: Hypoglycemia
  - St. John's Wort: Tyramine effect
- Common household plants
  - Water hemlock: Abdominal cramping, nausea, vomiting, intractable seizures
  - Jimsonweed: Anticholinergic toxidrome
  - Oleander: Digoxin-like cardiac conduction defects

Diagnosis

- All patients should be questioned about ingestion of herbal substances and vitamins
- Identification of the ingestant is the single most important action in determining the potential toxicity of a botanical ingestion
- Attempt to identify the ingested household plants or mushrooms via analysis of emesis, stool, and the site where ingestion occurred
- Though specific toxin testing is often possible, results are not readily available in the ED; further, one must know for what toxin to test
- Early involvement of a botanical specialist through the local poison center may be useful
- ED testing is generally directed at ruling out other causes of the patient's symptoms

Treatment

- Herbal agents
  - Toxicities should be managed based on the individual agent, pharmacologic interactions, and toxic symptoms
  - Symptomatic ingestions should be treated with multiple doses of activated charcoal
  - Herbals often interact with other drugs (e.g., significant interactions with warfarin)
- Common household plants
  - Supportive care and careful observation is sufficient in most cases
  - Symptomatic ingestions should be treated with multiple doses of activated charcoal
  - Specific ingestants may require antidotes (e.g., anticholinergics for jimsonweed, digoxin-specific antibody for oleander)

Disposition

- Early involvement of botanical specialists may be necessary
- Admit herbal toxicities with severe side effects
- All amatoxin mushroom and water hemlock ingestions should be admitted to an ICU for observation
- If amatoxin mushroom, water hemlock, and other potentially deadly ingestions are excluded, the patient may be discharged home if asymptomatic and volume-repleted after 6 hours

Environmental Emergencies

JEFFREY M. CATERINO, MD
H. WILLIAM ZIMMERMAN, MD
ROBERT DRIVER, MD
LORONE C. WASHINGTON, MD

164. Hypothermia

Etiology & Pathophysiology

- Core temperature <35°C caused by environmental exposure, decreased thermogenesis, impaired thermoregulation, or diminished ability to respond appropriately to the cold
  - –30–35°C: Increased metabolic output with tachycardia, hypertension, and tachypnea
  - –24–30°C: Slowing of body functions, decreased oxygen demand, altered mental status, bradycardia, hypotension, arrhythmias
  - –<24°C: Most organ systems shut down, may have asystole or Vfib
- High-risk in the elderly (impaired thermoregulation, mental status changes), neonates (large body surface area), alcohol/drug abusers
- Severe hypothermia protects organs from ischemia (i.e., at <20°C, cardiac arrest may be tolerated for hours without sequelae)
- Severely hypothermic myocardium is very irritable and is often refractory to conventional therapy (e.g., placing a central line, CPR, or even moving the patient may cause refractory Vfib)

Differential Dx

- Environmental exposure
- Mental status changes, preventing proper response to cold
- Sepsis
- Drug or alcohol abuse
- Hypothyroidism
- Hypopituitarism
- Hypoadrenalism
- Hypoglycemia
- CNS injury, CVA, or tumor
- Wernicke's encephalopathy
- Burns
- IV fluids

Presentation

- Cardiovascular effects
  - –Mild: tachycardia, hypertension
  - –Severe: bradycardia, decreased cardiac output, hypotension
  - –<30°C: Dysrhythmias
- CNS: Progressively decreasing mental status, ataxia, confusion, lethargy, coma; may have dilated and non-reactive pupils
- Pulmonary: Hypopnea, decreased peripheral O_2 release, bronchorrhea
- Renal: Diuresis and hypovolemia due to impaired tubule concentrating ability (ATN may ensue)
- Coagulopathy

Diagnosis

- Most thermometers only read to 34.4°C; specialized, low-reading thermometers may be required
- CBC may show increased hemoglobin due to hemoconcentration
- Check serum glucose, electrolytes, renal function (monitor for ATN), CPK (for rhabdomyolysis), PT/PTT, and DIC screen
- Coagulation studies (PT/PTT) may be normal despite the presence of a clinical coagulopathy (normal coagulation function may occur in the lab as blood is warmed)
- Consider checking plasma cortisol levels and obtaining blood cultures to rule out sepsis
- ABG: Metabolic acidosis with either respiratory acidosis (decreased ventilation) or alkalosis (decreased CO_2 production)
- ECG may show T wave inversions; prolongation of PR, QRS, or QT waves; J waves (Osborn waves) that appear as a hump at junction of the QRS and ST; and dysrhythmias (e.g., bradycardia, Afib/flutter, Vfib, asystole)
- Flat EEG occurs below 20°C

Treatment

- Hydrocortisone, thiamine, and antibiotics are standard therapy until the cause of the hypothermia is determined
- Treat arrhythmias by rewarming and ACLS protocols—the heart may be refractory to common treatments (e.g., defibrillation, atropine, antiarrhythmics, pacing); bretylium is the drug of choice as lidocaine may increase Vfib
- Passive rewarming (remove from cold, apply blankets) for hemodynamically stable patients with mild hypothermia
- Active external rewarming for moderate or severe cases (e.g., warming blankets, warm water immersion, room heaters); however, external rewarming initially warms the periphery, resulting in peripheral vasodilatation that may lead to hypotension or rewarming acidosis (lactic acid from tissues moves centrally)
- Active internal rewarming is indicated in severe cases or cardiac arrest to preferentially warm the heart and other vital organs (e.g., warmed O_2 administration; warmed IV fluids; GI, bladder, peritoneal, or pleural lavage; cardiopulmonary bypass)

Disposition

- Discharge patients with mild hypothermia
- Admit patients with moderate-severe hypothermia
- Mortality depends on etiology (e.g., sepsis carries a high mortality)
- Recovery has been documented with cardiac arrest as long as 6 hours due to the decreased metabolic demands of hypothermic tissues
- Death should not be declared until the patient is warmed to at least 30°C

165. Cold-Related Injuries

Etiology & Pathophysiology

- Factors affecting the severity of cold injury include temperature, clothing, duration of exposure, and humidity
- Chilblains (pernio): Chronic, intermittent skin inflammation due to persistent vasospasm following exposure to cold, damp conditions
- Trench foot: Neurovascular damage without ice crystal formation following prolonged foot exposure to cold, wet conditions
- Frostbite: Deep tissue damage (skin, muscle, subQ tissue) due to ice crystal formation; primarily on distal extremities, ears, nose, and face
  - Vasoconstriction initially occurs in response to cold temperatures
  - Extracellular ice crystal formation causes intracellular dehydration and hyperosmolarity, resulting in irreversible tissue damage
  - Reperfusion injury occurs with return of blood flow as free radical formation, intracellular edema, vascular leakage, inflammation, and thrombosis lead to necrosis and gangrene
- Frostnip: Superficial ice crystal formation and tissue injury

Differential Dx

- Non-freezing injuries
  - Frostnip (superficial frost-bite)
  - Chilblains (pernio)
  - Immersion foot ("trench foot" or "river rot")
- Freezing injuries (e.g., frostbite)
- Hypothermia

Presentation

- Chilblains: Skin lesions (erythema, plaques, edema, and nodules) progressing to ulcers, vesicles, and blisters; pruritus and paresthesias
- Trench foot: Cool, pale extremity with tingling, numbness, paresthesias, and cold sensitivity
- Superficial frostbite: Skin erythema, edema, hyperemia, pain, and numbness; may develop into blisters, bullae, or eschar
- Deep frostbite: Painful, dry, mottled, mummified skin; necrosis; and/or eschar formation; extremity appears yellow to white and waxy
- Frostnip: Transient numbness and paresthesias

Diagnosis

- Clinical diagnosis based on history and clinical picture

Treatment

- Chilblains: Affected skin should be rewarmed and elevated; nifedipine may prevent symptoms; topical or systemic steroids may speed resolution
- Trench foot: Keep extremity warm, dry, and elevated
- Frostbite
  - Treat systemic hypothermia and rehydrate with IV fluids
  - Avoid friction (*do not* rub with snow)
  - Remove wet or constrictive clothes
  - Field rewarming is rarely practical
  - Rapid and active rewarming of the affected areas by immersion in circulating water at 37–40°C for 10–30 minutes (until pliable with distal erythema)—premature termination of thawing is a common mistake
  - Debride clear blisters and apply topical aloe vera (decreases inflammation) and non-constrictive dressings
  - IV analgesia for intense pain associated with reperfusion
  - NSAIDs decrease arachidonic acid-mediated damage
  - Tetanus prophylaxis
  - Consider antibiotics for *Staphylococcus, Streptococcus*

Disposition

- Except for minor cases, all patients should be admitted for 24–48 hours to determine extent of injuries and address systemic hypothermia
- Final demarcation between viable and non-viable tissue may require 2–3 months
- Avoid all vasoconstrictive agents (including nicotine)
- Sequelae from frostbite injuries include intense pain, cold sensitivity, hyperhydrosis, and vasomotor paralysis, which may last for years
- Sensation will not return until healing is complete
- Surgical decisions regarding amputation are best deferred for 1–2 months

166. Heat-Related Illness

Etiology & Pathophysiology

- Illness may be due to increased internal heat production (e.g., infection, exertion) or decreased heat loss due to impaired sweating or rate of evaporation (e.g., warm ambient temperature with high humidity, dehydration)
- Heat edema: Vasodilatation results in peripheral pooling of fluid
- Heat rash ("prickly heat"): Rash due to blockage of sweat glands
- Heat syncope: Postural syncope due to heat-induced volume depletion and dehydration
- Heat cramps: Cramps occur due to Na^+ and K^+ loss in sweat
- Heat exhaustion: A more severe heat illness due to salt and water depletion that is associated with mildly elevated core temperatures
- Heat stroke: A life-threatening illness due to high core temperatures (>40°C) associated with failure of thermoregulatory control
- High-risk groups include infants, the elderly, and drug users

Differential Dx

- Heat syncope: Cardiac arrhythmia, CVA, pulmonary embolus, hypoglycemia
- Heatstroke: Bacterial infection, meningitis/encephalitis, sepsis, seizures, cerebral hemorrhage, thyroid storm, DKA, malignant hyperthermia, neuroleptic malignant syndrome, anticholinergic toxicity, alcohol withdrawal, salicylate overdose, cocaine, PCP, serotonin syndrome

Presentation

- Heat edema: Mild swelling and tightness of the extremities
- Heat rash: Pruritic, maculopapular rash in areas covered by clothing
- Heat syncope: Transient, postural loss of consciousness
- Heat cramps: Muscle cramps
- Heat exhaustion: Dizziness, weakness, malaise, light-headedness, N/V, tachycardia, tachypnea, diaphoresis (with normal mental status)
- Heat stroke: Altered mental status (irritability, confusion, ataxia, seizure, hallucinations, coma), high core temperature, tachycardia, anhidrosis, and hypotension

Diagnosis

- Heat edema, prickly heat, and heat cramps are clinical diagnoses
- Heat syncope should be evaluated as appropriate in patients with syncope; however, do not assume that heat was the actual cause of syncope
- Core temperature is often ≤40°C in heat exhaustion and >40°C in heat stroke
- Check CBC, electrolytes, LFTs, PT/PTT, CPK, and toxicology screen in severe cases of heat illness (in heat stroke, thrombocytopenia, hypokalemia, hypernatremia, hypocalcemia, elevated LFTs, or rhabdomyolysis may be present)
- Head CT may be required to rule out other disease processes in patients with mental status changes
- Lumbar puncture and blood cultures should be considered if infection cannot be ruled out

Treatment

- Antipyretics are ineffective in environmentally related heat illness (pyrogens are not the cause of the hyperthermia)
- Mild heat illness and heat exhaustion
  - Rest, remove from heat, and wear loose clothing
  - Aggressively replace lost fluids and electrolytes
  - Antihistamines for prickly heat
  - Support hose for heat edema (diuretics are ineffective)
- Heat stroke
  - May require intubation for decreased mental status
  - Aggressive volume replacement with IV fluids
  - Closely monitor core temperature
  - Methods of cooling include removal of clothing, evaporative cooling by spraying the patient with water and fanning, application of ice packs to groin and axillae, immersion in cool water, cold gastric lavage, and invasive cooling methods (e.g., peritoneal lavage, cardiopulmonary bypass)
  - Discontinue cooling at 39°C to prevent hypothermia
  - Treat shivering due to cooling with benzodiazepines

Disposition

- Other causes of hyperthermia must be ruled out—do not assume an illness is environmentally caused
- Discharge patients with heat exhaustion, heat syncope, heat cramps, or prickly heat
- Admit all patients with heatstroke
- Mortality of heatstroke is 10–25%, but is improved by rapid cooling
- Complications of heatstroke include rhabdomyolysis, CHF, liver injury, DIC, cerebral edema, liver failure, renal failure, hypoglycemia, lactic acidosis, and ARDS

167. High Altitude Illness

Etiology & Pathophysiology

- Barometric pressure decreases with increasing altitude—at high altitudes, oxygen concentration remains constant at 21% but the partial pressure of oxygen (21% of barometric pressure) decreases, resulting in hypobaric hypoxemia
- Hyperventilation ensues in an attempt to correct the hypoxemia; however, increases in respiratory rate are limited by the onset of respiratory alkalosis
- Additionally, in acute altitude illness fluid is retained secondary to sympathetic stimulation (i.e., increased ADH, renin, and angiotensin), which may result in pulmonary and cerebral edema
- Acclimatization occurs when the kidneys produce a compensatory metabolic acidosis (by excreting bicarbonate), allowing a further increase in respiratory rate to better compensate for hypoxemia
- Symptoms of altitude illness begin to occur at 8,000–10,000 feet elevation; at altitudes over 18,000 feet acclimatization is impossible

Differential Dx

- Acute mountain sickness (AMS): Rapid ascent prevents acclimatization
- High altitude pulmonary edema (HAPE): Non-cardiogenic edema due to fluid retention plus hypoxic pulmonary vaso-constriction
- High altitude cerebral edema (HACE): Neurologic deterioration following AMS or HAPE as hypoxia and fluid retention increase cerebral blood flow
- Worsening of pre-existing disease

Presentation

- AMS: Headache, fatigue, lightheadedness, nausea, anorexia, difficulty sleeping, irritability, and dyspnea
- HAPE: Symptoms of AMS plus dyspnea at rest, cough, peripheral cyanosis, and fever; exam reveals crackles, tachypnea, and tachycardia
- HACE: Symptoms of AMS and HAPE plus neurologic deterioration (cerebellar ataxia, seizures, altered mental status, nausea, vomiting, and/or focal neurologic deficits)

Diagnosis

- Clinical diagnoses based on symptom onset in the setting of a recent change in altitude
- ECG may show evidence of right heart strain, including right axis deviation and R waves in the precordial leads (due to hypoxic pulmonary vasoconstriction)
- Arterial blood gas reveals hypoxemia, respiratory alkalosis (increased pH with decreased pCO_2), and may show a compensatory metabolic acidosis (decreased HCO_3)
- Chest X-ray in HAPE shows patchy alveolar infiltrates, which differ from the diffuse cephalization pattern of cardiogenic pulmonary edema
- Head CT in HACE may show decreased space in the sulci (due to edema) or may be normal

Treatment

- Immediate descent and hyperbaric oxygen therapy is the definitive treatment for all altitude illnesses (hyperbaric chamber simulates descent but should only be considered a stopgap measure until descent can be arranged)
- Supplemental O_2
- Avoid narcotics and sedatives (may result in respiratory depression, which can worsen the hypoxemia)
- AMS
  - Symptomatic treatment with NSAIDs and anti-emetics
  - Acetazolamide aids in acclimatization by causing HCO_3 diuresis (aiding kidneys to produce metabolic acidosis)
- HAPE/HACE
  - Noninvasive positive pressure ventilation (CPAP or BiPAP) to provide respiratory support
  - IV dexamethasone to decrease edema
  - Consider nifedipine, loop diuretics, and morphine
- Prophylactic therapies for high altitude illness include acetazolamide, slow graduated ascent, and a high carbohydrate diet

Disposition

- Incidence and magnitude of symptoms depend on the rate of ascent, final altitude, and duration at altitude
- Symptoms occur in 25% of tourists to the western US and 67% of climbers on Mount Rainier
- Conditions are generally reversible if caught and treated early
- AMS is usually a self-limited illness with a peak in symptoms at 24–48 hours
- 60% of those with HACE who develop coma will die
- Significant and life-threatening symptoms may result from exacerbation of chronic medical conditions (e.g., COPD, coronary artery disease) when the patient is subjected to the stress of high altitudes

168. Dysbarism

Etiology & Pathophysiology

- Properties of gases include Boyle's law (volume of a gas varies inversely with pressure), Dalton's law (total pressure of gases equals the sum of their partial pressures), and Henry's law (the amount of gas dissolved in solution varies directly with pressure)
- Barotrauma: Direct tissue damage due to gas contraction/expansion in enclosed spaces following a pressure change (e.g., descent, ascent)
- Arterial gas embolism: A complication of pulmonary barotrauma; gas expansion causes rupture of pulmonary veins, allowing air into the circulation to form emboli
- Nitrogen narcosis: Elevated blood nitrogen levels occur due to high pressures, resulting in mental status changes
- Decompression sickness: High pressure (e.g., deep sea diving) increases tissue nitrogen content; rapid ascent then forces nitrogen out of solution, forming bubbles in the circulation that cause vascular occlusion, tissue injury, systemic inflammation, and organ damage

Differential Dx

- Barotrauma of descent (ear or sinuses)
- Barotrauma of ascent (lung, tooth, or GI)
- Arterial gas embolism
- Nitrogen narcosis
- Decompression sickness
- Trauma
- Hypoxia
- Hypercarbia
- Near drowning
- Hypothermia
- Marine animal bite
- Intracranial hemorrhage

Presentation

- Ear barotrauma: Pain, fullness, TM rupture, bloody drainage, vertigo
- Sinus barotrauma: Pain, pressure
- Pulmonary barotrauma: Dyspnea, chest pain, subQ emphysema
- Arterial embolism: Sudden loss of consciousness, CNS symptoms, paraplegia, cardiac ischemia
- Decompression sickness: Joint pain ("the bends"), skin rash, neurologic symptoms (paraplegia, paraparesis, bowel/bladder dysfunction, ataxia), subcutaneous emphysema, lung edema with cough and dyspnea
- Nitrogen narcosis: Mental status changes, loss of consciousness, and memory impairment

Diagnosis

- Diagnosis is made clinically based on history and exam
  - Type of diving and equipment
  - Number, time, and depth of recent dives
  - Amount (if any) of underwater decompression
  - Dive complications (marine animal envenomation, equipment malfunction)
  - Onset of symptoms—nitrogen narcosis occurs during the dive, arterial gas embolism occurs immediately after the dive (<10 minutes), and decompression sickness occurs >10 minutes after the dive
- Obtain CXR if there is any suspicion of pulmonary barotrauma (may show subcutaneous air, mediastinal air, or pneumothorax)
- Labwork may include CBC, electrolytes, and renal function
- Brain MRI may show evidence of air emboli but should not delay hyperbaric therapy

Treatment

- Pre-hospital air transport must fly below 1,000 feet and avoid pressurized planes to prevent worsening of symptoms
- Treat hypothermia with warming blankets and other means
- Administer 100% supplemental O_2 to force nitrogen from the blood and facilitate its removal from the body
- Intubate as needed for oxygenation and airway control—avoid high pressures and PEEP as they may increase the risk of arterial gas emboli
- IV fluids (normal saline) are generally required due to concurrent volume depletion
- Treatment of ear and sinus barotrauma includes antihistamines, decongestants (topical and oral), antibiotics for TM rupture, and avoidance of diving until congestion clears
- Arterial gas embolism and decompression sickness require immediate hyperbaric oxygen therapy (the recompression chamber will provide both oxygen and pressure); the patient should remain supine to prevent cerebral air embolism

Disposition

- Pressure is force per unit area—on the surface, pressure is 1 atmosphere pressure absolute (ATA); at 33 feet depth the pressure is 2 ATA, at 99 feet the pressure is 4 ATA
- Admit all patients with arterial gas embolism, decompression sickness, or nitrogen narcosis
- Observe other patients and discharge after 4–6 hours if they remain asymptomatic
- Arterial gas embolism may cause rapid death depending on the site of embolus
- Hyperbaric therapy can substantially improve outcomes if instituted early

169. Near Drowning

Etiology & Pathophysiology

- Drowning: Death from suffocation following submersion (>4000 deaths per year in the US)
- Near drowning: Survival after suffocation following submersion
- Secondary drowning: Death due to complications >24 hours after submersion
- After submersion, forced inspiration and vomiting occur due to rising $PaCO_2$ and diminishing PaO_2 levels; water and emesis are then aspirated
- Water and emesis in the alveoli cause direct alveolar flooding, breakdown of surfactant, and alveolar-capillary membrane damage
- End result is lung injury/edema, atelectasis, V/Q mismatch, and poor diffusion; leading to hypoxemia, hypercarbia, and respiratory failure
- Eventually, non-cardiogenic pulmonary edema develops due to direct lung injury, loss of surfactant, and inflammation
- Hypoxia and injury of neurologic, renal, and other organ systems occurs

Differential Dx

- Trauma
- Spinal cord injury (e.g., diving injury)
- Hypoglycemia
- Alcohol intoxication
- Drug ingestion
- Hypothermia
- Myocardial infarction
- Arrhythmia
- Electrolyte abnormality
- Seizure
- Syncope
- Child abuse

Presentation

- Peak incidence in infants, teenagers, and the elderly
- Presenting symptoms depend on the duration of immersion
- May be asymptomatic
- Respiratory symptoms may be mild (e.g., cough, dyspnea, tachypnea) or severe (e.g., respiratory distress and respiratory failure with associated hypoxemia, cyanosis, and altered mental status)
- Cardiac arrest
- The most feared complication is severe hypoxic brain injury
- Other complications include hypothermia, seizures, arrhythmias, bronchospasm, and hypotension

Diagnosis

- Perform a complete neurologic exam and Glasgow coma score
- CBC and electrolytes are usually normal but may be abnormal in ingestions of salt water or large volumes of fresh water
- Check glucose to rule out hypoglycemia
- Blood alcohol level and toxicology screen as indicated
- Arterial blood gas may reveal hypoxemia or a combined metabolic and respiratory acidosis
- Chest X-ray may show diffuse non-cardiogenic pulmonary edema or perihilar infiltrates
- ECG may show sequelae of acidosis or hypothermia
- C-spine X-rays may be necessary to clear the spine, especially in diving injuries

Treatment

- Maintain spinal precautions and assume a C-spine injury is present until proven otherwise
- Pre-hospital care should include C-spine precautions, CPR, supplemental oxygen, and establishment of an airway by intubation if necessary ("drainage" of the lungs or Heimlich maneuver is not helpful as there is typically only a minimal volume of water in the lungs)
- ED care is primarily supportive
    - Treat cardiopulmonary arrest per ACLS protocols
    - Ensure oxygenation and maintain airway (intubate for hypoxemia, poor respiratory effort, declining respiratory status, or inability to protect airway)
    - Treat hypothermia by warming
    - Sodium bicarbonate may be used in profoundly acidotic patients with hemodynamic instability
    - Antibiotics and steroids are *not* indicated for prophylactic pulmonary protection

Disposition

- The majority of patients who are alert or responsive to pain at presentation will survive without neurologic sequelae
- Even those patients who require CPR in the ED may have a good outcome (25% of children with GCS 3 survive with full neurologic recovery)
- Poor prognostic indicators include fixed dilated pupils, need for cardiac medications, and GCS <5
- Admit patients who require ventilatory support and those with moderate pulmonary symptoms (e.g., cough, dyspnea, tachypnea, hypoxemia)
- Discharge patients with minimal submersions who are asymptomatic or minimally symptomatic
- Long-term sequelae include ischemic encephalopathy, aspiration pneumonia, ARDS, and chronic lung disease

170. Lightning and Electrical Injuries

Etiology & Pathophysiology

- Types of electrical currents include household (110–220 volts), high-voltage (>600 volts), and lightning (1 million volts)
- Electron flow is measured in amps, which is directly proportional to flow and indirectly proportional to resistance (e.g., wet skin or water immersion results in less resistance and greater flow)
- Alternating current (AC) may cause muscle tetany, preventing the victim from letting go; direct current (DC) causes muscle contraction, which throws the victim off the source
- Household current is AC and causes half of all electrical deaths (due to ventricular fibrillation) but rarely causes deep tissue damage
- High voltage current is DC (power line, construction, or agricultural workers, MVAs) and often results in large amounts of soft tissue damage below normal-appearing skin
- Lightning is DC and causes asystole, but rarely causes deep tissue injury because it flows over, rather than through, the body

Differential Dx

- Thermal burn
- CVA
- Seizure
- Closed head injury
- Spinal cord injury
- Hypertensive encephalopathy
- Cardiac arrhythmia
- Cardiac ischemia/myocardial infarction
- Toxic ingestion
- Envenomation
- Hypoglycemia

Presentation

- Household current symptoms range from mild tingling to pain, local burns, tetanic contractions, dislocations, fractures, and Vfib
- High voltage/lightning injuries
  - Skin burns (entry/exit wounds)
  - Tissue damage below intact skin (severe in high voltage, minimal in lightning burns)
  - Respiratory arrest
  - Asystole/arrhythmias
  - CNS symptoms (e.g., confusion, coma, paresis, seizures, loss of consciousness, cerebral edema)
  - Compartment syndrome
  - Dislocations and/or fractures
  - Eye injury
  - Tympanic membrane rupture

Diagnosis

- ECG and cardiac monitoring are indicated in all electrical injury
  - High voltage or lightning strike may show asystole or ischemic changes (however, these are not due to acute coronary vessel closure)
  - Household current may cause ventricular fibrillation
- Household current injuries do not require testing beyond ECG
- CBC, electrolytes, renal function, CPK, CK-MB, and myoglobin should be ordered in high voltage and lightning injuries
- Head CT and C-spine films in patients with altered mental status
- Skin feathering (Lichtenberg figures) is a superficial, non-burn, fernlike skin marking that is pathognomonic for lightning strike
- Technetium[99] muscle scan to show areas of dead or damaged muscle is sometimes obtained before fasciotomy

Treatment

- Burn care should include administration of large fluid volumes due to 3rd spacing into damaged tissues (monitor for cerebral edema if CNS injury is suspected)
- Treat arrhythmias per ACLS protocols—prolonged CPR/ACLS may be effective in restoring rhythm
- High voltage/lightning injury
  - Immobilize spine and secure airway as needed
  - Administer IV antibiotics if muscle is injured
  - Fasciotomy/debridement may be required in the presence of deep tissue injury due to high voltage (rare in lightning injury)—indications for emergent fasciotomy include extensive deep limb burns, marked limb edema, and decreased distal pulses or nerve function
- Lightning injury triage is an exception to standard mass casualty protocols—ignore moving/awake victims and provide immediate care to non-moving patients who have reversible asystolic cardiac arrest and often have good neurologic recovery
- Watch for evidence of increased ICP in lightning strikes
- Treat rhabdomyolysis with IV fluids, alkalinization, diuretics

Disposition

- Both high and low voltage injuries may be fatal, primarily due to cardiac arrest
- Admit all high voltage injuries, all lightning injuries, and any household current injuries with systemic injury
- Discharge household injuries with minimal burns, normal ECG, and no ectopy on the monitor
- Complications of high voltage injury or lightning strike include arrhythmia, renal failure, infection/sepsis, neuropathy, amputation, cataracts, hearing loss, neurologic deficits (spasticity, confusion), pancreatitis, scarring, and depression
- Lightning current tends to pass over the body rather than through it, thereby causing much less deep tissue damage, compartment syndrome, rhabdomyolysis, and renal failure

171. Radiation Exposure

Etiology & Pathophysiology

- Effects of radiation exposure depend on the dose received and the type of radiation
- Radiation dose adsorbed is measured in rads and gray (1 Gy = 100 rads)
- Exposure may be internal (via inhalation, ingestion or through wounds/mucosa) or external (on skin or clothing)
- Types of radiation include γ-rays and X-rays (penetrate deep into the body), β-rays (moderate penetration), and α-rays (minimal penetration with damage only occurring if an emitter is inhaled or ingested)
- Nuclear weapon radiation may be confined to the radioactive device itself or may be widely distributed (local distribution from a "dirty bomb" or atmospheric distribution from a nuclear plant or nuclear weapon)
- Rapidly dividing cells are the most susceptible to radiation effects

Differential Dx

- Nuclear weapons
- Nuclear reactors (power plants, university research facilities)
- Spent nuclear fuel rods
- "Dirty bombs" (conventional explosives laced with a radioactive material that is spread upon detonation)
- Radiopharmaceutical agents
- Radiotherapy machines
- X-ray machines

Presentation

- Local exposure causes a radiation burn that appears days later as redness, blistering, and desquamation
- Prodromal phase of systemic exposures includes nausea, vomiting, diarrhea, and fatigue
- Latent phase is a symptom-free interval following the prodromal phase (length depends on the dose received—may last from hours to weeks)
- Illness phase occurs with GI, bone marrow, CNS, and/or cardiac symptoms

Diagnosis

- Geiger counter, dose rate meter, or radiation survey meter
- CBC changes occur within 48 hrs: Reveals decreased cell lines—anemia, thrombocytopenia, leukopenia, and/or lymphopenia
- Acute radiation syndrome may result from whole body exposure
    - 1 Gy: Nausea/vomiting
    - 2 Gy: Nausea/vomiting, bone marrow suppression
    - 6 Gy: Severe bone marrow failure
    - 10–30 Gy: Severe GI damage and interstitial pneumonitis for one week; further GI symptoms and sepsis after 2 weeks
    - >30 Gy: Nausea, vomiting, hypotension, ataxia, and convulsions; severe cardiovascular and CNS damage; death
- Hematopoietic syndrome: Bone marrow suppression may cause pancytopenia with infection, hemorrhage, and death
- GI syndrome: Mucosal damage causes fluid and electrolyte loss; sepsis may develop from systemic invasion of enteric flora
- Cardiovascular and CNS syndromes: Refractory hypotension and cerebral edema, universally fatal within 24–72 hours

Treatment

- Health care providers must wear mask, gown, and gloves to keep radiation exposure of medical personnel to <10 rads
- Administer IV fluids, antiemetics, and pain control
- Radiation burn: Local burn care (may require plastic surgery repair) and pain control with NSAIDs and narcotics
- External contamination: Remove and bag clothing; wash with soap and water
- Therapy for internal contaminations depends on the involved agent
    - Tritium: Copious IV fluids
    - Iodine: Potassium iodide
    - Cesium or strontium: Prussian blue and antacids to decrease GI uptake
    - Plutonium: Chelation therapy
- Inpatient care may include a bone marrow transplant in those with >8 Gy exposure; however, this may be a moot point, as patients frequently die from GI damage
- Hematopoietic growth factors are under investigation
- Other investigational medications include amifostene and androstenediol

Disposition

- Good disaster management is the key to improving survival and limiting exposure of health care providers and the general population to radiation
- Significant GI damage is virtually always fatal
- Lymphocyte count at 24 hours is a good indicator of prognosis
- Mortality is based on dose of radiation
    - 4 Gy: 50% without treatment will die
    - >6 Gy: 100% without treatment will die
    - 10–30 Gy: Vast majority die in 2–3 weeks even with therapy
    - >30 Gy: All die within 24–72 hours
- Exposed cells have an increased risk of malignant transformation
- Contact REACTS (Radiation emergency assistance center/training site) for questions and an emergency response team: (865) 576-1005

172. Dog, Cat, and Human Bite Wounds

Etiology & Pathophysiology

- The most common bite wounds in the ED are those from humans, cats, and dogs (but may be from any animal)
- Wound infection is common (80% of cat bites and 5% of dog bites become infected), especially with *Streptococcus, Staphylococcus,* or anaerobes (e.g., *Bacteroides*)
- Involved organisms may be suspected based on the type of bite
    - Cat bites: *Pasteurella, Moraxella, Neisseria*
    - Dog bites: *Capnocytophaga cynodegmi, Pasteurella*
    - Human bites: *Streptococcus viridans, Eikenella*
- *Pasteurella* infection is characterized by extremely rapid development and spread within 2–24 hours
- Risk of infection depends on the animal, wound location, type of wound, foreign bodies, delay to treatment, and co-morbid conditions

Differential Dx

Presentation

- Note location and size of injury
- Rule out joint involvement or tendon injury
- Dog bites usually result in crush or tear injuries
- Cat bites cause puncture wounds
- Human bites tend to be superficial
- Closed fist injury is a human bite wound that occurs over the dorsal 5th MCP joint when the fist strikes a mouth during an altercation (high rate of infection)
- Infected wounds present with erythema, warmth, discharge, swelling, lymphangitis, adenopathy, fever, and/or signs of flexor tenosynovitis

Diagnosis

- X-ray is indicated if associated fracture, osteomyelitis, or joint space involvement is suspected, in all closed fist injuries, and in most cat bites to rule out retained tooth fragments
- Wound culture is required if wound infection is present
- Blood culture should be considered in systemically ill patients

Treatment

- Administer tetanus toxoid if not up-to-date
- Wash copiously and debride as necessary
- Suture cosmetically significant wounds of the scalp, face, trunk, and proximal extremities
- Allow healing by secondary intention in wounds at a high risk of infection, puncture wounds, and hand wounds
- Antibiotics should be prescribed for all moderate-to-high risk wounds and for all distal extremity wounds
- Outpatient antibiotic regimens include amoxicillin/clavulanic acid alone or clindamycin plus either ciprofloxacin or TMP/SMX (or cefuroxime or doxycycline in cat bites)
- Inpatient IV antibiotic regimens include a penicillin/anti-penicillinase, cefoxitin, or a combination of clindamycin plus ciprofloxacin
- Rabies immunoprophylaxis for dog or cat bites includes rabies immune globulin (injected at wound site) plus vaccine
    - If the animal is healthy and can be observed for 10 days, treatment is only needed if the animal develops symptoms
    - If the animal is rabid, immediate treatment is required
    - If the animal is unknown, consult public health services

Disposition

- Consult hand surgery for any tendon injury, joint involvement, or fractures
- Admit patients with extensive or complicated infections (joint or tendon involvement), significant risk factors for serious infection, foreign body, infected closed fist injury, or failure to respond to antibiotics
- Discharge patients with no or minimal infection with follow-up in 24 hours
- Complications include wound infection, tenosynovitis, septic arthritis, osteomyelitis, sepsis, and exsanguination (due to large blood vessel injury)
- *Pasteurella* may cause sepsis, osteomyelitis, and septic arthritis
- *Capnocytophagia* may cause sepsis, DIC, renal failure, and endocarditis

173. Snakebite

Etiology & Pathophysiology

- 8,000 bites/year in the US with about 10 deaths
- Venomous snakes in the US include crotalids (hemotoxic venom), elapids (neurotoxic venom), and exotic species kept as pets or in zoos (mostly elapids)
- Elapid neurotoxic venom affects neuromuscular transmission
- Crotalid hemotoxic venom causes hemolysis, necrosis, DIC, and endothelial damage with vascular leakage, decreased intravascular volume, and hemorrhage
- Crotalids cause 98% of all US bites; they strike once, inject venom, and release; 25% of bites do not have associated envenomation
- Coral snake elapids do not inject venom; they chew prey causing a venom exposure; >50% have no envenomation
- Exotic elapids usually inject venom
- Risk of systemic effects depends on snake type, amount of venom injected, bite location, and the health status of the victim

Differential Dx

- Crotalids (pit vipers) include rattlesnakes, copperheads, cottonmouth/water moccasins; characterized by a facial pit, elliptical pupils, and triangular head
- Coral snakes are the only indigenous US elapids; red bands bordered by yellow ("red on yellow kill a fellow, red on black venom lack"), round head, and round pupils
- Exotic elapids include cobras, Australian brown snakes, tiger snakes, taipans, death adders

Presentation

- Crotalids
  - Puncture marks (may have 1–4)
  - Local symptoms (pain, swelling, erythema, necrosis, edema, ecchymoses)
  - Systemic symptoms (weakness, N/V, numbness/tingling, perioral paresthesias, bruising, tachycardia, shock, death)
- Coral snakes
  - Multiple, painless small wounds
  - Local symptoms of numbness, and fasciculations
  - Systemic symptoms of slurred speech, weakness, CN palsies, dysphagia, diplopia, diaphoresis, respiratory paralysis, and death

Diagnosis

- Identify the type of snake if possible
- Determine seriousness of envenomation
  - None: Puncture wound with no to minimal pain/tenderness
  - Mild: Pain and tenderness at the bite site; perioral paresthesias
  - Moderate: Local symptoms, systemic symptoms, and mild coagulopathy
  - Severe: Severe symptoms of the entire extremity, severe systemic symptoms, and coagulopathy
- Labs may be abnormal in crotalid bites but are usually normal with the neurotoxic coral snake venom
  - CBC may reveal hemolysis
  - PT/PTT, DIC screen reveal coagulation abnormalities
  - Renal function may reveal acute renal failure
  - CPK may be elevated if rhabdomyolysis is present
  - Electrolytes and LFTs may be abnormal
- Do not handle dead snakes as reflex biting may occur

Treatment

- Avoid incision/suction (increased risk of infection), electric shocks, and tourniquets (increased ischemia)
- Avoid excessive activity and immobilize the extremity
- Constriction band at 20 mmHg is used to obstruct superficial venous flow and slow venom spread
- Venom extractor device may be helpful only if applied within 5 minutes of bite
- Supportive care may include intubation, IV fluids, pressors, blood products as needed, and tetanus prophylaxis
- Crotalid antivenom should be administered within 24 hours of bite if systemic symptoms, coagulopathy, or significant or progressive localized injury is present
  - Antivenom (Crotalidae) Polyvalent (ACP) is highly antigenic (allergic, anaphylactic, and serum sickness reactions in up to 50%); a trial skin test or premedication with antihistamines is recommended in most patients
  - Cro-fab antivenom is now the preferred agent as it causes fewer side effects than ACP
- Coral snake antivenin should be administered in all bites
- Antivenom for other exotic snakes may be held at local zoos

Disposition

- Poison control centers and local zoos are good sources for exotic snake information
- If crotalid envenomation occurs, observe for at least 12 hours to ensure that there is no local progression or development of coagulopathy
- Neurotoxic elapid bites should be observed for 24 hours as onset of symptoms may not occur for up to 12 hours; treat early with antivenom, before venom binding to nerve sites occurs
- Admit all patients with systemic symptoms

174. Arthropod Bites

Etiology & Pathophysiology

- Stings and bites may cause severe life-threatening sequelae due to venom toxicity or allergic reactions
- Most patients only develop local symptoms
- Hymenoptera (e.g., bees, hornets, wasps, yellow jackets, ants)
  - May cause a local reaction, systemic toxic reaction (due to envenomation from multiple stings), or anaphylaxis (IgE-mediated)
  - African honeybees ("killer bees") and fire ants are aggressive and are known for causing large numbers of stings at a time
- Brown recluse (*Loxosceles recluse*) bite results in local vasoconstriction and ischemia and/or systemic symptoms
- Black widow (*Latrodectus*) injects a neurotoxic venom that causes acetylcholine release at neural and neuromuscular junctions
- Scorpion bites by US species cause minimal symptoms (except *C. exilicauda,* which may cause cholinergic symptoms via a neurotoxin)

Differential Dx

- Snakebite
- Other arachnids (ticks, scabies, chiggers)
- Other spider species (tarantula, Hobo spider)
- Fleas
- Lice
- Mosquitoes/flies
- Reduviid bugs (e.g., bed bugs)
- Blister beetles
- Caterpillars
- Tetanus
- Dystonic reaction
- Hypocalcemia

Presentation

- Local symptoms (see diagnosis)
- Hymenoptera systemic toxicity: Diarrhea, N/V, syncope, headache, DIC, weakness, renal failure, death
- Hymenoptera anaphylaxis: Urticaria, edema, bronchospasm, airway obstruction, pruritus, hypotension, shock, death
- Brown recluse: Fever, chills, N/V, myalgia, hemolysis, petechiae, DIC
- Black widow: Muscle spasms, severe pain, rigid abdominal or back muscles, HTN, paralysis, shock, respiratory failure, death
- Scorpion: Respiratory failure, HTN, motor hyperactivity, drooling, impaired vision

Diagnosis

- Identify spider types
  - Brown recluse: Small (2 cm); violin shaped mark on thorax
  - Black widow: Larger (5 cm); red hourglass on abdomen (only the female can penetrate human skin)
- Localized bite characteristics
  - Hymenoptera: Pain, erythema, pruritus
  - Brown recluse: A small erythematous area that heals in most patients; some patients have severe pain, erythema, and a blister that develops into necrosis with eschar (up to 20 cm in diameter)
  - Black widow: Immediate pain and erythema with a "target" lesion; localized dull crampy pain and numbness
  - Scorpion: Small painful erythematous area; localized weakness and numbness
- CBC, electrolytes, renal function, PT/PTT, and DIC screen may be ordered if systemic toxicity is suspected

Treatment

- Tetanus prophylaxis in patients who are not up-to-date
- Hymenoptera: Remove stingers, apply ice, supportive care
  - Systemic toxicity: Supportive care only
  - Anaphylaxis: IV epinephrine, antihistamines and H2 blockers, aerosolized β-agonists, and treatment of hypotension with IV fluids, dopamine, & norepinephrine
- Brown recluse: Supportive care and pain control
  - Antivenom is not available
  - Large lesions may require surgical debridement
  - Transfusion with red cells and clotting factors as needed
- Black widow: Supportive care and pain control
  - Administer antivenom in patients with shock, children, elderly, pregnancy, or refractory symptoms
  - Benzodiazepines for muscle relaxation
  - Nitroprusside for severe hypertension
- Scorpion: Supportive care
  - *C. exilicauda* antivenom is available for severe cases
  - Benzodiazepines for muscle spasms
  - Atropine for cholinergic hyperactivity

Disposition

- Admit any patient with persistent systemic signs and symptoms
- Discharge patients with resolution of symptoms or local reactions only
- Hymenoptera: Systemic toxicity is caused by multiple stings at once; anaphylaxis is much more common and may be due to only one sting, but may cause death within minutes
- Brown recluse bites may progress to DIC, renal failure, and death
- Black widow and scorpion bites can cause respiratory muscle spasm with respiratory failure and death
- Patients with severe hymenoptera allergy should be given epinephrine syringes (Epi-pen or Ana-kit) to carry and wear a medic-alert bracelet

175. Marine Injuries

Etiology & Pathophysiology

- Marine predators (e.g., sharks, barracuda, moray eels, giant grouper, alligators, crocodiles) may produce severe, life-threatening wounds
- Sedentary marine fauna, such as coral, barnacles, crabs, and invertebrate shells, may cause injury by incidental contact
- Coelenterates have specialized stinging cells (nematocysts), which contain venom that is directly toxic and may cause anaphylaxis
- Echinodermata have sharp venomous spines, which may become retained foreign bodies
- Other marine envenomations may be due to sponges (spicules cause contact dermatitis), sea snakes (neurotoxic venom), cone shells (neurotoxic venom), stingrays, spiny fish (scorpionfish and stonefish contain venom as strong as a cobra), and octopi
- Bacterial superinfection with marine pathogens may occur (e.g., vibrio species, *Streptococcus, Staphylococcus,* gram negatives, *Mycobacteria marionum, B. fragilis, C. perfringens, E. rhusopathiae*)

Differential Dx

- Sharks
- Coelenterates (e.g., Portuguese man-of-war, jellyfish, fire coral, sea nettles, sea anemones, true corals)
- Echinodermata (e.g., starfish, sea urchins, sea cucumbers)
- Stingrays
- Spiny fish (lionfish, scorpionfish, stonefish, catfish, toadfish)
- Seabathers' eruption
- Swimming pool granuloma
- Fish handler's disease

Presentation

- Predators: Large irregular wounds with injury to underlying structures
- Fauna: Superficial abrasions
- Coelenterates: Pruritic, painful, erythematous, raised eruptions, which may be in linear interlacing arrays and may blister
- Echinodermata: Severely painful puncture wounds with a surrounding irritant dermatitis, local muscle pain, retained foreign body
- Spiny fish: Severe pain, erythema
- Sponges: Local contact dermatitis that may progress to desquamation
- Sea snakes: Fang marks, systemic symptoms with paralysis

Diagnosis

- Focus on the history of the injury, including the geographical location of the event, identification of the offending animal, and the length of time since the encounter
- Obtain plain X-rays to identify foreign bodies if an echinodermata, spiny fish, or sea snake injury is suspected
- CBC, PT/PTT, LFTs, and urinalysis should be ordered if systemic symptoms are present
- Systemic effects of marine envenomation due to coelenterates (Portuguese man-of-war and box jellyfish), echinodermata, spiny fish, or sea snakes may include weakness, nausea/vomiting, diarrhea, vertigo, headache, diaphoresis, syncope, hypotension, anaphylaxis, bronchospasm, respiratory arrest, and death

Treatment

- General wound care should include copious irrigation with removal of foreign bodies, pain control, tetanus prophylaxis, and empiric antibiotics (3rd generation cephalosporin or a quinolone)
- Coelenterates
  - Coepiously irrigate with saline (hypotonic solutions may cause discharge of the nematocysts)
  - Apply 5% acetic acid (vinegar), isopropyl alcohol, olive oil, papain, or urine to deactivate the nematocysts
  - After deactivation, remove nematocysts by application of a flour, talc, or baking soda paste and shaving the area
  - Box jellyfish antivenom is available
- Echinodermata and spiny fish: Hot water immersion should provide symptomatic relief; irrigate and explore for retained spines or foreign bodies
- Sea snakes: Sea snake or crotalidae antivenom should be administered
- Systemic symptoms may require fluids, vasopressors, or intubation

Disposition

- Discharge patients who do not have systemic symptoms with wound care instructions and appropriate follow-up
- Individuals with mild systemic complaints may be observed for 8 hours and discharged
- Admit patients with unstable vital signs, severe systemic symptoms, moderate systemic symptoms that do not resolve, significant comorbidities, or antivenom treatment
- Puncture wounds warrant delayed closure and close follow-up
- India-Pacific box jellyfish has high mortality (20%) due to hypotension and paralysis

176. Mushroom Ingestions

Etiology & Pathophysiology

- Mushrooms are spore-forming fungi that are usually non-toxic
- Toxic mushrooms are classified based on the timing and nature of symptoms they cause
    - GI irritants (e.g., *C. molybdites*): Rapid onset of GI symptoms
    - *Amanita phalloides* (death cap): Hepatotoxicity due to amatoxins and phallotoxins; onset of symptoms 4–6 hours after ingestion
    - *Amanita muscaria*: Causes a muscarinic reaction
    - *Amanita pantherina*: Neurotoxin rapidly causes CNS hyperactivity
    - *Gyromitra*: Gyromitrin toxin metabolites cause CNS hyperactivity (by decreasing GABA) and hepatotoxicity
    - *Cortinarius orellanus*: Results in renal toxicity after 3–20 days
    - Psilocybin (hallucinogenics): Hallucinogenic symptoms
    - Coprinus (inky cap): Disulfiram-like reactions

Differential Dx

- Gastroenteritis
- Bacterial food poisoning
- Heavy metal poisoning (e.g., lead, mercury)

Presentation

- GI irritants: Early onset (1–2 hours) of N/V, diarrhea, abdominal pain
- *A. phalloides:* Late onset (4–12 hrs) of GI symptoms; hepatic failure results in 48–72 hrs
- *A. muscaria*: Cholinergic symptoms—SLUDGE (salivation, lacrimation, urination, diaphoresis, GI upset, emesis)
- *A. pantherina*: Rapid onset of intoxication, dizziness, seizures, and anticholinergic symptoms
- *Gyromitra*: Delayed onset (6–24 hrs) of GI symptoms, ataxia, seizures, delirium, hepatic failure
- *Cortinarius*: Renal failure
- Psilocybin: Hallucination, euphoria

Diagnosis

- Diagnosis is generally clinical
- Patients at risk of toxic ingestion include children (most common), foragers (e.g., naturalists, migrant workers, immigrants), and those who seek hallucinogenic experiences
- Mushroom identification should be undertaken by an experienced mycologist using spore print, spore chromatography, and other testing—identification from books or pictures may be misleading
- Amatoxin-containing mushrooms may be identified with a Meixner test: A drop of HCl is added to the dried liquid mushroom extract; blue color change is positive for amatoxins
- Serum radioimmunoassay is also available
- Gastric aspirate or vomitus may be sent for spore identification
- Check electrolytes, glucose, BUN/creatinine, LFTs, and PT/PTT

Treatment

- Perform GI decontamination with activated charcoal in all mushroom ingestions
- GI irritants require only supportive care with rehydration, antiemetics, and electrolyte repletion
- *A. phalloides*: Silibinin, penicillin G, and hyperbaric oxygen may be used in addition to activated charcoal
- *A. muscarina* reactions: IV fluids and atropine to counteract cholinergic hyperactivity
- *A. pantherina*: Benzodiazepines or barbiturates for CNS hyperactivity
- *Gyromitra*: Pyridoxine and benzodiazepines in those with CNS symptoms
- *Cortinarius*: Hydration and monitoring of urine output and possible hemodialysis; steroids are controversial
- Psilocybin (hallucinogenics): Quiet surroundings and benzodiazepines or barbiturates for agitation
- Disulfiram reaction: Avoid alcohol; administer norepinephrine for severe hypotension and propranolol for tachycardia

Disposition

- Outcomes are predicted by onset of symptoms—early symptom onset indicates minimal toxicity, late onset of symptoms may indicate severe or potentially fatal toxicity
- Discharge patients with early onset of GI symptoms (1–2 hours) with follow-up labs in 24 hours
- Admit patients with late developing symptoms, laboratory abnormalities or a known ingestion of *Amanita, Gyromitra,* or *Cortinarius*
- Full recovery is expected following ingestion of early GI irritants, *A. muscarine, A. pantherina,* and psilocybin
- 30% of *A. phalloides* and *Gyromitra* ingestions result in death
- Persistent renal dysfunction may occur following *Cortinarius* ingestion

Terrorism and Disaster Medicine

CHRISTOPHER R. CARPENTER, MD
SCOTT KAHAN, MD

177. Disaster Medicine

Etiology & Pathophysiology

- A disaster is declared when an event causes injuries of such severity and/or patient volume that normal health care systems are overwhelmed
- Natural disasters have claimed about 3 million lives worldwide over the past two decades with 800 million more adversely affected
- Goal of disaster medicine is to direct limited resources to the greatest number of victims
- National Disaster Medical System (NDMS) coordinates care (among Dept of Defense, FEMA, Dept of Health & Human Services, and others) and provides assistance in areas overwhelmed by disasters (e.g., by evacuating patients who cannot be cared for to appropriate areas)
- Disaster Medical Assistance Teams (DMAT) are formed by NDMS to act as rapid-response medical and support personnel

Differential Dx

- Natural disaster
- Airline crash
- War
- Bombings
- Weapons of mass destruction (nuclear, chemical, biological)
- Environmental accidents
- Disease pandemics

Presentation

- Most patients arrive in ED within 90 minutes of a disaster
- Less severely injured arrive first by EMS-independent means and may delay treatment of the more critically injured patients who arrive shortly thereafter
- Anticipate problems (e.g., supply shortages, loss of communications, overcrowding, power failure, hospital damage)
- Most lives saved are within the first two days after the disaster

Diagnosis

- Victims may require decontamination prior to entering the ED—do not allow ED staff to become incapacitated by exposure to toxic agents
- Immediate health concerns include aspiration, burns, smoke inhalation, blast injuries, crush injuries, hypothermia, radiation exposure, and loss of medication
- Delayed health concerns include diarrhea, food or water shortage, measles, meningitis, pulmonary edema, wound infections, homelessness, and population shift

Treatment

- First responder
  - Personal safety is the first responsibility
  - Identify damages, urgent needs, and available resources
- Emergency Department Triage Categories
  - Red: Life-threatening condition which can be stabilized with immediate care (e.g., hypoxia)
  - Yellow: Decompensation will occur if injury is untreated but a sixty-minute delay should be tolerated (e.g., stable penetrating trauma)
  - Green: Patient will remain stable even if untreated for hours (e.g., contusions, minor lacerations)
  - Black: Unresponsive patient without spontaneous ventilation or circulation or with a severe injury not expected to survive—do not waste resources on these patients while salvageable patients decompensate

Disposition

- Hospital space should be functionally divided
  - Disaster command
  - Decontamination
  - Triage
  - Registration
  - Patient care
  - Pre-op
  - Surgery
  - Morgue
  - Family waiting
  - Public relations
- Patient care stations should be established and may include resuscitation, major illness/injury, and primary care

178. Chemical Weapons

Etiology & Pathophysiology

- Nerve agents: Tabun (GA), sarin (GB), soman (GD), GF, and VX gases inhibit acetylcholinesterase, resulting in accumulation of acetylcholine in nerve synapses and syndromes of cholinergic excess
- Incapacitating agents: Mace (chloroacetophenone), tear gas (ortho-chloro-benzalmalonitrile) and pepper spray (coleoresin capsicum) irritate exposed mucosa and skin
- Pulmonary agents (choking agents): Chlorine and phosgene cause airway damage/irritation
- Vesicants (blister agents): Sulfur mustard and Lewisite produce irreversible cutaneous damage to skin, eyes, and respiratory mucosa within minutes of exposure

Differential Dx

- Nerve agents
  - Gastroenteritis
  - Organophosphate exposure
  - Seizure disorder
  - Sepsis
- Respiratory distress
  - Asthma exacerbation
  - Hypersensitivity reaction
  - Pulmonary infection
- Skin irritation
  - Caustic exposure
  - Hypersensitivity reaction

Presentation

- Nerve agents: SLUDGE mnemonic for cholinergic excess (salivation, lacrimation, urination, diarrhea, gastric distress, and emesis); large exposures cause seizures and bradycardia; miosis usually indicates a lethal dose
- Incapacitating agents: Extreme pain in eyes, skin, and upper respiratory tract
- Pulmonary agents: Airway burning/irritation and non-cardiogenic pulmonary edema within 8 hours of exposure
- Vesicants: Skin blisters, eye damage, respiratory tract irritation/damage

Diagnosis

- Diagnosis depends primarily on clinical presentation—only the military has tests/monitors to rapidly determine the presence of most chemical weapons
- Nerve agents: Recognize SLUDGE toxidrome; erythrocyte acetylcholinesterase level can be measured to document exposure and monitor recovery
- Incapacitating agents: Recognize intentional/accidental exposure and irritation of exposed organs
- Pulmonary agents become low-lying gases due to their high density; phosgene smells of sweet hay; symptoms correlate directly with level of activity during exposure
- Vesicants have low mortality but incapacitate victims for 1–4 months following exposure
  - Mustard produces pruritic erythema within one day of exposure, while airway injury typically manifests within 6 hours—urinary thiodiglycol level may be elevated
  - Urinary arsenic levels may be elevated after Lewisite exposure

Treatment

- Medical staff should use protective garments (MOPP gear) and decontaminate victims immediately
- Decontamination site should be isolated from the ED; use either soap and water or diluted hypochlorite (household bleach) solution
- Intubation may be necessary for respiratory muscle weakness or direct lung damage due to exposures
- Nerve agent exposures require IV therapy to reverse effects
  - IV atropine competitively inhibits acetylcholine
  - IV pralidoxime reactivates acetylcholinesterase
  - Diazepam prevents seizures
- Incapacitating agent exposures are self-limited; remove patient from environment and irrigate copiously
- Pulmonary agent exposures should be treated with supplemental O_2 oxygen, strict bed rest, inhaled β-agonists (e.g., albuterol), NSAIDs, and IV steroids
- Vesicant exposures generally only require supportive care; parenteral dimercaprol may be administered within 2 hours of Lewisite exposure

Disposition

- Nerve agents: Optimum observation time following exposure is not well defined; intubated patients may require days of supportive care prior to extubation; death usually occurs in minutes
- Pulmonary agents: Patients with pulmonary edema within 6 hours of exposure are unlikely to survive; those with normal pulmonary exam 12 hours after exposure may be discharged home; those with mild cough require re-evaluation every 1–2 hours
- Vesicants: Initial ventilatory support is usually only required by those with pre-existing airway disease; however, as time passes more patients can be expected to require intervention

179. Biological Weapons

Etiology & Pathophysiology

- Made from biological organisms or the products of biological organisms and disseminated via aerosol sprays, explosives, or food/water contamination
- Biological agents are attractive because they are easy to acquire, easy to use, inexpensive, invisible and odorless, have a long incubation period to allow spread of agent, and are difficult to identify
- See associated entries for anthrax and smallpox
- *C. botulinum* produces a potent, lethal toxin that irreversibly prevents acetylcholine release, causing muscle paralysis
- Plague *(Yersinia pestis)* causes 3 forms of disease (bubonic, pneumonic, and septicemic) with high person-to-person transmission; 100% mortality for pneumonic plague if untreated
- Hemorrhagic fever viruses (Ebola, Hantavirus, and Dengue fever)
- Other potential biological weapons include tularemia, brucellosis, cholera, Q fever, viral encephalitis

Differential Dx

- Coagulopathy
- Pneumonia
- Endocarditis
- Food poisoning
- Chemical agent
- Gastroenteritis
- Meningitis
- PCP/AIDS
- URI
- Varicella (chickenpox)
- Viral syndrome
- Guillain-Barré syndrome
- Myasthenia gravis
- Vector-borne diseases

Presentation

- Botulism: Difficulty speaking, ptosis, diplopia, dysphagia, and weakness with eventual paralysis and respiratory failure
- Plague: Fever, chills, headache, malaise, purulent inguinal lymphadenitis (bubonic form), sepsis, pneumonia
- Hemorrhagic fever: Prodromal malaise, fever, headaches, and abdominal pain followed 3–5 days later by petechiae and diffuse bleeding (some variants, such as Hantavirus, have renal involvement)

Diagnosis

- *If you do not think about it, you will not find it*—the initial presentations may be vague but awareness of unusual patterns should trigger further inquiry
- Recognize epidemiologic clues to biological weapon attacks
  –Presence of an unusually large number of patients with similar symptoms (particularly young, healthy patients)
  –Many unexplained deaths
  –Disease refractory to standard therapy
  –Historical similarities between cases (e.g., same food, plane)
  –Dead or dying animals in the community
  –Atypical illness for a population or age group
- Botulism: Assays are available for toxin in serum
- Plague: CSF, sputum, or lymph node aspirates reveal bipolar "safety pin"-shaped organisms
- Hemorrhagic fever: Diagnostic assay and genetic sequencing are not readily available in the ED; leukopenia and DIC are common

Treatment

- Gown, gloves, and HEPA-filter mask should be worn by all health care personnel
- Decontamination via removal of clothing and soap and water wash is probably sufficient for inhaled biological agents
- Patient must remain in isolation
- Vaccines have variable efficacy (available for anthrax, plague, yellow fever, tularemia, and some causes of hemorrhagic fever; smallpox vaccine supplies are being replaced following the attacks of 2001)
- Botulism: Treat with antitoxin and supportive care
- Plague: Streptomycin, tetracycline, doxycycline, ciprofloxacin, and chloramphenicol are also useful if given within 24 hours of the onset of pulmonary symptoms
- Hemorrhagic fever: Aggressive volume/pressure support, IV ribavirin for Hantavirus, supportive care for Ebola

Disposition

- Early involvement of health department, poison control center, and law enforcement officials can quickly mobilize available resources and prevent panic and further dissemination of the agent
- Isolated cases and first presenters may be missed due to non-specific presentations; however, as numbers and severity increase, the likely etiology will quickly become apparent
- Early public health response is essential to containment and management
- In a suspected biological attack, the FBI, county health department, local hospitals, and CDC should be immediately alerted

180. Anthrax

Etiology & Pathophysiology

- Caused by *Bacillus anthracis,* a gram positive spore-forming rod
- *B. anthracis* is ubiquitous in soil—naturally occurring anthrax is a disease of domesticated animals with human cases resulting only by contact with infected animals or animal products (human-to-human transmission is very rare); virtually unknown in Western countries that immunize livestock
- Weaponized anthrax are highly lethal spore forms that are relatively easy to produce and stable in the environment; developed in weapons programs by countries and autonomous groups (e.g., Aum Shinrikyo sect, known for the 1995 Tokyo subway sarin gas attack)
- Cutaneous anthrax (>95% of cases): Introduction of spores into subepidermal tissue through a skin lesion (e.g., cut, scrape)
- Pulmonary anthrax: Inhalation of airborne spores; highly lethal (99% mortality without treatment, 80% mortality even with treatment)
- Gastrointestinal: Ingestion of spores, usually in contaminated foods

Differential Dx

- Cutaneous anthrax
  - –Erysipelas
  - –Boil
  - –Syphilis
  - –Cellulitis
- Pulmonary anthrax
  - –Pneumonia
  - –Bronchitis
  - –Influenza
- GI anthrax
  - –Gastroenteritis/food poisoning
  - –Acute abdomen of various etiologies
  - –Streptococcal pharyngitis

Presentation

- Cutaneous anthrax erupts 3–4 days after infection: Painless, reddish papules, becoming vesicles; eventually a black eschar develops; systemic symptoms may occur
- Pulmonary anthrax: Influenza-like prodrome (fever, chills, fatigue, HA, cough, myalgias) followed by sudden onset of dyspnea, cyanosis, and mental status changes; may progress to coma and death
- GI anthrax: Nausea, vomiting, fever, abdominal pain, dysentery, hematemesis, and sepsis
- Oropharyngeal infection: Sore throat, dysphagia, fever, mucosal lesions, and lymphadenopathy

Diagnosis

- History of exposure and clinical presentation
- Chest X-ray in pulmonary anthrax reveals a widened mediastinum due to enlarged mediastinal lymph nodes and may show diffuse patchy infiltrates
- Hypoxemia in pulmonary anthrax
- Definitive diagnosis by isolation of bacteria from cutaneous vesicles, sputum, vomitus, feces, and/or ascites fluid
- Bacteria on gram stain are large, encapsulated, gram-positive rods often with a central vacuole; non-motile; non-hemolytic
- Blood cultures may be positive in any form of anthrax
- No screening test is available; nasal swabs or serology should only be used in symptomatic patients or for epidemiologic reasons

Treatment

- Begin antibiotics promptly—in pulmonary anthrax, antibiotics are usually only effective if begun before onset of symptoms
  - –IV ciprofloxacin is first line therapy
  - –Doxycycline alone or penicillin plus streptomycin are acceptable alternatives
  - –There are some engineered strains of anthrax with resistance to both doxycycline and penicillin
- Post-exposure prophylaxis with oral ciprofloxacin or doxycycline plus anthrax vaccine
- Vaccine is available for those at high risk or with confirmed exposure; those on prophylactic antibiotics should receive vaccine prior to the discontinuation of antibiotic therapy
- Intubation and ventilatory support may be necessary in pulmonary anthrax

Disposition

- All forms of anthrax may be fatal
  - –Cutaneous: Usually self-limited; few deaths if treated
  - –Pulmonary: Mortality is 99% without treatment and 80% with treatment
  - –GI: May result in sepsis, shock, and death (with or without treatment)
- Meningitis and sepsis are dangerous complications of all three forms of anthrax; nearly 100% of secondary meningitis cases are fatal
- Estimated 3 million deaths if aerosolized anthrax were to be released over Washington, D.C.

181. Smallpox

Etiology & Pathophysiology

- Caused by a variola virus that infects only humans
- Highly infectious, especially early in the disease
- Spread only by person-to-person transmission via respiratory droplets
- Virus then spreads from the respiratory tract to blood, internal organs, and skin, with an asymptomatic incubation period of about 2 weeks following exposure
- Epidemics throughout history have been devastating
- Routine vaccination ended in 1972 and smallpox was eliminated from the world in 1977—the only known stocks of smallpox are kept at the CDC in Atlanta and in a lab in Russia; however, other labs in Russia and possibly other countries may have access to the virus
- Smallpox has the potential to be one of the most devastating bio-weapons (highly infectious, fast-spreading, long prodromal phase, often lethal, minimal available vaccine supplies, and community immunity has been lost since the cessation of routine immunizations)

Differential Dx

- Chickenpox
- Influenza

Presentation

- Initial symptoms include high fever, myalgias, fatigue, headache, and backache; nausea and vomiting may be present
- Rash follows 2–3 days later
    - Especially prominent on face, extremities, and mucous membranes of mouth and nose
    - Progresses from reddish macules to papules to pus-filled vesicles to crusting scabs
    - All lesions appear in the same stage of development (as opposed to chickenpox)
    - Scabs fall off in 3–4 weeks, leaving pitted scars
- Blindness may occur

Diagnosis

- Primarily diagnosed by identification of the characteristic rash by trained personnel
- Distinguish rash from chickenpox
    - Chickenpox lesions tend to be more superficial
    - Chickenpox lesions are more prominent on the trunk than on the face or extremities
    - Chickenpox lesions virtually never occur on the palms or soles
    - In chickenpox, lesions of various stages exist together; whereas in smallpox, lesions in each area are at the same stage of development

Treatment

- Patients should be isolated until rash/scabs disappear
- There is no proven effective treatment; antivirals (cidofovir and IV ribavirin) are being studied
- Supportive care should include IV fluids, analgesics, antipyretics
- Antibiotics for secondary bacterial infections
- Vaccine will prevent disease and diminish the severity of illness in exposed individuals
    - The available vaccine is made of live vaccinia virus, which is closely related to the variola virus
    - Must be administered within 4 days of exposure (before rash develops)
    - Contraindicated in pregnancy, immunosuppression or immunocompromise, or history of eczema
    - May have severe side effects, including death
- Vaccinia immune globulin is indicated in exposed individuals within 3 days of exposure

Disposition

- Most patients recover; however, death occurs in up to 30% of cases (there are engineered forms of smallpox that are more lethal)
- Deep scars may remain ("pockmarks")
- Infection control procedures are essential to contain outbreaks
    - Decontamination of instruments, clothing, and bedding
    - Protective clothing and masks for medical personnel
    - Vaccines for those at risk
- Currently, vaccination of first responders and certain health care professionals is being considered

Psychiatric Emergencies

AMY SMOOKLER, MD

182. Acute Psychosis

Etiology & Pathophysiology

- Dysfunctional behavior or thought processes with the presence of delusions, hallucinations, and disorganized speech or behaviors
- Differentiate organic (medical) from functional (psychiatric) causes
- Medical conditions are a common cause of psychosis
  - Endocrine disorders (e.g., thyroid or adrenal abnormalities)
  - Liver or renal failure
  - Neurologic (e.g., meningitis, hemorrhage, seizure, CVA, tumors)
  - Hypoglycemia or electrolyte abnormalities
  - Hypertensive emergency
  - Trauma (e.g., intracerebral bleed, closed head injury)
  - Hypoxia
  - Infection (e.g., HIV, sepsis, UTI, pneumonia, meningitis, Lyme)
  - Drugs (steroid use, therapeutics, drugs of abuse, withdrawal states)
  - Deficiency states (e.g., vitamin B_{12}, thiamine, folate)

Differential Dx

- Dementia
- Delirium
- Psychiatric causes
  - Schizophrenia
  - Schizophreniform disorder
  - Schizoaffective disorder
  - Delusional disorder
  - Due to a medical condition
  - Due to substance abuse
  - Brief psychotic disorder
  - Mania or bipolar disorder
  - Depression with psychotic features
  - Postpartum psychosis

Presentation

- Delusions (fixed false beliefs)
- Hallucinations (alterations in sensorium)
- Severe behavioral changes
- Decreased social interaction
- Poor hygiene
- Bizarre behaviors (e.g., rocking, staring)
- Difficulties in goal-directed activity and communication, reflecting disorganized thinking
- May have symptoms/signs of organic disease
- Patients may present in catatonia

Diagnosis

- Complete history and physical exam is essential to differentiate functional versus organic disease
- Suspicion of medical illness based upon vital signs, physical exam, or history should be thoroughly evaluated
- Acute medical illness may exacerbate psychosis; thus, medical illness must be ruled out even in patients with a history of psychiatric disease
- Background information on the patient's prior level of functioning should be obtained if possible
- Obtain lab work as necessary, possibly including head CT, alcohol level, drug screen, electrolytes, CBC, LFTs, BUN/creatinine, and tests of endocrine function

Treatment

- Treat underlying medical disorders, if present
- Antipsychotic medications may be used, depending on the degree of agitation and symptomatology: IV/IM haloperidol, IM risperidone, or droperidol
  - Antipsychotics may cause arrhythmias (especially droperidol), dystonic reactions, akathisia, seizures, or neuroleptic malignant syndrome
  - If an acute dystonic reaction occurs secondary to antipsychotic use, stop the drug and administer IV/IM benztropine or diphenhydramine
- Benzodiazepines (e.g., midazolam) are effective sedatives, especially in the acutely intoxicated (e.g., alcohol, cocaine) or withdrawing patient
- Physical restraints are often required to manage violent patients

Disposition

- Many acutely psychotic patients will require admission, either because they are a danger to themselves or others or due to underlying medical illness requiring inpatient treatment
- Outpatient therapy is reasonable if organic causes are ruled out or treated, if the patient is not a danger to self or others, and if appropriate follow-up is available
- If the patient refuses treatment but is deemed unable to understand the risks and benefits of their decision, they must be detained to ensure their safety

183. Mood Disorders

Etiology & Pathophysiology

- Mood disorders include depression, bipolar disorder, dysthymia, and cyclothymia
    - Major depression: Depressed mood or loss of interest in daily activities lasting at least two weeks, associated with other symptoms, and causing impairment in functioning
    - Bipolar disorder (manic-depression): Alternating episodes of depression and mania
    - Dysthymic disorder: Chronic depressed mood on most days for at least 2 years; other symptoms are rarely present
- Extremely common (up to 15% of the population)
- Risk factors include female sex, family or personal history, and coexisting illness
- Pathophysiology may include abnormal activity of norepinephrine and dopamine, hormonal abnormalities (e.g., cortisol), genetic predisposition, and psychological issues

Differential Dx

- Delirium
- Dementia
- Psychosis (e.g., schizophrenia)
- Adjustment disorder
- Personality disorder
- Drug intoxication/withdrawal
- Normal bereavement
- Medication-induced mood disorder
- Medical illness (e.g., coronary ischemia, malignancy, neurologic disease, or endocrine problems, such as hypothyroidism)

Presentation

- Depression: Hopelessness, apathy
- Mania: Extreme elation, irritability, grandiosity
- Psychomotor agitation (e.g., hand wringing, fidgeting, pacing, and pressured speech) may be seen in both mania and depression
- Psychomotor retardation during depressive episodes (e.g., slowed thoughts and movements, slurred speech, slumped posture)
- Poor concentration, excessive guilt, suicidal ideation, and delusions in severe depression
- Increased or decreased sleep or appetite and sexual dysfunction

Diagnosis

- Criteria for diagnosis of major depressive episode: Five or more of the following symptoms in the same two-week period
    - Depressed mood
    - Anhedonia (lack of pleasure)
    - Insomnia or increased sleep–Fatigue
    - Weight loss, weight gain, or change in appetite
    - Psychomotor agitation or retardation
    - Feelings of worthlessness or guilt
    - Poor concentration or indecisiveness
    - Recurrent thoughts or plan of death or suicide
- Criteria for diagnosis of a manic episode: At least two weeks of an abnormally elevated or irritable mood with 3 of the following: Grandiosity (inflated self-esteem), decreased need for sleep, pressured speech, distractibility, flight of ideas or racing thoughts, increase in goal-directed activity (e.g., spending all night working on a new project), increased risk-taking behavior (e.g., shopping sprees, sexual encounters)

Treatment

- Medical diseases must be ruled out or appropriately treated
- Secure a safe environment, including the presence of a security guard
- Chemical and physical restraints may be required in manic, aggressive patients
- Depression: A variety of antidepressants are available; however, most require several weeks for effect; cognitive-behavioral therapy has been shown to be as effective as pharmacologic therapy
- Bipolar disorders require IV/IM haloperidol or benzodiazepines for acute treatment of mania
    - Long-term therapies may include mood stabilizers (e.g., lithium, valproate, carbamazepine); as with antidepressants, these agents generally take several weeks for effect

Disposition

- Suicidal or homicidal patients must be detained until appropriate psychiatric evaluation has been completed
- Admit depressed patients who are suicidal or homicidal, those unable to care for themselves, and those without a support network or adequate follow-up
- Manic patients will often require admission, since they are engaging in risky or life-threatening behaviors
- Overall lifetime risk of suicide in depressed patients is 15%
- Risk factors for suicide include family or personal history of suicides or attempts, co-existing substance abuse, poor social situation, underlying medical illness, increasing age, and male gender

184. Panic Attacks and Conversion Disorder

Etiology & Pathophysiology

- Conversion disorder: A somatoform disorder in which psychological stress is unconsciously transformed into physical symptoms (e.g., visual loss, focal neurologic deficits, pseudoseizure)
  - No underlying pathophysiologic explanation
  - Often considered a defense mechanism for dealing with unpleasant thoughts or situations
- Panic disorder: A chronic, relapsing form of anxiety disorder characterized by recurrent panic attacks (episodes of severe anxiety with associated physical symptoms)
  - Etiologies may include genetic and biochemical factors, a deficit of the inhibitory neurotransmitter GABA, and/or overabundance of sympathetic or serotonin activity in the locus ceruleus
  - May be a learned response from internal physical cues

Differential Dx

- Conversion disorder: Seizure, CVA/TIA, multiple sclerosis, SLE, myositis, Lyme disease, depression, cerebral bleed or mass lesion, hypochondriasis
- Panic disorder: Hypoglycemia, hyperthyroidism, cardiac ischemic or arrhythmia, mitral valve prolapse, COPD, asthma, pulmonary embolus, migraine, caffeine/nicotine/drug use or withdrawal, Cushing's syndrome, pheochromocytoma, steroid use, domestic violence

Presentation

- Conversion disorder
  - Presents with one or more dramatic symptoms of abrupt onset
  - Symptoms may not correspond to expected anatomic distributions of known lesions
- Panic disorder
  - Recurrent, intermittent panic attacks followed by persistent anticipatory anxiety (fear of recurrence), fear of the implications of the attacks, or change in behavior due to the attack (usually avoidance)
  - Often associated with depression
  - Agoraphobia is often present

Diagnosis

- Conversion disorder criteria for diagnosis
  - Stressful event precedes a physical impairment or distress
  - Deficit of voluntary motor control or sensation
  - Not intentional and not explainable by an organic cause
  - Often results in (but not limited to) pain or sexual dysfunction
- Panic disorder criteria for diagnosis
  - Recurrent, intermittent, unexpected panic attacks followed by persistent anticipatory anxiety, fear of implications of attacks, or change in behavior due to the attack (e.g., avoidance)
- Panic attacks require at least four of the following:
  - Heart palpitations
  - Shortness of breath
  - Nausea/GI distress
  - Numbness or tingling
  - Fear of losing control
  - Chest discomfort
  - Trembling/shaking
  - Sweating, chills, or hot flashes
  - Dizziness/faint feeling
  - Fear of dying
  - Depersonalization (not feeling a part of one's own body)

Treatment

- Conversion disorder
  - Avoid illegitimatizing the patient's complaints (e.g., accusing them of "faking")
  - Remove stressors and develop coping strategies to deal with perceived symptoms
  - Reassurance that no life-threatening event will happen
  - Avoid ordering tests or consulting specialists as this reinforces the behavior and may worsen the problem
  - Pharmacologic agents include lorazepam and amobarbital
- Panic disorder
  - Reassure that nothing life-threatening is occurring
  - Avoid caffeine, nicotine, and drug use
  - Benzodiazepines are used to treat acute symptoms in severe, persistent, or frequent attacks
  - Antidepressants can control symptoms but do not work acutely
  - Psychiatric counseling, especially cognitive-behavioral therapy

Disposition

- Use laboratory testing and imaging as needed to rule out organic causes
- Suicidal or homicidal patients should be admitted
- Both disorders can usually be treated on an outpatient basis, assuming adequate follow-up can be arranged
- Potential for abuse/dependence with benzodiazepines—avoid long-term use and avoid short-acting agents due to greater risk of dependence and rebound anxiety

185. Eating Disorders

Etiology & Pathophysiology

- Anorexia nervosa: Inadequate intake of nutrition associated with decreased body weight, intense fear of obesity, distorted body image, and amenorrhea
- Bulimia nervosa: Episodic binge eating followed by purging (via vomiting, diuretics, laxatives, or excessive exercise), feeling of lack of control over eating, and excessive focus on body image
- Etiology is multifactorial, including genetic factors, biochemical factors (decreased serotonin and noradrenaline stimulation), hormonal factors, cultural factors (i.e., "thin is ideal" in Western society), a feeling of lack of control (more commonly in anorexia), poor self-image and need for approval
- Affects 5–10% of adolescent females; <1% of adolescent males
- Age of onset is most commonly from adolescence through the fourth decade of life

Differential Dx

- Psychiatric illnesses
  - Depression (e.g., poor appetite, weight loss)
  - Schizophrenia (e.g., paranoia revolving around food)
- Medical illnesses
  - Hyperthyroidism
  - Diabetes mellitus
  - Addison's disease
  - Chronic diarrhea
  - Inflammatory bowel disease
  - Chronic mesenteric ischemia
  - Superior mesenteric artery syndrome

Presentation

- Anorexia
  - Body weight <85% of normal
  - Amenorrhea
  - May also present with binging and purging
- Bulimia
  - Often normal or overweight
  - Dental caries/loss of enamel
  - Salivary/parotid enlargement
  - Dry mucous membranes
  - Esophageal irritation
  - Scars on knuckles (due to repeated induction of vomiting)
  - Amenorrhea
- Stress or compression fractures due to excessive exercise, osteoporosis

Diagnosis

- CBC may reveal anemia and leukopenia
- Electrolyte abnormalities are common (especially hypokalemia)
- Increased amylase
- Hypoglycemia
- Acid-base disturbances may be present
  - Metabolic acidosis occurs in anorexia (due to starvation ketosis) and in bulimia with excessive use of laxatives or exercise
  - Hypokalemic, hypochloremic metabolic alkalosis occurs in bulimia with vomiting or diuretic use
- ECG may reveal arrhythmias associated with electrolyte abnormalities
- CXR may show atelectasis or pneumonia due to respiratory muscle atrophy
- GI pathology may include Mallory-Weiss tears, esophageal rupture, hematemesis, esophageal irritation, constipation, and post-binge pancreatitis

Treatment

- Correct electrolyte abnormalities
- Long-term psychiatric and nutritional therapy
- Bulimia usually responds to counseling and antidepressants
- Anorexia nervosa
  - Counseling
  - Appetite stimulants, such as cyproheptadine (Periactin), have some beneficial effect
  - Gradually reintroduce food
  - May need parenteral nutrition (TPN) due to atrophy of gut mucosa and diminished production of enzymes
  - Careful correction of chronic metabolic derangements is essential as too rapid correction may result in serious adverse consequences
  - Trials of amitriptyline, clomipramine, pimozide, and chlorpromazine may be beneficial

Disposition

- Criteria for admission
  - Serious depression with suicidality
  - Major complications (i.e., GI bleed, severe electrolyte abnormalities)
  - Non-supportive family situation
  - Failures of outpatient treatment
  - Weight loss >30% over 3 months
- Discharge if duration of illness <3 months, weight >70% of ideal, stable and motivated patient and family, good outpatient monitoring with arranged therapy
- Depression is a common underlying component of eating disorders
- Mortality is 2–18%
- Deaths occur due to suicide, electrolyte abnormalities, cardiac arrhythmia, or infection
- Up to 50% have persistent disease

186. Withdrawal Syndromes

Etiology & Pathophysiology

- Drug dependence: A physiologic state in which a decrease in drug administration results in withdrawal symptoms and tolerance
- Drug addiction: Continued use of drugs despite detriment to self, others, and/or society
- Alcohol activates inhibitory GABA receptors in the CNS, causing sedation
  - Chronic ethanol use results in downregulation of GABA
  - When ethanol is removed, a lack of GABA inhibition results in an excitatory state
- Sedative/hypnotics (e.g., benzodiazepines, barbiturates) activate GABA when drug is present; withdrawal results in excitatory state
- Opioid withdrawal results from upregulation of cAMP following chronic usage

Differential Dx

- CNS trauma
- CNS infection
- Hyperthyroidism
- Sepsis
- Heat stroke
- Hypoglycemia
- Hyperglycemia
- Drug intoxication (e.g., cocaine, amphetamines)
- Acute abdomen
- Anticholinergic syndrome
- Acute schizophrenia

Presentation

- Alcohol withdrawal: Agitation, tremulousness, N/V, insomnia, tachycardia, fever
  - May progress to hallucinations, confusion, and seizures
  - Delirium tremens (DTs): Severe episodes of gross tremor, HTN, fever, tachycardia, and severe confusion and disorientation
- Sedative/hypnotics: HTN, tremors, tachycardia, diaphoresis, fever, seizures
- Opioids: Lacrimation, rhinorrhea, mydriasis, sweating, yawning, piloerection, restlessness, insomnia, N/V, and/or abdominal pain; mental status is normal

Diagnosis

- Do not assume symptoms are from withdrawal unless other medical illnesses have been ruled out
- Laboratory tests to rule out other causes of symptoms or sequelae of withdrawal (CBC, electrolytes, renal and liver function, PT/PTT/INR, and workup for infections)
- Head CT for unexplained mental status changes
- Lumbar puncture if meningitis/encephalitis cannot be ruled out
- Classification of alcohol withdrawal
  - Minor (six or more hours after use): Course tremor, increased autonomic tone, sleep disturbance, and anxiety
  - Major (>24 hours after use): More extreme symptoms of increased excitatory tone, hallucinations (but without confusion), and risk of seizures
  - Delirium tremens (>72 hours after use) is the extreme end of the spectrum of increased autonomic tone; associated with significant confusion, altered sensorium, and disorientation

Treatment

- Alcohol withdrawal
  - IV glucose, IV fluids, thiamine (administer prior to glucose to prevent Wernicke's encephalopathy), magnesium, and folate
  - Benzodiazepines (e.g., lorazepam) are administered to enhance GABA activity, sedate the patient, and decrease the incidence of seizures and delirium tremens
  - Barbiturates may also be administered
  - Clonidine or β-blockers may decrease symptoms but do not treat withdrawal (may even mask progression)
  - Butyrophenones (e.g., haloperidol) are not preferred as they may decrease the seizure threshold; however, haloperidol plus lorazepam has been proven safe
- Sedative/hypnotic withdrawal is treated with a slow taper of long-acting benzodiazepines or barbiturates
- Opioid withdrawal is treated with methadone (a long-acting opioid) or other opiates to decrease symptoms
  - Clonidine is effective for mild opioid withdrawal

Disposition

- Alcohol withdrawal
  - A medical emergency requiring admission
  - May progress from mild withdrawal to major withdrawal to DTs
  - Mortality of delirium tremens is 15%
  - Patients exhibiting signs of delirium tremens require admission to an ICU
- Sedative/hypnotic withdrawal may result in life-threatening seizures; admission is generally warranted
- Opioid withdrawal is not life-threatening; however, often requires admission for symptoms such as persistent nausea and vomiting

Obstetric-Gynecologic Emergencies

MELORA J. TROTTER, MD

187. Vaginal Bleeding

Etiology & Pathophysiology

- Estrogen causes proliferation of the endometrium; progesterone stabilizes the endometrium
- Menorrhagia: Menses >7 days or >80 mL blood loss
- Metrorrhagia: Vaginal bleeding outside normal menses
- Menometrorrhagia: Excessive bleeding outside menses
- Dysfunctional uterine bleeding: Irregular bleeding due to anovulation in the absence of organic disease (persistent estrogen production without the presence of balancing progesterone, results in eventual shedding of the proliferative endometrium); causes include polycystic ovary syndrome, obesity, adolescence, perimenopause, stress, excessive exercise
- Ovulatory bleeding: Abnormal bleeding despite normal cycles (e.g., structural or cancerous lesions, fibroids, OCPs, endometriosis)

Differential Dx

- Normal menses
- Pregnancy
- Anovulation
- Infection
- Endometriosis/adenomyosis
- Medication (OCP)
- Atrophic vaginitis
- Fibroids
- Malignancy (cervix, uterus)
- Coagulopathy
- Endocrine disorder
- Trauma/abuse
- Foreign body

Presentation

- Irregular periods suggest anovulation or perimenopause
- Pelvic pain may be present in endometriosis, fibroids, trauma, or infection (e.g., PID)
- Fever, vaginal discharge, nausea, and vomiting suggest infection
- Obesity and hirsutism suggest polycystic ovary syndrome
- Dyspareunia suggests endometriosis or infection
- Bleeding or easy bruising suggest coagulopathy
- Enlarged/tender adnexa or uterus suggests fibroids
- Smaller nodules suggests endometriosis

Diagnosis

- β-hCG to exclude pregnancy
- CBC and type and screen in moderate to heavy blood loss
- PT/PTT for patients with other sites of bleeding, those currently on anticoagulation therapy, or those with persistently heavy periods (suspicious for von Willebrand's disease)
- Speculum exam to determine lower versus upper genital tract bleeding; findings may include adenoma, polyps, condyloma, lacerations, ecchymosis, or foreign bodies
- Cultures of vaginal secretions for *Gonorrhea, Chlamydia,* and trichomonas
- ED ultrasound will identify intrauterine or ectopic pregnancies; formal OB/GYN ultrasound is needed to identify an enlarged uterus, fibroids, uterine blot clot, enlarged adnexa, or endometrial thickening
- CT and MRI are generally not useful

Treatment

- Hemodynamically unstable patients should receive immediate fluid resuscitation and blood transfusions; persistent bleeding may require dilatation and curettage or hysterectomy
- Hemodynamically stable patients should receive hormone therapy to stabilize the endometrium
  - Severe bleeding: IV or oral estrogen alone, then add progesterone once the bleeding stops
  - Mild-moderate bleeding: Oral contraceptives (the estrogen-progestin combination takes effect more slowly than estrogen alone)
  - Minimal bleeding: Progesterone alone for 10 days to stabilize the immature endometrium
  - After the endometrium is stabilized and bleeding stops, therapy is withdrawn allowing a withdrawal bleed that imitates normal menses
- Chronic management for repetitive bleeding may include oral contraceptives, NSAIDs (decreases uterine blood flow), clomiphene, or danazol

Disposition

- Admit patients with hemodynamic instability or severe blood loss
- Follow-up with OB/Gyn for most causes of vaginal bleeding
- Appropriate counseling in cases of sexual abuse
- Unopposed estrogen increases the risk of endometrial hyperplasia and cancer—suspect endometrial cancer in any post-menopausal female with vaginal bleeding

188. Vulvovaginitis

Etiology & Pathophysiology

- Vaginitis: Inflammation of the vagina and vulva
  - Bacterial vaginosis (BV) is the most common cause of vaginitis; due to overgrowth of *Gardnerella vaginalis;* associated with preterm labor, premature rupture of membranes, and endometritis
  - *Candida* vaginitis: Second most common cause of vaginitis; due to yeast, most commonly *Candida albicans*
  - Trichomoniasis: A sexually transmitted disease caused by the protozoan *T. vaginalis;* may predispose to preterm labor and premature rupture of membranes
  - Atrophic vaginitis: Mucosal atrophy due to decreased estrogen in postmenopausal women
- Cervicitis: Inflammation of the cervix (without ascending spread to the upper genital tract), commonly due to *Neisseria gonorrhoeae* or *Chlamydia trachomatis*

Differential Dx

- Atrophic vaginitis
- Bacterial vaginosis
- Candida vaginitis
- Trichomonas vaginalis
- Cervicitis
- Pelvic inflammatory disease
- Genital herpes
- Urinary tract infection
- Vaginal foreign body
- Behcet's syndrome
- Collagen vascular disease
- Contact vulvovaginitis
- Pinworms

Presentation

- Vaginal irritation
- Dyspareunia
- BV: Thin, white, foul smelling ("fishy-smelling") discharge
- Candida: Thick, white, chunky "cottage cheese" discharge; pruritus; dysuria
- Trichomoniasis: Foul smelling, purulent, yellowish discharge
- Atrophic vaginitis: Soreness, spotting, scant discharge
- Contact vulvovaginitis: Intense pruritus, swelling
- Cervicitis: Vaginal discharge

Diagnosis

- Identify offending agent: Urinalysis, wet mount (*Trichomonas*), gram stain (*Gardnerella*), KOH prep (*Candida*), gonococcus and chlamydia cultures, and consider syphilis testing
- BV: Vaginal pH >4.5, "clue cells" on microscopy, positive "whiff" test (foul odor with KOH)
- *Candida:* Vaginal pH 4.0–4.5, pseudohyphae and yeast buds on KOH microscopy; "strawberry cervix" due to punctate hemorrhages
- Trichomoniasis: Vaginal pH 5.0–6.0; motile trichomonads and many PMNs on microscopy
- Atrophic vaginitis: May have vaginal petechiae or ecchymoses; few or no vaginal folds
- Contact vulvovaginitis: Erythematous and edematous vulva and vagina, ulcerations, possible secondary *Candida* infection
- Cervicitis: Cervical motion tenderness, cervical erythema; no abdominal or adnexal tenderness

Treatment

- BV: Metronidazole for 7 days or as a 2 g single dose (contraindicated during the 1st trimester of pregnancy); alternatives include metronidazole gel and clindamycin cream or tab
- Candida: Fluconazole for a single dose or topical antifungals for 3 days
- Trichomoniasis: Metronidazole 2 g single dose
- Atrophic vaginitis: Topical vaginal estrogen for 1–2 wks
- Contact vulvovaginitis: Avoid the offending agent (e.g., soap, bubble bath, latex condoms, perfumes); cool sitz baths or topical steroids may help symptomatically
- Cervicitis: Treat for both gonococcus and chlamydia (single dose therapy is sufficient)—treat as PID if there is any question of abdominal or adnexal tenderness
  - Azithromycin 2 g single dose (however, seldom used because it usually induces vomiting)
  - 3rd generation cephalosporin or fluoroquinolone (single dose) for gonorrhea, plus either azithromycin (single dose) or doxycycline (for 7 days) for chlamydia

Disposition

- Outpatient therapy for all patients
- BV: Patients treated with metronidazole should be advised to avoid alcohol due to disulfiram-like reactions
- *Candida*: In cases of recurrent infections, rule out the presence of HIV and diabetes mellitus, treat partners, and obtain cultures to isolate potentially resistant organisms (e.g., *Candida glabrata*)
- Trichomonas: All sexual partners should be treated; re-infection is common
- Atrophic vaginitis: Bleeding in a postmenopausal patient requires OB/Gyn referral for Pap smear to rule out endometrial cancer
- All patients should have OB/Gyn follow-up in 48 hours

189. Pelvic Inflammatory Disease

Etiology & Pathophysiology

- Ascending infections of the female upper reproductive tract (uterus, fallopian tubes, pelvic structures), including endometritis, salpingitis, and tubo-ovarian abscess
- Affects 1 million women in the US each year
- The most common cause of pelvic pain in nonpregnant women
- The majority of cases are due to *Neisseria gonorrhoeae* and *Chlamydia trachomatis;* other causative organisms include *Mycoplasma hominis, Ureaplasma urealyticum,* enteric gram-negative rods, and anaerobes
- Predisposing factors include multiple sexual partners, history of STDs, age <25, use of intrauterine device, frequent vaginal douching
- Complications include ectopic pregnancy and infertility (both due to scarring of the fallopian tubes), chronic pelvic pain, tubo-ovarian abscess, and Fitz-Hugh-Curtis syndrome (perihepatic gonococcal infection)

Differential Dx

- Cervicitis/urethritis
- Appendicitis
- Ectopic pregnancy
- Endometriosis
- Ovarian torsion
- Nephrolithiasis
- Diverticulitis
- Pyelonephritis
- Spontaneous or septic abortion
- Bacterial vaginosis
- Trichomonas
- Candida vaginitis

Presentation

- Fever
- Vaginal discharge
- Irregular vaginal bleeding
- Pelvic pain and/or abdominal pain
- Dysuria
- Nausea and/or vomiting
- Dyspareunia
- Symptoms occur more frequently following menstruation

Diagnosis

- PID is a clinical diagnosis that generally does not require imaging studies, except to rule out other pathology
- CDC criteria (90% sensitive) for PID include the presence of lower abdominal pain/tenderness, cervical motion tenderness, and adnexal tenderness
- Criteria not required but supportive of the diagnosis include nausea/vomiting, temperature >101°F (38.3°C), dyspareunia, abnormal cervical or vaginal discharge, culture evidence of *C. trachomatis* or *N. gonorrhoeae,* and elevated ESR or CRP
- Labs should include urinalysis, wet mount, gram stain, cervical cultures for gonococcus and chlamydia, and urine pregnancy test
- Transvaginal ultrasound is used to rule out ectopic pregnancy and may show pelvic fluid (suggesting PID) or tubo-ovarian abscess
- Abdominal CT may show pelvic fluid, tubo-ovarian abscess, ovarian cyst, or other pathology
- Laparoscopy is the gold standard for diagnosis; however, it is rarely done except to rule out and treat surgical disease

Treatment

- Maintain a low threshold for diagnosis and antibiotic treatment due to the potentially serious sequelae
- Requires a 14 day, 2-drug course of antibiotics covering *N. gonorrhoeae, C. trachomatis,* anaerobes, and gram negatives
- Outpatient regimens
  - IM single dose ceftriaxone plus doxycycline for 14 days
  - IM single dose 3rd generation cephalosporin and oral probenicid plus doxycycline for 14 days
  - IV single dose azithromycin followed by oral azithromycin for 7 days and metronidazole for 14 days
  - Ofloxacin plus metronidazole for 14 days
- Inpatient regimens—begin IV dosing until the patient improves for 24 hours, followed by oral therapy to complete a 14 day course
  - Doxycycline plus either cefotetan or cefoxitin
  - Azithromycin plus metronidazole
  - Clindamycin plus gentamycin followed by doxycycline
  - Ofloxacin plus metronidazole
  - Ampicillin/sulbactam plus doxycycline

Disposition

- Admit patients who are severely ill or toxic, pregnant, suspected to be non-compliant (e.g., adolescent, substance abuser), HIV positive, suspected to have a tubo-ovarian abscess, outpatient therapy failures, unable to tolerate oral medications, or uncertain diagnosis
- Patients who are discharged should have follow-up within 72 hours
- All sexual partners within the previous two months should be examined and treated prior to resuming intercourse
- 95% cure rate with antibiotics
- 10% infertility rate following 1 episode; 40% infertility rate after 3 episodes

190. Ovarian Pathology

Etiology & Pathophysiology

- Ovarian cysts: Result from follicles that neither ovulate nor regress
  - Rupture of an ovarian follicle causes sudden pelvic pain and may result in peritoneal irritation from fluid or blood
  - Follicular cyst is a smaller cyst (~2 cm) that ruptures during ovulation (mid-cycle); pain dissipates over 1–2 days
  - Corpus luteal (hemorrhagic) cyst is a larger cyst (up to 10 cm) that ruptures just prior to menses; may cause hemorrhage and, rarely, shock; symptoms similar to ectopic pregnancy
- Ovarian torsion: Twisting of the ovary on its vascular pedicle, resulting in ischemia and infarction; increased risk with ovarian mass
- Tubo-ovarian abscess (TOA): Abscess of the ovary, fallopian tube, or broad ligament; often due to anaerobic bacteria and commonly associated with PID; may cause irreversible damage and infertility

Differential Dx

- Appendicitis
- Ectopic pregnancy
- Endometriosis
- Mittelschmertz
- Pelvic inflammatory disease
- Cervicitis
- Endometritis
- Menstrual cramps
- Uterine fibroids (leiomyoma)
- Adenomyoma
- Nephrolithiasis
- Urinary tract infection
- Pyelonephritis
- Diverticulitis

Presentation

- Abdominal or pelvic pain
  - Usually unilateral
  - May be sharp and sudden (e.g., torsion, rupture of cysts) or dull with gradual onset (e.g., stretching of capsule around a cyst, TOA)
  - Ovarian torsion: Sudden, severe pain out of proportion to exam, radiating from groin to flank
- Vaginal bleeding or discharge
- Nausea/vomiting
- Rectal pain from fluid in cul-de-sac
- Syncope
- Fever in TOA and torsion
- Hypotension/shock may occur in luteal cysts and TOA

Diagnosis

- Abdominal exam: Often tender; peritoneal signs (e.g., rebound, guarding, rigidity) occur with torsion or hemorrhagic luteal cysts
- Speculum exam: May see pus from the cervical os with TOA
- Bimanual exam: Cervical motion tenderness occurs with TOA, torsion, and some cysts; adnexal mass and/or tenderness may be present with any ovarian pathology
- Urine β-hCG to rule out intrauterine and ectopic pregnancy
- Urinalysis to rule out UTI
- WBC and ESR may be elevated in TOA or torsion
- U/S may show a unilateral cyst, TOA, or fluid in the cul-de-sac
- Doppler U/S in torsion may reveal an enlarged ovary and decreased blood flow
- Abdominal/pelvic CT will identify most cases of torsion and TOA and rule out other pathology (e.g., nephrolithiasis)
- Laparoscopy/laparotomy may be required for definitive diagnosis of torsion or TOA

Treatment

- Treat shock with IV fluids and blood as needed—patients in shock require emergent surgery
- Pain management as appropriate for severity
- Consult OB/Gyn or surgery if peritoneal signs are present
- Ovarian cysts: Manage pain with NSAIDs and narcotics; operative intervention in cases of shock
- Ovarian torsion: Emergent surgical repair
- TOA: IV antibiotics to cover *N. gonorrhoeae, C. trachomatis,* and anaerobes
  - Doxycycline plus either cefotetan, cefoxitin or ampicillin/sulbactam
  - 2nd generation quinolone plus metronidazole
  - Clindamycin plus gentamycin plus doxycycline
  - Surgery is required if peritoneal signs are present or abscess persists after antibiotics

Disposition

- In general, admit patients with unclear etiologies or if unable to tolerate oral intake
- Follicular cyst: Discharge home with NSAIDs
- Luteal cyst: Often require admission for hemodynamic observation, especially if patient is anemic or has a large amount of blood in the pelvis
- Torsion: Admit for emergent surgery
- TOA: Admit for IV antibiotics and counseling about the risks of infertility (near 100%) and ectopic pregnancy; sexual partners should be treated

191. Complications of Pregnancy

Etiology & Pathophysiology

- Hyperemesis gravidarum: 1st trimester nausea and intractable vomiting with ketonemia, dehydration, and >5% weight loss; may be caused by elevated β-hCG levels (e.g., twins, molar pregnancy)
- HELLP syndrome: A syndrome with high mortality (up to 25%) that causes *H*emolysis, *E*levated *L*iver enzymes, *L*ow *P*latelets, and often hypertension; possibly caused by endothelial injury with resulting vasospasm and platelet activation; often complicates pre-eclampsia
- Amniotic fluid embolus (AFE): A dangerous complication (maternal/fetal morbidity and mortality is 80%) that occurs during delivery, miscarriage, amniocentesis, trauma, or spontaneously
- Rh immunization: Rh(−) mom is exposed to fetal Rh(+) blood (just 0.1 mL of fetal RBCs are needed to sensitize the mother); formation of Rh antibodies occurs, which may endanger future pregnancies
- Thromboembolic disease: Pregnancy is a hypercoagulable state with 5 times increased risk of DVT and possible pulmonary embolus

Differential Dx

- Gastroenteritis
- Ectopic pregnancy
- Molar pregnancy
- Pulmonary embolus
- Preeclampsia/eclampsia
- Acute abdominal pain (e.g., appendicitis, cholecystitis, hepatitis, pancreatitis, PUD, GERD)
- UTI/pyelonephritis
- Superficial phlebitis
- Morning sickness
- DKA
- ITP/TTP

Presentation

- Hyperemesis: Nausea, persistent vomiting, and symptoms of dehydration
- HELLP: RUQ or epigastric pain/tenderness, nausea/vomiting, fatigue, hypertension
- AFE: Dyspnea, shock, seizures, bleeding diathesis
- Rh immunization is asymptomatic
- Thromboembolic disease: Signs of DVT (e.g., painful or swollen leg, Homan's sign) and/or PE (e.g., dyspnea, tachypnea, chest pain)

Diagnosis

- Hyperemesis: Hypokalemia; ketonuria on urinalysis; check LFTs, amylase, and lipase to rule out other causes of vomiting
- HELLP: Thrombocytopenia, decreased RBCs, and schistocytes on CBC; elevated LFTs, bilirubin, and LDH; decreased haptoglobin; proteinuria on urinalysis; consider abdominal ultrasound to rule out gallbladder disease
- AFE: A clinical diagnosis (or diagnosed at autopsy) with hypotension, hypoxemia on ABG, and coagulopathy (↑ PT/PTT)
- Rh immunization: Kleihauer-Betke test is positive in large maternal exposures to fetal blood (e.g., blunt abdominal trauma), but may be negative in smaller exposures (e.g., pregnant patient with vaginal bleeding, ectopic pregnancy, induced or spontaneous abortion, amniocentesis); therefore, treat all Rh(−) patients with any suspected exposure to fetal blood
- Thromboembolic disease: Perform appropriate workup for DVT/PE (lower extremity Doppler is usually the first test, V/Q scan is preferred over spiral CT in pregnancy)

Treatment

- Hyperemesis: Avoid oral intake; consider symptomatic treatment with antiemetics (metoclopramide is the only category B agent, others are category C); rehydrate with 5% glucose in normal saline or LR until urine dipstick becomes negative for ketones; correct electrolytes
- HELLP: Delivery is the only definitive therapy; supportive care includes correction of coagulopathy, hydralazine for HTN, platelet/RBC transfusions, and magnesium for coexisting preeclampsia/eclampsia
- AFE: Deliver fetus immediately, correct coagulopathy, and provide supportive care of ABCs
- Rh immunization: Administer anti-D immune globulin (e.g., Rhogam) to all Rh(−) mothers with any concern of exposure to fetal blood
- Thromboembolic disease: Anticoagulate with IV heparin (warfarin is absolutely contraindicated in pregnancy); some patients may require an IVC filter

Disposition

- Hyperemesis: Most patients require admission (e.g., persistent vomiting, electrolyte abnormalities, weight loss >10% of pre-pregnancy weight); discharge if tolerating clears and ketonuria resolves; recurs in 25% of patients
- HELLP: Admit all patients; complications include placental abruption, renal failure, ARDS, cerebral edema, GI bleed, and subcapsular liver hematoma
- AFE: High mortality, especially during the first hour; remaining patients will likely progress to ARDS and LV dysfunction
- Rh immunization: Discharge following treatment
- Thromboembolic disease: Admit for IV heparin

192. Ectopic Pregnancy

Etiology & Pathophysiology

- Any pregnancy outside the uterine cavity—in most cases, implantation occurs in the fallopian tube but may also occur in the cervix, abdominal cavity, or on the ovary
- Eventually the pregnancy ruptures and causes maternal hemorrhage
- 2nd leading cause of maternal death
- Risk factors include PID, tubal ligation or other fallopian tube surgery, IUD use, fertility medications, cigarettes, and prior ectopic pregnancy
- Incidence has been increasing due to increased rates of PID
- Presentation is variable—consider the diagnosis in any reproductive age woman
- Previous tubal ligation *does not* rule out the possibility of ectopic pregnancy
- Heterotopic pregnancy: An intrauterine pregnancy occurs simultaneously with an ectopic pregnancy

Differential Dx

- Intrauterine pregnancy
- Molar pregnancy
- Heterotopic pregnancy
- Spontaneous abortion
- UTI/pyelonephritis
- Appendicitis
- Renal colic
- Pelvic inflammatory disease
- Ovarian cyst or abscess
- Ovarian torsion
- Endometriosis

Presentation

- Signs and symptoms are generally non-specific
- Abdominal pain and tenderness, ranging from mild to severe
- Vaginal bleeding or passage of tissue
- Nausea and vomiting
- Syncope or pre-syncope
- Amenorrhea (5–12 weeks)
- Adnexal mass and/or tenderness
- Hypotension and/or orthostasis
- Tachycardia

Diagnosis

- Obtain a urine β-hCG to confirm pregnancy, then measure serum quantitative β-hCG (ectopic pregnancies have lower than expected concentrations)
- Ultrasound is often diagnostic—absence of intrauterine pregnancy given sufficient β-hCG levels is an ectopic pregnancy until proven otherwise
  - Absence of intrauterine pregnancy (IUP)
  - May show an extrauterine mass or free pelvic fluid
  - Transvaginal U/S should show IUP if β-hCG >1500
  - Transabdominal U/S should show IUP if β-hCG >5000
- Serum progesterone may be useful at <10 weeks (progesterone <5 suggests ectopic pregnancy, >25 is usually an IUP)
- Culdocentesis is used if ultrasound is unavailable and the patient is unstable—0.3–10 cc of non-clotting blood diagnoses ectopic
- Laparoscopy is both diagnostic and therapeutic; used if ultrasound is non-diagnostic and suspicion persists
- Check Rh status in all patients

Treatment

- Treatment varies depending on dates, size of pregnancy, and hemodynamic stability of the patient
- Hemodynamically unstable patients should receive normal saline and blood via two large bore IVs; check PT/PTT to rule out bleeding disorders; obtain emergent OB/Gyn consultation for surgery
- Methotrexate is sometimes used to induce a medical abortion (80–90% effective); serum β-hCG should be followed every 2 days to assure resolution of pregnancy; used only in consultation with OB/Gyn
- Surgical resection and control of bleeding via laparoscopy or laparotomy is the most common treatment and is the treatment of choice in hemodynamically unstable patients
- If the diagnosis is unclear and the patient is stable, OB/Gyn sometimes recommends serial β-hCG measurement every two days (doubles every 2 days in IUP; increases more slowly in ectopic pregnancy)
- Rh($-$) patients should receive anti-D immune globulin (Rhogam)

Disposition

- High suspicion for ectopic pregnancy is necessary given its high mortality and the availability of effective therapy
- Obtain OB/Gyn consultation in all proven or suspected ectopic pregnancies
- Following OB/Gyn consultation, discharge low-risk patients and those treated with methotrexate; obtain repeat serum β-hCG in 2 days
- Admit all patients who are hemodynamically unstable, at risk of non-compliance, or require surgery
- A low β-hCG level may not be benign (ruptures have been reported at levels as low as 10)

193. Vaginal Bleeding in Pregnancy

Etiology & Pathophysiology

- 1st trimester bleeding occurs in 20% of pregnancies; 50% of cases will result in miscarriage
  - Threatened abortion: Bleeding with a closed cervical os
  - Inevitable abortion: Open cervical os associated with bleeding or the presence of fetal tissue
  - Incomplete abortion (partial passage of embryo): Cervical os or vagina contains products of conception (POCs)
  - Complete abortion: All POCs are expelled and the os is closed
- 2nd and 3rd trimester bleeding
  - Placenta previa: Placenta is implanted over the cervical os
  - Gestational trophoblastic disease (molar pregnancy): Presence of chorionic villi (placental tissue) with no or minimal fetal tissue
  - Placental abruption: Enlarging hematoma tears placenta from the uterus; increased in HTN, smoking, cocaine, preeclampsia, trauma
  - Vasa previa: Fetal bleeding into the uterus due to torn veins

Differential Dx

- Ectopic pregnancy
- Threatened abortion
- Inevitable abortion
- Incomplete abortion
- Complete abortion
- Molar pregnancy
- Placenta previa
- Placental abruption
- Trauma/abuse
- Bloody show
- Uterine rupture
- Vasa previa

Presentation

- 1st trimester abortion: Bleeding, abdominal cramping/pain, and/or passage of tissue
- Molar pregnancy: Large uterus, hyperemesis, pre-eclampsia
- Placenta previa: Painless bleeding; 20% have contractions
- Abruption: Sudden onset of abdominal pain, contractions, and vaginal bleeding; may have shock and symptoms of DIC; amount of bleeding may be underestimated due to trapping of blood behind the placenta
- Vasa previa: Painless, small volume bleed without maternal symptoms

Diagnosis

- Quantitative β-hCG (very high in trophoblastic disease, low in spontaneous abortion) and Rh factor in all patients
- Type and screen, baseline hemoglobin, and coagulation studies
- 1st trimester bleeding
  - Pelvic exam to assess for the presence of fetal tissue and for cervical os opening
  - Ultrasound is used to confirm intrauterine pregnancy and to visualize abortions (small uterine size, lack of gestational sac, no heart activity) or molar pregnancy (large uterus, "snowstorm" pattern)
  - Send any tissue for pathologic analysis
- 2nd and 3rd trimester bleeding
  - Pelvic exam is contraindicated until placenta previa is ruled out by U/S
  - Ultrasound is >95% sensitive for placenta previa but frequently misses abruption
  - Fetal monitor—distress may be the only sign of vasa previa

Treatment

- Fluid and blood resuscitation as necessary for hypotension
- Fetal monitoring if >20 weeks gestational age
- Anti-D immune globulin (Rhogam) in all Rh(−) patients
- 1st trimester abortion: Generally do not require intervention; dilatation and curettage may be necessary for continued bleeding due to retained products
- Molar pregnancy requires dilatation and curettage
- Placenta previa:
  - Mild bleeding requires only admission and monitoring
  - Shock, severe bleeding, or hemodynamic instability requires emergent C-section
  - Tocolytics may be used to decrease uterine irritability
- Placental abruption
  - Replace blood products, correct coagulopathy and DIC
  - Urgent vaginal delivery of stable patients
  - Emergent C-section delivery if the fetus or mother is unstable
- Fresh frozen plasma may be necessary for patients with DIC

Disposition

- Threatened abortion: May be discharged if blood pressure is stable with follow-up β-hCG in 48 hours (doubling of level indicates pregnancy is still viable)
- Inevitable abortion: Discharge if stable with OB/Gyn follow-up; may require dilation and evacuation
- Molar pregnancy: Most patients are admitted; there is a 15% risk of choriocarcinoma, even after dilatation and curettage
- Placenta previa: Admit to obstetrics to monitor course and possibly deliver fetus
- Abruption: Admit all patients; high risk of significant maternal/fetal morbidity and mortality; complications include DIC (very high risk) and amniotic fluid embolus
- Vasa previa has a 75% fetal mortality

194. Hypertension in Pregnancy

Etiology & Pathophysiology

- HTN in pregnancy increases the risk of preterm delivery, IUGR, hepatic rupture, placental abruption, and fetal and maternal death
- Risk factors for hypertension in pregnancy include multiple gestations, molar pregnancy, diabetes, primigravida, extremes of age, and personal or family history of hypertension
- Chronic HTN: Elevated blood pressure prior to pregnancy or occurring before the 20th week of pregnancy
- Chronic HTN with pre-eclampsia: Patient with hypertension prior to pregnancy who then develops pre-eclampsia or eclampsia
- Transient HTN: New onset of HTN without pre-eclampsia symptoms
- Pre-eclampsia: HTN, edema, and proteinuria that occur during pregnancy; likely secondary to a placental abnormality causing vasospasm and fluid retention
- Eclampsia: Pre-eclampsia symptoms followed by seizures; may occur from the 12th week of gestation through the 10th postpartum day

Differential Dx

- Chronic HTN
- Secondary HTN (e.g., Cushing disease, hyperaldosteronism, pheochromocytoma, renovascular)
- HELLP syndrome
- Hydatidiform mole
- Cocaine or amphetamine use
- Meningitis/encephalitis
- Epilepsy
- Physiologic edema of pregnancy
- Central venous thrombosis
- Intracranial hemorrhage

Presentation

- Edema
- Rapid weight gain
- Frontal headache
- Visual changes (e.g., scotoma)
- Oliguria
- Loss of consciousness
- Seizures
- Tinnitus
- Tachycardia
- Nausea/vomiting
- Hematemesis
- Hepatomegaly
- RUQ or epigastric pain suggests HELLP syndrome

Diagnosis

- Diagnostic criteria for preeclampsia (all 3 must be present)
    - Blood pressure ≥140/90 or a rise in systolic BP by 30 mmHg or diastolic BP by 15 mmHg above baseline; diagnosis requires 2 elevated pressures at rest, taken 6 hours apart
    - Edema resulting in a 5 lb weight gain within 1 week
    - Proteinuria of 1+ on urine dipstick or 300 mg/24 hrs
- Obtain CBC (rule out hemolysis), liver function tests (rule out HELLP syndrome), renal function tests, and coagulation profile (PT/PTT)
- Ultrasound may show intrauterine growth retardation, fetal distress, oligohydramnios, or molar pregnancy
- Head CT may be used in patients who do not respond to magnesium treatment in order to rule out other pathologies

Treatment

- Pre-eclampsia
    - Bed rest in the left lateral decubitus position
    - Acetaminophen for headache
    - Continuous fetal monitoring
    - Avoid IV fluids (will worsen edema)
    - IV magnesium sulfate infusion decreases blood pressure and the seizure threshold—frequently check for evidence of magnesium toxicity (e.g., hyporeflexia)
- Severe pre-eclampsia or eclampsia
    - Magnesium for seizures (benzodiazepines are less effective)
    - Definitive therapy is delivery of fetus
- Blood pressure control is indicated in chronic HTN or in pre-eclampsia if diastolic BP remains >110 mmHg after administration of magnesium
    - First line therapy is hydralazine or methyldopa; labetalol or nipride may be used in refractory cases
    - Contraindicated antihypertensive medications include ACE inhibitors, thiazides, and propranolol

Disposition

- Pre-eclampsia may still occur up to 10 days after delivery
- OB/Gyn consultation is mandatory
- Majority of pre-eclamptic patients are admitted; occasionally, reliable patients with good follow-up and mild disease will be discharged after consultation with OB/Gyn
- Eclamptic patients are always admitted for IV medications
- Complications of pre-eclampsia or eclampsia include seizure, placental abruption, intracerebral hemorrhage, DIC, HELLP syndrome, pulmonary edema, liver hemorrhage, renal failure, death

195. Emergency Delivery

Etiology & Pathophysiology

- Labor is defined as the presence of contractions, cervical dilatation and effacement, and fetal descent preceding delivery
- Preterm labor begins before 37 weeks gestational age; risk factors include dehydration, multiple gestations, and infections
- Breech presentation occurs in 4% of term deliveries, may preclude vaginal delivery, and increases the risk of fetal distress
- Rupture of membranes usually occurs during labor; however, it may abnormally precede labor (premature rupture of membranes)
- Meconium is potentially infectious amniotic fluid
- Shoulder dystocia: Shoulder entrapment at the pubis during delivery
- Prolapsed cord: Umbilical cord protrudes into the vagina, where it may be compressed by the presenting fetus and cause fetal hypoxia
- Nuccal cord: Umbilical cord becomes wrapped around the neck of the fetus

Differential Dx

- UTI
- Vulvovaginitis
- Braxton-Hicks contractions/ "false labor" (short, irregular contractions without cervical changes or fetal descent)
- Placental abruption
- Placenta previa

Presentation

- Change or increase in vaginal discharge
- Bloody show (small volume of bloody fluid)
- Contractions increasing in frequency, intensity, and duration
- Low back pain
- Rupture of membranes may be described as "a gush of fluid" from vagina
- Pelvic pressure

Diagnosis

- Monitor maternal vital signs and fetal heart rate
- Monitor uterine contractions to rule out Braxton-Hicks contractions
- Sterile speculum exam to confirm rupture of membranes
    - Rupture is associated with pooling of fluid in the vagina, positive nitrazine test (paper turns blue due to pH >7.0), and ferning on a glass slide
    - Consider cultures to rule out infectious causes of preterm labor and chorioamnionitis (e.g., Group B strep, STDs)
    - Note the presence of meconium (thick, greenish fluid)
    - May see cord prolapse, fetal foot, or fetal breech
- Sterile digital exams to check cervix for dilatation, effacement (thinning), and fetal station
- Speculum or digital exam is *contraindicated* if any bleeding is present—must first rule out placenta previa by ultrasound
- Ultrasound may be used to determine presenting part and fetal position

Treatment

- Uncomplicated delivery
    - Extend and deliver the head; suction nose and mouth
    - Check for nuchal cord and reduce if present
    - Rotate the head by 90° and deliver shoulders
    - Double clamp and cut cord; care for infant as necessary
    - Deliver placenta by applying gentle traction
- Breech delivery
    - Deliver buttocks and then each leg one at a time
    - Allow torso to freely slide out (traction may entrap arms)
    - Rotate, deliver anterior arm, then repeat for other arm
    - Keep body parallel to floor (prevent neck extension and airway obstruction); deliver head via suprapubic pressure
- Shoulder dystocia: May require episiotomy, bladder drainage, maternal knee-to-chest, suprapubic pressure, corkscrew maneuver, or posterior shoulder delivery
- Prolapsed cord: Push presenting part off cord back into the cervix; hold in place until emergent C-section is performed
- Preterm labor: Steroids for fetal lung maturity and consider tocolytics (Mg^{3+} or β-agonists) to delay labor if <35 weeks

Disposition

- If possible, emergent transfer to labor and delivery is preferred; however, fetal distress may require emergent delivery in the ED
- Admit all patients
- Infant resuscitation must be performed as needed; consult the NICU for premature infants
- C-section is required for incomplete breech or footling presentations, prolapsed cord, placenta previa, and placental abruption
- Tocolysis in preterm labor should only be undertaken after consulting with OB/Gyn

196. Postpartum Complications

Etiology & Pathophysiology

- Postpartum hemorrhage: >500 mL of blood loss within 6 weeks after delivery (most cases occur within 24 hours of delivery)
  - Uterine atony (most common): Uterine muscle fails to contract
  - Lacerations (increased risk with forceps delivery and macrosomia)
  - Retained products: Portion of placenta stays attached to the uterus
  - Uterine inversion: Uterus prolapses into vagina (increased risk in multiple gestations and VBAC)
  - Uterine rupture (increased in multiple gestations, prior C-section)
- Postpartum cardiomyopathy (PPC): Idiopathic biventricular heart failure that occurs within days to weeks after delivery
- Endometritis: Bacterial infection of endometrium, often associated with PROM, prolonged labor, frequent pelvic exams, and C-section
- Lacational mastitis: Breast infection secondary to ductal obstruction
- Pulmonary embolus, HELLP syndrome, and pre-eclampsia/eclampsia also may occur postpartum

Differential Dx

- Hemorrhage: Normal bleeding from placental separation, normal lochia, birth trauma, coagulopathy (especially von Willebrand's disease)
- PPC: Pulmonary embolus, hypothyroidism, pre-eclampsia
- Endometritis: Hyperthyroidism, pneumonia, UTI, septic thrombophlebitis, local wound infection, intra-abdominal abscess

Presentation

- Hemorrhage: Vaginal bleeding, incisional bleeding, abdominal pain, tachycardia, tachypnea, shock
- PPC: Fatigue, edema, dyspnea (at rest or on exertion), cough, orthopnea, chest pain, S_3, crackles on lung exam (symptoms may be mild to severe)
- Endometritis: Foul smelling vaginal discharge, fever, abdominal pain/tenderness
- Mastitis: Warm, painful, erythematous breast

Diagnosis

- Postpartum hemorrhage: Obtain CBC, PT/PTT, and type/cross
  - Atony: Soft, "boggy" uterus with bleeding seen from cervix
  - Lacerations: Seen on speculum exam
  - Retained products: May be palpable on exam; uterus is globular and firm; ultrasound may show a uterus filled with blood or the presence of placenta
  - Uterine inversion: Mass visible in vagina on exam; unable to palpate uterus
  - Uterine rupture: Difficult to diagnose; may see fetal distress and severe bleeding during labor; ultrasound may be helpful
- PPC: CXR shows cardiomegaly and vascular congestion; ECG often shows arrhythmias; echocardiogram is diagnostic
- Endometritis: Fever and leukocytosis; obtain GC and chlamydia cultures; consider blood cultures
- Mastitis: Fever, tender breast, erythema

Treatment

- Hemorrhage: Provide standard resuscitation therapy (e.g., two large bore IVs, urgent type and cross, transfusions as needed, correct coagulopathy)
  - Atony: Manual uterine massage and IV oxytocin; if these fail, use methylergonovine and/or prostaglandin F2a (Hemabate); surgical intervention may be necessary
  - Lacerations: Repair with absorbable suture
  - Retained products: Manually remove retained products; persistently retained products require dilatation and curettage for removal
  - Inversion: Manually replace uterus (terbutaline and magnesium will help relax uterus but the procedure may require anesthesia); once replaced, administer oxytocin to cause uterine contraction and prevent bleeding
  - Rupture: Delivery with operative repair or hysterectomy
- PPC: Diuretics, fluid restriction, afterload reduction (e.g., ACE inhibitor), digoxin as needed, and anticoagulation
- Endometritis/mastitis: Empiric treatment with PCN/antipenicillinase or gentamycin plus clindamycin

Disposition

- Postpartum hemorrhage: Virtually all patients are admitted
- Lacerations: May be discharged
- PPC is often life-threatening (50% mortality at one year and survivors often have persistently decreased LV function); admit all patients; 30% will develop DVT or PE
- Endometritis: Admit for IV antibiotics
- Mastitis patients may be discharged with instructions for sufficient analgesia, warm or cold compresses, and continued breast feeding or pumping (hastens recovery)
- Consider septic pelvic thrombophlebitis in patients with persistent spiking fevers without source

197. Sexual Assault

Etiology & Pathophysiology

- Rape is a legal term, not a medical diagnosis—requires carnal knowledge, non-consent, and compulsion or fear of great harm
- Experts report that 1 in 5 women are raped in their lifetimes; however, few victims report the crime
- Men, as well as women and children, are victims of sexual assault
- Law enforcement will use evidence obtained from the original exam to prosecute offenders, including DNA evidence, glycoprotein p30, acid phosphatase, and presence of sperm
- Gonorrhea and chlamydia are the most commonly transmitted STDs
- Risk of contracting HIV depends on the type of intercourse—it is difficult to determine the need for post-exposure HIV prophylaxis as the assailant is usually unavailable for testing; the decision must be made based on local epidemiology, known characteristics of the assailant, and the wishes of the victim

Differential Dx

- Non-sexual assault
- Domestic violence
- Child abuse
- Diagnoses associated with sexual assault include transmission of STDs, risk of pregnancy, soft tissue injuries, orthopedic injuries, intracranial hemorrhage, and tracheal or laryngeal injuries secondary to choking

Presentation

- History of the assault should include when, where, number of assailants, weapons used, type of assault (e.g., fondling, type of penetration), whether ejaculation occurred (and where), condom use, loss of consciousness, and drug or alcohol use
- Past gynecologic history should include when consensual intercourse last occurred and what birth control is regularly used
- Determine if the patient urinated, defecated, bathed, changed clothes, ate, drank, or douched following the assault
- Examine for associated injuries

Diagnosis

- Ensure patient comfort throughout the exam to prevent further psychological injury; a chaperone should be present
- Obtain consent before beginning the evidence collection kit; collecting evidence does not mean that prosecution must occur
- Evidence kit ("rape kit") is completed by following step-by-step instructions for collection of evidence
- Photograph injuries when possible
- Examine (including a pelvic exam) and treat associated injuries
- Toluidine swab on vaginal mucosa will reveal tears (turns blue)
- Use a Wood's lamp to fluoresce semen stains
- Urine β-hCG to determine preexisting pregnancy
- Gonorrhea and chlamydia cultures, wet mount, HIV-ELISA test (determines baseline HIV status)
- Flunitrazepam (Rohypnol, the "date-rape drug") level if ingestion is clinically suspected

Treatment

- Treat traumatic injuries appropriately
- STD prophylaxis for gonorrhea, chlamydia, trichomonas, and bacterial vaginosis are recommended
  - Gonorrhea: Single dose of IM ceftriaxone, oral quinolone, or oral cefixime
  - Chlamydia: Single dose of oral azithromycin or 10 days of doxycycline, erythromycin, or ofloxacin
  - Trichomonas/bacterial vaginosis: Single dose of oral metronidazole
  - Hepatitis B: If patient has not previously been immunized, give the first of three doses of vaccine; consider hepatitis B immune globulin in high-risk cases
  - HIV testing should be done as an outpatient following counseling; may consider prophylaxis via zidovudine plus lamivudine for 28 days
  - Antibiotics differ if the patient is pregnant
- Pregnancy prophylaxis (if β-hCG is negative): Ethinyl estradiol/levonorgestrel 2 tablets in the ED and 2 tablets 12 hours later (must begin within 72 hours of assault)

Disposition

- Counseling should begin in ED by a social worker or local crisis center
- Ensure that patient has a safe place to go to upon discharge and arrange follow-up counseling
- Follow-up in 1–2 weeks for pregnancy testing, cervical culture, and hepatitis B vaccine
- Rape kit, including clothing worn during the assault; samples of hair, saliva, blood, nails; and oral, vaginal, and anal swabs should be given directly to law enforcement personnel or locked-up until they arrive (must maintain the chain of evidence)
- Must report any assaults on minors to legal authorities; some states also mandate reporting of adult sexual assaults

Pediatric Emergencies

NIHAR BHAKTA, MD

198. Fever Without Source

Etiology & Pathophysiology

- Infants 0–36 months old presenting with fever (rectal temperature >38°C) but without obvious source of fever after careful history and physical—20% of childhood fevers have no apparent cause
- Majority of children have a self-limited viral infection that resolves without sequelae; however, serious bacterial infections (e.g., meningitis, pyelonephritis, pneumonia, "occult bacteremia") must be ruled out
- Most common bacterial causes include *S. pneumoniae, Group B Streptococcus, N. meningitidis, H. influenzae* type B, *Listeria,* and *E. coli*
- Practice guidelines vary significantly based on age
- The incidence of occult bacteremia has decreased dramatically with the introduction of the *H. influenzae* and *S. pneumoniae* vaccines—well-appearing infants who have received both are at very low risk for invasive bacterial disease

Differential Dx

- Viral syndrome
- Occult bacteremia
- Occult pneumonia
- Occult UTI or pyelonephritis
- Meningitis
- Osteomyelitis
- Pneumonia
- Otitis media
- Gastroenteritis
- Endocarditis
- Rheumatic fever
- Malaria
- Tuberculosis
- Post-vaccination fever

Presentation

- Fever
- Lethargy/decreased activity
- Toxic appearance
- Irritability
- Decreased crying and/or eye contact
- Social withdrawal
- Pallor
- Vomiting/diarrhea
- Abnormal vital signs
- Weight loss
- Rash

Diagnosis

- <30 days old
    - All patients require CBC, blood/urine culture, LP, and CXR
- 30–90 days old
    - All require CBC, urinalysis, and blood/urine cultures
    - Low-risk patients may then be discharged home +/− LP
    - High-risk patients require LP and admission for IV antibiotics
- 3–36 months old
    - If toxic-appearing: Full workup and IV antibiotics
    - Non-toxic appearing and temperature <39°: Discharge
    - Non-toxic and temperature >39°: Urinalysis and CBC prior to discharge; consider blood cultures and empiric antibiotics
- Criteria for "low-risk"
    - Appears well, is previously healthy, has no chronic illness
    - WBC count 5,000 to 15,000; normal differential
    - Urinalysis: Negative gram stain, LE, and nitrites; <5 WBC
    - CSF: <8 WBC/mm^3, no organisms
    - Stool: <5 WBC/hpf

Treatment

- Begin empiric antibiotic therapy immediately for all infants <30 days old
    - Broad-spectrum antibiotics (ampicillin and cefotaxime/gentamycin) until all cultures are negative
    - Coverage includes *Listeria, E. coli,* and *Group B Strep*
- 30 to 90 days
    - High risk or toxic-appearing: IV cefotaxime or ceftriaxone until cultures are negative
    - Low risk: May discharge without antibiotics or may administer single dose IM ceftriaxone (if giving antibiotics, LP should be performed first to prevent possible confusion from partially treated meningitis)
- 3–36 months old
    - Toxic-appearing infants should receive IV antibiotics (e.g., ceftriaxone or cefotaxime)
    - Well appearing with temperature <39°: No treatment
    - Well appearing with temperature >39°: Consider empiric ceftriaxone/cefotaxime, especially if they have not received the *S. pneumoniae* vaccine

Disposition

- Infants <30 days old with fever require admission and antibiotics for at least 48 hours, pending culture results
- Infants >30 days and <3 months should be admitted if they have any high risk criteria or have unsure follow-up
- Infants 3–36 months old may be discharged home if the patient is clinically well, labs are normal, and follow-up can be ensured
- All infants with fever without source require re-evaluation in 24–48 hours
- Follow-up is critical; therefore, social issues should be evaluated (i.e., reliability of the parents to assess their child, access to phone and hospital, ease of communication if culture is positive)

199. Apnea

Etiology & Pathophysiology

- Apnea: Cessation of airflow lasting longer than 30 seconds
- Apparent life-threatening event (ALTE): Apnea, color change, choking or gagging, or a change in muscle tone during an event that the caretaker believes to be life threatening (occurs in 5% of infants)
- Etiologies may include infection (e.g., sepsis, meningitis, RSV), aspiration, airway obstruction, GERD, asphyxia, seizure, intracranial hemorrhage, drug or narcotic ingestion, immature respiratory center (prematurity), anemia (especially if <28 days), hypoglycemia, inborn errors of metabolism, arrhythmia, child abuse, Munchausen by proxy
- Detailed history may determine the etiology and chance of recurrence
  - Was patient awake or asleep?
  - Was there a change in color?
  - Was event related to feeding?
  - Was or is there a fever?
  - Atypical eye/limb movement?
  - Need for intervention (e.g., CPR) to resolve the episode?
  - Was there respiratory effort?
  - History of GERD or seizures?
  - Duration of episode?

Differential Dx

- Periodic breathing (respiratory pattern with repeated occurrence of three or more central apnea episodes in 20 seconds)
- Breath-holding spells (expiratory apnea and hypoxia following an unpleasant stimulus that may cause loss of consciousness or seizure—recovery occurs with a loud gasp after stimulation)
- Sudden Infant Death Syndrome (SIDS)

Presentation

- Central apnea: Complete absence of respiratory effort (most common cause of apnea)
- Obstructive apnea: The infant makes a respiratory effort, but no airflow occurs secondary to airway obstruction (most often associated with GE reflux)
- Mixed apnea: A combination of central and obstructive apnea
- Signs of increased ICP, abnormal heart sounds/rhythms, inadequate chest wall movement, abdominal distension, ruddy appearance (polycythemia), or pallor (anemia) may be present

Diagnosis

- History and physical exam
- Cardiorespiratory monitoring for all patients
- Rule out sepsis via blood, urine, and CSF cultures in appropriate patients (including all patients <2 months old)
- Laboratory studies are selected based on clinical suspicion
  - CBC may suggest infection, anemia, or polycythemia
  - Serum glucose, electrolytes, calcium, BUN/Cr, and ammonia to rule out a metabolic abnormality
  - Arterial blood gas to rule out acidosis and hypoxia
- CXR, ECG, and/or echocardiogram if suspect heart/lung disease
- Head CT if intraventricular hemorrhage is suspected
- Abdominal X-ray to evaluate for necrotizing enterocolitis
- Nasopharyngeal swab to evaluate for pertussis and RSV if URI symptoms are present
- Further studies may include EEG, swallowing evaluation, evaluation for GERD, and lumbar puncture

Treatment

- Resuscitation as necessary if the infant shows signs of shock (e.g., abnormal breathing, poor peripheral perfusion, hypotension)
- Continuous positive airway pressure (CPAP) and/or mechanical ventilation may be necessary
- Consider empiric broad-spectrum antibiotics if initial laboratory studies suggest bacterial infection or if etiology cannot be identified (especially in infants <28 days old)
- Treat underlying etiologies as necessary
  - Transfusion with packed red blood cells if patient is anemic (hematocrit <20% without symptoms or HCT <25% with symptoms and/or oxygen requirement)
  - Caffeine for apnea of prematurity
  - Reflux precautions (e.g., head up, prone position, small-volume feeds, thickened feedings, pharmacologic treatments) for GERD
  - Benzodiazepines or barbiturates for documented seizures
  - Glucose or calcium if needed

Disposition

- Most important goal in the ED is to determine if an ALTE has actually occurred
- Admission is required for nearly all patients
- Admit to PICU any infant who requires resuscitation or is <28 days old with persistent symptoms
- Discharge may be acceptable in a minority of infants, usually with home apnea monitoring, after consulting with the pediatrician
- An ALTE may increase the likelihood of SIDS

200. Pharyngitis and Otitis Media

Etiology & Pathophysiology

- Pharyngitis: Inflammation of the mucous membranes of the pharynx and tonsils due to infection, allergy, or trauma
  - Viral pharyngitis (especially adenovirus, EBV, influenza, parainfluenza) is the most common overall cause
  - *Streptococcus pyogenes* (Group A β-hemolytic streptococcus) is the most common treatable cause (may also cause serious invasive disease, such as toxic shock syndrome and necrotizing fasciitis)
- Otitis media: Infection of the middle ear due to clogging of the eustachian tubes (especially in infants with predisposing anatomy)
  - Common causes include *S. pneumoniae, M. catarrhalis, H. influenzae* (non-typable strain) and any respiratory virus
  - Neonatal disease may also be caused by *E. coli, Klebsiella, Enterobacter,* group B streptococci, and *S. aureus*
  - Risk factors include day-care, secondhand smoke, past history

Differential Dx

- Pharyngitis
  - Sinusitis
  - Respiratory irritants
  - Caustic ingestions
  - Lymphoma/leukemia
  - Diphtheria
- Otitis media
  - Otitis externa
  - Upper respiratory infection
  - Sinus infection
  - Dental pain
  - Gastroenteritis
  - Urinary tract infection
  - Otitis media with effusion

Presentation

- Streptococcal pharyngitis
  - Classic presentation: Sore throat, fever, tonsillar exudate, enlarged cervical lymph nodes, and *lack* of cough/rhinorrhea
  - Other symptoms may include headache, vomiting, and abdominal pain, scarlitiniform sand-paper rash
  - Children ages 4–12 years
- Otitis media
  - Often preceded by URI
  - Ear pain, pulling at ear
  - Ear discharge, poor hearing
  - Fever
  - Irritability, vomiting in infants
  - Especially children 6–18 months

Diagnosis

- Strep pharyngitis must be distinguished from viral pharyngitis to prevent unnecessary antibiotic use
  - If 3 or more of the classic signs are present and patient is >10 years old, treat for strep pharyngitis without further testing
  - Patients with none or 1 of classic signs do not require testing
  - Strep rapid antigen test is used in equivocal cases; a positive test confirms diagnosis but sensitivity is only 50–85%, so all negative tests should be sent for culture
  - Strep culture is the gold standard
  - Other screening tests used in atypical presentations include CBC, Monospot test (for EBV), and gonococcal throat culture
- Otitis media is a clinical diagnosis
  - Immobility of the tympanic membrane on insufflation
  - May see effusion behind the TM (bulging, loss of bony landmarks) and TM erythema
  - Tympanocentesis is not used in the ED and is only necessary in some cases of neonates, severe pain, or failure of therapy

Treatment

- Analgesia and antipyretics (e.g., acetaminophen, NSAIDs)
- Strep pharyngitis (treat for 10 days)
  - Penicillin V is the drug of choice
  - Other possible agents include amoxicillin, macrolides, or single dose IM benzathine penicillin
  - Treat all patients who have a positive rapid strep test
  - Defer treatment on patients with negative rapid tests until culture proves positive
  - In patients >10 years old with a classic clinical presentation, begin treatment without further testing
- Otitis media (treat for 10–14 days)
  - Children <10: First-line is high-dose amoxicillin (80 mg/kg/day), single dose IM ceftriaxone, or cefprozil
  - Refractory cases: Amoxicillin/clavulanic acid, cefuroxime, cefpodoxime, or azithromycin
  - Children >10: First-line is amoxicillin, amoxicillin/ clavulanate, cefuroxime, or single dose IM ceftriaxone
  - Widespread drug resistance exists (especially among *S. pneumoniae, M. catarrhalis*)

Disposition

- Admit only complicated pharyngitis
- Children are infectious for 24 hrs after the initiation of therapy
- Symptoms should improve in 48–72 hours after starting antibiotics
- Complications of strep include airway obstruction, peritonsillar abscess, Ludwig's angina (submandibular abscess), rheumatic fever (in untreated cases), post-strep glomerulonephritis (not prevented by treatment)
- Otitis media may result in recurrent or persistent infections
- Fluid may persist behind the ear for weeks to months
- Complications of otitis media include chronic suppurative otitis media, mastoiditis, hearing loss, subdural empyema, meningitis, facial paralysis, brain abscess

201. Bronchiolitis

Etiology & Pathophysiology

- Inflammation of the small bronchi and bronchioles, resulting in respiratory distress
- Most cases are due to respiratory synctial virus (RSV)
  - Transmission via respiratory droplets and close contact
  - Invades nasopharyngeal epithelial cells and spreads to the lower respiratory tract, causing sloughing of dead bronchial cells and increased mucus production
  - Plugging and obstruction of airways, atelectasis, and hyperinflation then occur, resulting in hypoxemia, increased work of breathing, and respiratory distress
- Other potential pathogens include parainfluenza, influenza, adenovirus, rhinovirus, chlamydia, and *Mycoplasma pneumoniae*
- May develop secondary bacterial pneumonia
- Very common cause of respiratory distress/hospitalization in infants
- More common and severe in premature and younger infants (<4 mo)

Differential Dx

- Asthma exacerbation
- Pertussis
- Croup
- Bacterial or viral pneumonia
- Aspiration pneumonitis
- Congestive heart failure
- Vascular ring
- Foreign body aspiration
- Chlamydia pneumonia
- Cystic fibrosis

Presentation

- Audible wheezing
- Dyspnea
- Tachypnea
- Cough, rhinitis, and congestion
- Poor feeding
- Lethargy
- Low-grade fever
- Increased work of breathing (chest retractions, neck muscle use, paradoxical abdominal movement)
- Wheezes and rhonchi on exam
- Nasal flaring and discharge
- Dehydration
- Hypotension may occur
- Severe disease (10–20% of cases) may result in grunting, apnea, cyanosis, and respiratory failure

Diagnosis

- Primarily a clinical diagnosis based on history and physical exam
- Nasopharygeal swab and testing for RSV or other common viral pathogens confirms disease
  - Immunofluorescent antibody testing
  - ELISA testing
  - Culture (rarely obtained)
- Chest X-ray is obtained for ill-appearing children (not necessary in mild disease)
  - Hyperinflation and peribronchial cuffing
  - May have scattered, patchy atelectasis and consolidation (difficult to rule out pneumonia)
- Consider workup for bacterial infection (blood cultures, lumbar puncture, U/A) if RSV is not confirmed, if patient is ill-appearing, and in all patients <30 days old
- Pulse oximetry may reveal hypoxemia, but is nonspecific
- CBC may show leukocytosis with left shift or bandemia

Treatment

- No proven therapy exists except supportive care
- Supplemental O_2 to achieve saturations greater than 92%
- IV hydration and antipyretics
- Nebulized albuterol may achieve bronchodilation; however, it is not effective in all patients and should only be used if a clinical response to therapy is observed
- Nebulized racemic epinephrine may be superior to albuterol and should be used in ill patients not responsive to albuterol
- Aerosolized ribavirin (an antiviral) may be considered in extremely ill children with underlying cardiac or pulmonary conditions
- Respigam (RSV immune globulin) and palivizumab (RSV monoclonal antibody) may be administered prophylactically to exposed high-risk patients (e.g., premature infants, CF)
- Consider antibiotics if suspect bacterial pneumonia (though extremely unlikely)
- Corticosteroids and nebulized ipratropium have not been proven effective
- Patients with severe recurrent apnea or respiratory failure will require assisted ventilation

Disposition

- Criteria for admission
  - Hypoxia (room air pulse ox <93%)
  - Tachypnea (greater than 1.5 × normal respiratory rate)
  - Dehydration (i.e., patients unable to feed secondary to tachypnea)
  - Any apneic events
  - Severe underlying disease
  - Age <6 weeks
  - Hospitalize even moderately ill patients as they may quickly decompensate
- Criteria for discharge
  - Pulse ox >93% on room air
  - Near-normal respiratory rate after therapy
  - Able to tolerate oral intake
  - Stable social setting
  - Primary care follow-up available

202. Whooping Cough

Etiology & Pathophysiology

- A severe lower respiratory tract infection caused by *Bordetella pertussis* (a non-motile gram negative coccobacillus)
- A whooping cough-like syndrome may also be caused by *Bordetella parapertussis*, *Bordetella bronchiseptica*, *Mycoplasma pneumoniae*, *Chlamydia trachomatis*, *Chlamydia pneumoniae*, or adenovirus
- Transmission occurs from person-to-person via respiratory tract secretions (nearly 100% of non-immune household contacts of affected patients will develop disease)
- Incubation period is 7–21 days
- >1000 cases per year in the US
- May occur at any age with greatest incidence in children <1 year old
- Vaccine administered as part of childhood immunization (DPT) provides waning (over ~10 years) immunity

Differential Dx

- Viral URI
- Habit cough (cough tic)
- Asthma
- Bronchiolitis
- Bacterial pneumonia
- Cystic fibrosis
- Tuberculosis
- Foreign body aspiration
- Bacterial tracheitis
- GERD

Presentation

- Three stages of pertussis infection
  - Catarrhal stage (1–2 weeks): Mild upper respiratory tract symptoms (low fever, cough, coryza)
  - Paroxysmal stage (2–6 weeks): Severe paroxysms of cough with characteristic inspiratory stridor ("whoop"), occasionally followed by vomiting
  - Convalescent phase (2–4 weeks): Symptoms gradually lessen (cough may persist for months)
- Infants <6 months: Whoop is often absent; apnea and cyanosis present
- Adolescents and adults: URI-type syndrome with persistent cough but without a whoop

Diagnosis

- Diagnosis is typically clinical
- Helpful clues in the history include history of apnea or cyanosis, history of cough worsening in severity and forcefulness, or family member with a persistent cough
- CBC: Leukocytosis with predominant lymphocytosis
- CXR: Perihilar infiltrates or "shaggy" right heart border
- Nasopharyngeal culture is the gold standard for diagnosis but is not 100% sensitive
- Direct fluorescence antibody test of nasopharyngeal secretions is available in some centers

Treatment

- Macrolides (e.g., erythromycin, azithromycin, clarithromycin) for 14 days are recommended for all patients with proven pertussis
- Infants less than 1 year of age and other patients with potentially severe disease often require hospitalization for supportive care of apnea, cyanosis, coughing paroxysms, and vomiting/dehydration
- Hospitalized patients should be isolated for 5 days after initiation of antibiotic therapy
- No clear benefit of corticosteroids or albuterol
- All household and other close contacts (e.g., daycare) should receive prophylaxis with erythromycin
- Close contacts < age 7 should receive pertussis immunization according to recommended schedule

Disposition

- Infants <1 year of age with suspected pertussis infection must be admitted and monitored for apnea
- Complications include pneumonia, otitis media, apnea, seizures, encephalopathy, pneumothorax, and dehydration (due to inability to feed during coughing spells or due to post-tussive emesis)
- The incidence of all complications is greatest in infants <1 year of age
- Fever during the paroxysmal or convalescent phase suggests secondary bacterial infection
- Antibiotic treatment will limit transmission; however, treatment will not shorten duration of illness if given beyond the catarrhal phase (i.e., must be given before whoop appears)
- May return to daycare 5 days after initiation of antibiotic therapy

203. Laryngotracheobronchitis (Croup)

Etiology & Pathophysiology

- Infection and inflammation of subglottic tissues and/or tracheal mucosa (does not affect the pulmonary bed)
- Airway edema causes luminal narrowing and airflow obstruction, resulting in stridor, cough, hoarseness, and respiratory distress
- Generally a benign, self-limited disease that occurs in children 6 months to 3 years of age; however, 20–30% of children require hospitalization and 1–3% require intubation
- Most commonly of viral origin: Parainfluenza is the most common cause (60% of cases); other viruses include RSV, adenovirus, and influenza
- Person-to-person transmission via respiratory droplets or fomite exposure (then spreads from nasopharynx to the larynx and trachea)
- Seasonal peak in late fall/early winter

Differential Dx

- Foreign body aspiration
- Laryngomalacia
- Tracheomalacia
- Epiglottitis
- Bacterial tracheitis
- Subglottic stenosis
- Vascular ring
- Laryngeal web
- Laryngitis
- Angioneurotic edema
- Peritonsillar abscess
- Retropharyngeal abscess

Presentation

- Prodrome: 1–5 days of nonspecific URI symptoms (cough, congestion, sore throat) progressing to fevers
- No signs of toxicity (as opposed to epiglottitis or bacterial tracheitis)
- Characteristic "bark-like" cough, hoarseness, and inspiratory stridor (symptoms worse at night)
- Patients with mild disease may have normal lung exam (± wheeze)
- Mild-to-moderate disease presents with stridor following agitation, without respiratory distress
- Severe disease results in respiratory distress (stridor at rest, nasal flaring, retractions, poor air exchange, mental status changes)

Diagnosis

- Croup is a clinical diagnosis
- Radiographic studies are usually not necessary for diagnosis, but a PA neck film may show non-specific findings
   - Steeple sign: Pointed subglottic tracheal air shadow (narrowing of laryngeal air column due to mucosal edema) 5–10 mm below the vocal cords on frontal neck films
   - Ballooning: Overdistention of the hypopharynx during inspiration on lateral neck films
   - May rule out other causes (e.g., epiglottitis, foreign body)
- Clinical croup score is sometimes used to identify the severity of croup (score based on inspiratory breath sounds, stridor, cough, retractions and flaring, and cyanosis)
- Pulse oximetry may (rarely) reveal hypoxemia
- CBC may show leukocytosis

Treatment

- Administer IV fluids and antipyretics as needed
- Humidified air (either cool mist or hot steam) will decrease upper airway inflammation and ameliorate symptoms; an excellent home therapy for mild croup
- Nebulized epinephrine may be used in moderate-to-severe viral croup to decrease laryngeal mucosa edema (via vasoconstriction) and improve stridor and respiratory distress; however, obstruction may return after medication wears off (approximately 2 hours)
- Corticosteroids or nebulized budesonide are also used to decrease laryngeal mucosa edema (dexamethaxone has been shown to improve symptoms and decrease the need for hospitalization and intubation)
- Heliox (mixture of helium and oxygen) improves air flow and decreases work of breathing—may prevent intubation
- Endotracheal intubation is required in patients with severe airway obstruction (i.e., increasing stridor, retractions, cyanosis, signs of exhaustion, altered mental status) and/or patients who fail to respond to the above treatments
- Antibiotics are not indicated

Disposition

- Decision to hospitalize should be made after 3–4 hours of ED observation
- Criteria for discharge include no stridor at rest, normal air entry, normal color/no hypoxia, normal level of consciousness, able to tolerate oral intake, parents able to return child to ED if symptoms worsen, and at least 4 hours since last epinephrine treatment
- Follow-up is required in 24–48 hours
- If patient fails to improve after 5–7 days, other causes (e.g., bacterial infection, measles) should be considered
- Complications include bacterial tracheitis due to *S. aureus, H. influenzae, S. pneumoniae,* or *M. catarrhalis* (acute onset of respiratory compromise that mimics epiglottitis is bacterial tracheitis until proven otherwise)

204. Epiglottitis

Etiology & Pathophysiology

- An acute airway emergency with high morbidity and mortality
- Caused by bacteria or viruses that result in edema and cellulitis of the epiglottis
- Bacterial causes include *Streptococcus pneumoniae, Moraxella catarrhalis, H. influenzae* type B, *H. parainfluenzae,* and *Pseudomonas*
- Viral causes include herpes simplex virus, parainfluenza viruses, varicella-zoster virus, and Epstein-Barr virus
- Incidence of epiglottitis has decreased significantly since the introduction of the HiB vaccine, with *Streptococcus* becoming the most common cause
- Typically occurs during ages 2–7 but may occur at any age (even adults)

Differential Dx

- Bacterial tracheitis
- Croup
- Peritonsillar abscess
- Retropharyngeal abscess
- Uvulitis
- Foreign body aspiration
- Diphtheria
- Mononucleosis
- Thermal/chemical airway burn
- Trauma to airway
- Laryngeomalacia
- Severe pharyngitis
- URI in a child with upper airway disease (e.g., subglottic or tracheal stenosis)

Presentation

- Abrupt onset of high fever (>40°C) with rapid development of sore throat, hoarse voice, dysphagia, and respiratory distress (marked stridor with subcostal and supraclavicular retractions)
- Toxic appearance with irritability and anxiety
- Cherry red, swollen epiglottis
- Patients tend to assume a characteristic tripod position in order to optimize airway diameter (sit erect with chin hyperextended, mouth wide open, and body leaning forward)
- Cyanosis may occur
- Absence of cough

Diagnosis

- Patients are at risk for acute airway compromise at any time during the evaluation—if highly suspected, the patient should immediately proceed to surgery for bronchoscopy and intubation
- Laboratory evaluation should be done only if the airway is definitively patent or has been stabilized
- Lateral neck X-ray shows a swollen epiglottis ("thumb print sign"), thickened aryepiglottic folds, dilation of the hypopharynx, and/or a swollen retropharyngeal space
- Chest X-ray may reveal associated pneumonia
- Direct fiberoptic visualization should only be performed if prepared to intubate
    - Classically, visualization of the airway in the OR will determine the etiology of the patient's respiratory distress
    - If the epiglottis is red and inflamed, the diagnosis is confirmed
- CBC may show leukocytosis
- Blood and epiglottic cultures should be obtained

Treatment

- Avoid agitating the child (*do not* place IV, examine the throat, or draw cultures) as this may cause acute airway closure
- Treatment is first surgical then medical
    - Evaluation and securing of airway is critical in patients with suspected epiglottitis
    - Endotracheal intubation should be done by the most experienced expert available (generally ENT surgery or anesthesia); if endotracheal intubation cannot be performed, tracheostomy should be performed
    - If diagnosis is strongly suspected, proceed to surgery to visualize the airway and intubate the child
- Administer supplemental O_2
- IV antibiotics should include ampicillin plus cefotaxime
- There is no proven efficacy of corticosteroids

Disposition

- All patients must be admitted to a PICU
- Someone experienced at intubation and surgical airways should accompany the patient at all times
- Transfer patients to another facility if ENT or pediatric ICU support is not available
- Sequelae may include acute respiratory failure, sepsis/shock, pneumothorax, tracheal stenosis, cerebral anoxic injury, and/or death
- Mortality may be as high as 10%; however, if airway is secured immediately, mortality is closer to 1%
- Cyanosis is associated with poor prognosis

205. Pneumonia

Etiology & Pathophysiology

- Lower respiratory tract infection of the lung parenchyma, resulting in inflammation, alveolar exudates, and consolidation
- Viral pneumonia is more common in all age groups except neonates
- Neonatal pneumonia is often bacterial (*Group B Strep, E. coli, Klebsiella, S. aureus, Pseudomonas aeruginosa, H. influenzae, S. marcescens*)
- Infants: Viral or bacterial (*S. pneumoniae, H. influenzae, Chlamydia*)
- School age/adolescents: Viral or bacterial (*S. pneumoniae, S. aureus, H. influenzae, Group A Strep, B. pertussis, Mycoplasma pneumoniae*)
- Specific etiology is often not determined; however, identification of pathogens may lead to diagnosis of underlying problems (e.g., *P. carinii* in AIDS patients, *P. aeruginosa* in cystic fibrosis patients)
- Conditions predisposing to pneumonia include cerebral palsy, cystic fibrosis, seizures, congenital immune deficits, aspiration risks, and anatomic abnormalities

Differential Dx

- Reactive airway disease/asthma
- Bronchiolitis
- Aspiration
- Inhalation of toxin
- Drug reaction
- Tumors (primary or metastatic)
- Cystic fibrosis
- Pulmonary sequestration
- Congenital heart disease/CHF (tachypnea with normal lung exam in patients <6 mo is heart disease until proven otherwise)
- Atelectasis
- Pleural effusion

Presentation

- "Typical" pneumonia is characterized by acute or subacute onset of fever, dyspnea, and productive cough
- Signs of respiratory distress may be present (e.g., tachypnea, flaring, grunting, retractions, accessory muscle use, dyspnea)
- Apnea
- Cyanosis
- Pleuritic chest pain
- Abdominal pain
- Lethargy/ill appearance
- Auscultation findings: Crackles, tachypnea, decreased and tubular breath sounds, fremitus, wheezing, egophony, dullness to percussion

Diagnosis

- History and physical exam suggest the diagnosis; however, lung exam may be unrevealing
- Pulse oximetry may reveal hypoxemia
- Chest X-ray: Consolidation/infiltrates are diagnostic
  - Viral, mycoplasma, and Chlamydia: Diffuse infiltrates
  - Bacterial: Lobar consolidation
  - May also see atelectasis, effusion, or peribronchial thickening
- CBC: Leukocytosis with left shift in many cases
- Blood cultures are positive in 10–15% of patients with *S. pneumoniae* and *S. aureus* pneumonias
- Sputum cultures may identify the organism, but are usually difficult to obtain and not very helpful
- Fluorescent antibody tests for Chlamydia and pertussis and viral antigen tests for RSV exist but are rarely used
- Consider HIV testing in young patients with repeated pneumonia

Treatment

- Administer supplemental O_2
- IV fluids are often needed for rehydration due to poor oral intake and increased insensible losses (due to fever and tachypnea)
- Neonates require IV antibiotic therapy: Ampicillin, nafcillin, or vancomycin plus either cefotaxime or gentamycin
- Infants and children
  - Inpatient therapy: IV erythromycin plus cefuroxime or cefotaxime
  - Outpatient therapy: Any macrolide or erythromycin/sulfisoxazole for 10 days
- Consider congenital *Chlamydia trachomatis* pneumonia in infants less than 6 months old
- Cystic fibrosis patients will likely require double coverage against *Pseudomonas* (e.g., gentamycin plus ceftazidime)
- Bronchodilators may be used in patients with significant wheezing

Disposition

- Criteria for discharge
  - Pulse oximetry >94% on room air
  - Able to tolerate oral medications and oral intake
  - Absence of respiratory distress at rest
  - No history of apnea
  - Age >3 months
  - Able caregivers
- Patients that do not satisfy the above criteria require hospitalization for IV medications and close observation
- Complications include sepsis, effusion/empyema, dehydration, pneumothorax, and respiratory failure
- In neonates and immunocompromised patients, untreated or incompletely treated pneumonia may be fatal

206. Congenital Heart Disease

Etiology & Pathophysiology

- Lesions may result in cyanosis (due to mixing of oxygenated and deoxygenated blood) or CHF (due to increased pulmonary blood flow); some are dependent on a patent ductus arteriosus to maintain systemic flow (usually closes by 1 month of age)
- Cyanotic lesions include
  - Tricuspid atresia
  - Transposition of the great vessels (presents at 1 week old—aorta arises from RV and pulmonary artery arises from LV)
  - Tetralogy of Fallot (presents before age 4 with VSD, RV outflow obstruction, RV hypertrophy, and overriding aorta)
  - Truncus arteriosus (single arterial trunk arises from the heart)
- Lesions resulting in CHF include ventricular septal defect (the most common cardiac defect), patent ductus arteriosus, hypoplastic LV, and coarctation of the aorta
- Acyanotic syncope may occur with critical aortic stenosis

Differential Dx

- Cyanosis/CHF
  - Respiratory infection (croup, pneumonia, bronchiolitis)
  - Sepsis   —Anemia
  - Hypothyroid   —Arrythmias
  - Myocarditis/pericarditis
  - Cardiomyopathy
  - Methemoglobinemia
  - Inborn metabolic disease
- Ductal-dependent lesions
  - Aortic stenosis/coarctation
  - Hypoplastic left ventricle
  - Transposed great vessels
  - Tricuspid atresia

Presentation

- May present in cardiogenic shock (especially if ductal-dependent): Cyanosis, cool periphery, poor capillary refill, and hypotension
- Cyanosis: Tachypnea (earliest sign), tachycardia, feeding intolerance, characteristic murmurs, pallor, mottling
- CHF: Irritability, weak cry, poor feeding, diaphoresis with feedings or prolonged feeding, failure to thrive, exam findings (crackles, tachypnea, tachycardia, murmurs, hepatomegaly)
- In older children, CHF presents as exercise intolerance, chronic cough, weight gain/loss

Diagnosis

- Auscultation: Pathologic murmurs are often holosystolic, diastolic, >2/6 intensity, or radiating
- Arm BP > leg BP in coarctation of the aorta
- Hyperoxia challenge test: Confirms suspicion of hypoxic or cyanotic cardiac lesions if PaO_2 does not rise with administration of 100% O_2 (hypoxia persists due to persistent mixing of oxygenated blood with deoxygenated blood)
- ECG: Evaluate rhythm and chamber size (e.g., LV hypertrophy)
- Chest X-ray should be obtained in all patients
  - Evaluate size/shape of the heart
  - Evaluate pulmonary vasculature for congestion due to left to right shunt or LV failure
  - Right-sided aortic arch is seen in Tetralogy of Fallot, transposition of great vessels, and tricuspid atresia
- Echocardiogram (with Doppler) is diagnostic for most lesions

Treatment

- Ductal-dependent lesions (usually present in the first 14 days of life) require immediate, life-saving reopening of the ductus arteriosus
  - IV prostaglandin E1 infusion is administered if pulse oximetry is <70% (side effects include apnea and hypotension)
  - Surgery provides definitive therapy for these lesions
- TET spell: Hypercyanotic episode in Tetralogy of Fallot
  - Decreased systemic vascular resistance (SVR) or increased cardiac output causes increase of right-to-left shunt across the large VSD, resulting in large amounts of deoxygenated blood entering the systemic circulation
  - Resistant to oxygen therapy because of right-to-left shunt
  - Therapy requires increasing SVR (knee-chest position, morphine, IV phenylephrine drip, ketamine sedation)
- Treatment of CHF is similar to adult care
  - Preload reduction (e.g., loop diuretics)
  - Afterload reduction (e.g., ACE-inhibitors, nitroprusside, nitroglycerin)
  - Positive inotropes (e.g., dopamine, digoxin)
  - May ultimately need surgical correction of cardiac defect

Disposition

- All neonates with newly diagnosed congenital heart disease should be admitted and referred to a center with Pediatric Cardiology specialists
- Any patient with an obstructive left-sided lesion requires admission to a PICU and urgent cardiothoracic surgery
- Patients with CHF exacerbation are usually admitted

207. Abdominal Pain

Etiology & Pathophysiology

- A frequent complaint in all pediatric age groups
- Multiple etiologies exist
- True emergencies must be promptly identified in the ED
  - Infants: Child abuse, pyloric stenosis, hernia, volvulus, sepsis, intussusception
  - Children: Appendicitis, hernia, DKA, child abuse, intussusception
  - Adolescents: Appendicitis, ectopic pregnancy, DKA, PID, testicular or ovarian torsion

Differential Dx

- Gastroenteritis
- Constipation
- Appendicitis   • Sepsis
- Pancreatitis   • Peptic ulcer
- Splenic rupture   • Trauma
- Sickle cell crisis   • DKA
- Renal colic   • Toxins
- Incarcerated hernia
- Malrotation with volvulus
- Testicular/ovarian torsion
- Respiratory illness (URI, otitis media, pneumonia, pharyngitis)
- Urinary tract infection
- Ectopic pregnancy
- Pelvic Inflammatory Disease

Presentation

- Presentation depends both on age of patient and specific etiology
- Note onset, course, duration, intensity, and radiation of pain
- Note exacerbating factors (e.g., eating, movement)
- Note improving factors (e.g., lying still, passing stool)
- Associated symptoms may include fever, N/V, diarrhea, headache, hematochezia, hematemesis, polyuria/polydipsia
- Peritoneal signs suggest a surgical emergency
- Do not forgo rectal, genital, and pelvic exams

Diagnosis

- Children often cannot differentiate emotional stress from somatic pain; thus, while referring to abdominal pain, they may actually be indicating fear, anxiety, nausea, hunger, or urge to defecate
- Initial tests may include electrolytes (dehydration, vomiting, diarrhea), urinalysis (UTI, DKA), and urine β-hCG (pregnancy)
- CBC is nonspecific and insensitive—rarely aids in diagnosis
- Chest X-ray may diagnose pneumonia or perforation
- Abdominal X-ray is rarely helpful, but may show a "double bubble" sign in volvulus or free air in perforation
- Abdominal CT is the test of choice for appendicitis and renal colic
- Barium or air enema may be diagnostic of and therapeutic for intussusception
- Ultrasound is used to evaluate pyloric stenosis, appendicitis, testicular torsion, intussusception, and volvulus
- Barium swallow is the test of choice for malrotation/volvulus

Treatment

- Surgical emergencies include appendicitis, intussusception, malrotation with volvulus, incarcerated hernia, ectopic pregnancy, and ovarian/testicular torsion
  - In patients with potential surgical emergencies, avoid oral intake, ensure large bore IV access, and begin IV fluids
- Administer appropriate analgesia—there is no evidence that pain management will "mask" signs of abdominal disease
  - Narcotic pain medicines are appropriate if the child has significant pain
  - Avoid aspirin in febrile children due to the risk of developing Reye syndrome
- Further treatment depends on specific etiology

Disposition

- All patients with surgical or medical emergencies require admission
- Patients require frequent evaluation of vital signs and repeat physical examinations to determine if they are clinically stable for discharge
- A period of observation may be necessary in unclear cases—consider observation for 23 hours with close monitoring of vital signs, laboratory results, and physical examination
- Patients may be discharged if pain resolves, serious conditions are ruled out, the parents are reliable, and good follow-up care is available

208. Pyloric Stenosis

Etiology & Pathophysiology

- Congenital hypertrophy of the muscular layers of the pylorus, resulting in gastric outlet obstruction
- Post-feeding vomiting due to gastric outlet obstruction leads to dehydration, electrolyte abnormalities, and weight loss
- Etiology is unknown
- Incidence of 3 per 1000 live births
- Males are affected 4 times more often than females
- Up to 50% have a family history
- Usually presents at 2–8 weeks of age; however, may present as late as 5 months

Differential Dx

- Overfeeding
- Food allergy
- GERD
- Acute gastroenteritis
- Pyloric atresia
- Lower GI obstruction (e.g., malrotation with volvulus, inguinal hernia)
- Infection (e.g., UTI, sepsis)
- Child abuse
- Appendicitis
- Congenital adrenal hyperplasia
- Inborn error of metabolism

Presentation

- Nonbilious, projectile vomiting shortly after feeding
- Infant continues to remain vigorous and attempts to feed
- Dehydration
- The classic physical finding is a palpable, olive-shaped epigastric mass
- Peristaltic waves (gastric waves) may be seen across the abdomen prior to vomiting

Diagnosis

- History and physical is strongly suggestive
- Abdominal X-ray may show a dilated stomach; also used to rule out other causes of bowel obstruction
- Abdominal ultrasound is the best diagnostic test (sensitivity >90%): Shows increased pyloric muscle thickness (>4 mm) or length (>16 mm)
- Upper GI series is used if ultrasound is negative but high clinical suspicion still exists: Will show a "string sign" of contrast in the pyloric channel, suggesting narrowing of the pylorus
- Electrolyte abnormalities may include hypochloremic metabolic alkalosis, hyponatremia, and hypokalemia

Treatment

- Correct electrolyte abnormalities and dehydration with normal saline solution plus 5% dextrose with added potassium
- Pylorotomy surgery is the definitive therapy

Disposition

- All patients require admission for IV fluids until pylorotomy is performed
- If unable to obtain ultrasound quickly, admit the patient for rehydration until further imaging can be performed to evaluate for pyloric stenosis
- Most infants recover from the surgery without sequelae

209. Gastroenteritis

Etiology & Pathophysiology

- Intestinal inflammation that results in diarrhea and vomiting
- Most commonly viral (30–40% of cases), affecting the proximal small bowel: Rotavirus, enteric adenovirus, enteroviruses, astrovirus, calicivirus, Norwalk virus
- Bacterial pathogens generally affect the colon (via mucosal invasion, cytotoxic cell death, disruption of mucosal cell function, or toxin release resulting in excessive water secretion): *E. coli, Campylobacter jejuni,* Shigella, Salmonella, *Staphylococcus aureus,* Vibrio, Yersinia, Clostridium, *Bacillus cereus, Listeria*
- Parasites include *Giardia, Cryptosporidium,* and *E. histolytica*
- Dysentery (bloody or mucousy diarrhea): Yersinia, Campylobacter, Shigella, Salmonella, E. coli O157, Clostridium, *C. difficile*
- Up to 30 million cases per year in the US
- Transmission may be fecal-oral, foodborne, waterborne, or via respiratory droplets

Differential Dx

- Antibiotic-induced gastroenteritis
- Overfeeding
- Inflammatory Bowel Disease (<9 years old)
- Intoxication
- Cystic fibrosis
- Intussusception
- Hemolytic-Uremic Syndrome
- Pyloric stenosis (<4 months)
- Lactose intolerance
- Malabsorption syndromes
- Hirschsprung's disease (<1 month)

Presentation

- Nausea and vomiting
- Diarrhea (watery, mucoid, and/or bloody)
- Dehydration may present as weight loss, dry mucosa, poor skin turgor, sunken eyeballs or fontanel, poor capillary refill, decreased tears, decreased urine output, lethargy, hypotension
- Constipation in early stages
- Abdominal cramps and tenderness
- Tenesmus
- Fever may or may not be present
- Prostration, malaise, anorexia, lethargy
- Headache

Diagnosis

- Clinical diagnosis
- Check CBC and chemistries if suspect dehydration, electrolyte imbalances or hypoglycemia
- Fecal leukocytes may indicate a bacterial infection (often present in invasive *E. coli,* Shigella, and Campylobacter infection)
- Imaging studies should be done if there is vomiting without diarrhea (looking for obstruction, volvulus, or possibly increased intracranial pressure)—do not assume an infectious cause in these patients
- Additional evaluation may be necessary if the child appears toxic, has dysentery, and/or is febrile
  - Stool culture for bacteria (may guide antibiotic choice)
  - Stool for rotavirus enzyme (Rotazyme)
  - Stool for ova and parasites (if chronic symptoms)
  - Stool for *C. difficile* toxin (in patients with recent antibiotics)
- Blood cultures may be helpful in infants if invasive bacterial disease is suspected (they are at increased risk of bacteremia)

Treatment

- Most cases are self-limited; the goal of therapy is to keep the patient well hydrated until symptoms resolve
  - Attempt oral rehydration in most cases; use commercial oral rehydration solutions that have appropriate electrolyte concentrations
  - IV rehydration in severely ill patients or those who fail oral therapy: Normal saline or lactated Ringer's solution to replace losses plus maintenance requirements plus ongoing losses over 24 hours with ½ in the first 8 hours
- Correct electrolyte abnormalities (children are at high risk of hypoglycemia)
- Antibiotics are generally not indicated, except in some bacterial diseases
  - Administer if <6 months old, if appears septic, if severe dysentery, or if immunocompromised
  - With certain *E. coli* strains, there is increased risk of hemolytic-uremic syndrome if antibiotics are used
- Avoid opiates, anticholinergics, or absorbents in children
- Antiemetics or anti-motility agents are also not recommended in children

Disposition

- Most patients can be discharged
- 10% of patients become dehydrated (life-threatening in 1%)
- Discharge to home if able to tolerate oral rehydration and have good follow-up; re-examine in 24 hours
- Criteria for admission
  - Greater than 5–10% dehydration
  - Unable to tolerate oral intake
  - Persistent vomiting
  - Shock
  - Evidence of Hemolytic-Uremic syndrome
- Complications include hypoglycemia, hyper- or hyponatremia, colonic perforation, toxic encephalopathy, seizures, sepsis, and Hemolytic-Uremic syndrome

210. Intussusception

Etiology & Pathophysiology

- Invagination of a proximal segment of bowel into a more distal segment
- As the associated mesentery gets dragged into the "telescoped" bowel, venous engorgement, edema, and bowel ischemia occur
- Symptoms are due to ischemia and small bowel obstruction
- Occurs in children <3 years old
- Most common abdominal emergency in infancy
- Most common cause of obstruction in infants 3 months to 3 years old
- In 5–10% of cases, there is a pathological lead point (a mass that is dragged via peristalsis into distal bowel); typical lead points include polyps, Meckel's diverticulum, hematomas due to Henoch-Schonlein purpura, hypertrophied lymphoid tissue (viral infection), and hemangiomas
- If occurs in children >9 years old, suspect a malignant lead point
- Occurs at the ileocolic junction in almost 90% of cases

Differential Dx

- Gastroenteritis
- Meckel's diverticulum
- Volvulus
- Adhesions
- Incarcerated hernia
- Polyps
- Foreign body aspiration
- UTI
- Incarcerated malrotation
- Hirschsprung's disease
- Tumors (lymphoma)
- Parasitic infection (enterobius)
- Henoch-Schonlein purpura
- Appendicitis
- Pyloric stenosis

Presentation

- Classic triad in 20%: Vomiting, pain, bloody stool ("currant jelly")
- Typical patient is a previously healthy infant with sudden onset of severe, intermittent colicky abdominal pain
- Bouts occur in 15–20 minute intervals, associated with pallor, straining, inconsolable crying and drawing up legs
- Between episodes, the patient may look comfortable
- Clear or bilious emesis
- Sausage-shaped, palpable mass in the RUQ
- May present only with altered mental status or with fever

Diagnosis

- Early diagnosis is crucial to avoid necrosis of the bowel, perforation, and peritonitis
- History and physical are highly suggestive of the diagnosis
- Stool guaiac is positive in the majority of cases
- Abdominal X-ray may reveal an intestinal obstruction pattern, an empty sigmoid or rectum, a soft tissue density surrounded by a crescent of gas in the area of intussusception (target sign), or free air due to perforation
- Contrast enema (air or barium) is the gold standard for diagnosis and may also be therapeutic
    - Shows a filling defect or cupping in the area where the contrast cannot be advanced
    - Classic finding on barium enema is a "coil spring" appearance as contrast is trapped in folds of the bowel
- Diagnosis may also be made by abdominal CT or ultrasound

Treatment

- Avoid oral intake
- NG tube for abdominal decompression
- Aggressive IV fluid resuscitation to correct dehydration (due to vomiting and third spacing into the intestinal wall and lumen)
- Obtain pediatric surgery consultation prior to attempted reduction
- Contrast enema for reduction
    - Air contrast is used more often than barium due to a lower risk of chemical peritonitis if perforation occurs
    - Risk of perforation is 1–3%
    - 80–90% success rate
- Enema is contraindicated (due to high risk of perforation) if there are symptoms present >12 hours, free air, peritoneal signs, or signs of shock
- Surgery is indicated if enema is unsuccessful, enema is contraindicated, or if intussusception recurs
- Broad-spectrum IV antibiotics are administered if perforation is suspected

Disposition

- The child may appear well between episodes
- Will progress to bowel ischemia, bowel death, and shock within 24 hours
- Usually fatal if the diagnosis is missed
- All patients require admission, even if the intussusception has been successfully reduced in the ED
- There is a 10% risk of recurrence after non-operative reduction, usually within 24 hours of the initial reduction

211. Appendicitis

Etiology & Pathophysiology

- Obstruction of the appendiceal lumen leads to inflammation, distension, vascular compromise, infection, ischemia, and ultimately rupture with peritonitis
- Obstruction is most often caused by a fecalith; other causes include swollen lymphoid follicle, pinworm, carcinoid tumor, or foreign body
- Perforation is the most concerning complication; may occur as early as 8–24 hours after symptom onset
- Appendicitis is the most common atraumatic surgical abdominal disorder in children 2 years or older
- Much rarer in children <2 years old
- Males have a lifetime risk of 8.6% and females a risk of 6.7%

Differential Dx

- Gastroenteritis
- Constipation
- Peptic ulcer
- *Yersinia enterocolitica*
- Intestinal obstruction
- Intussusception
- Mesenteric adenitis
- Urinary tract infection
- Pelvic Inflammatory Disease
- IBD exacerbation
- Diabetic ketoacidosis
- Torsion of testes or ovary
- Renal colic or pyelonephritis
- Ectopic pregnancy
- Lower lobe pneumonia
- Sepsis

Presentation

- Fever
- Anorexia, nausea/vomiting
- Abdominal pain
  - Classically, periumbilical pain that migrates to the right lower quadrant (McBurney's point)
  - Increases with movement
  - Young children often present with poorly localized pain
- Decreased bowel sounds
- Perforation: Toxic-appearance; rigid, distended abdomen; RLQ tenderness/guarding/rebound; decreased bowel sounds; shock
- Psoas sign: Pain upon hip extension
- Obturator sign: Pain with external rotation of the hip

Diagnosis

- Close observation and a high index of suspicion are essential
- The history and physical exam is characteristic; however, diagnosis is extremely difficult in children less than age 4, with 75% having perforation at the time of diagnosis
- CBC may show leukocytosis with left shift, but is often normal
- Urinalysis may show sterile pyuria (WBCs without bacteria) due to ureteral irritation from the inflamed appendix
- Ultrasound and abdominal CT are the best imaging tests for diagnosis; however, neither definitively rules out appendicitis
- Abdominal X-ray is rarely helpful
  - May show a RLQ fecalith or appendiceal gas
  - May show free air if perforation is present
  - May show acute scoliosis, due to psoas muscle spasm
- Misdiagnosis occurs in 10% of all cases

Treatment

- Avoid oral intake
- Hydration (normal saline) to correct volume depletion
- Correct electrolyte abnormalities
- Broad-spectrum, triple antibiotic therapy with IV ampicillin, gentamycin, and clindamycin
- IV analgesia as needed
- Emergent appendectomy (open or laparoscopic) is the definitive treatment

Disposition

- All patients with definite appendicitis will be admitted for appendectomy and IV antibiotics
- Patients with suspected appendicitis should be observed in the hospital for at least 24 hours while undergoing serial abdominal exams +/− CBCs
- Patients with low likelihood of disease and good follow-up may be discharged, with re-examination in 12–24 hours
- Delay in diagnosis increases the risk of perforation, sepsis, and shock
- 25–30% of cases in children are perforated at the time of surgery

212. Bacterial Meningitis

Etiology & Pathophysiology

- Bacterial meningitis often occurs secondary to bacteremic seeding of the meninges
  - <1 month of age: Group B Strep, *E. coli*, *Listeria*
  - 1 to 2 months: *H. influenzae* type B, *E. coli*, *S. pneumoniae*, Group B Strep
  - 2 months to 6 years: *S. pneumoniae*, *N. meningitidis*, *H. influenzae* type B
  - >6 years: *S. pneumoniae*, *N. meningitidis*
- Risk factors include respiratory infections, VP shunt, mastoiditis, head trauma, immunodeficiency, hemoglobinopathy
- Viral causes include enteroviruses, mumps, HSV, arboviruses, HIV, poliovirus, VZV, parainfluenza, EBV, CMV, adenovirus, parvovirus
- Immunocompromised patients: *Pseudomonas, Serratia, Proteus*
- Fungal, mycobacterial, and aseptic (drug-induced) cases also occur

Differential Dx

- Viral encephalitis
- Migraine
- Brain abscess or tumor
- Head injury
- Toxic ingestion
- Subdural empyema
- Leukemia
- Systemic Lupus Erythematosus
- Kawasaki's disease
- Subdural hematoma
- Subarachnoid hemorrhage
- Sinusitis
- Mollaret's syndrome

Presentation

- Fever and meningeal signs occur in 85% of patients, but may be absent in the very young
- Common symptoms include headache, neck stiffness, fever, vomiting, photophobia, arthralgia, myalgia
- Altered level of consciousness (e.g., lethargy, irritability) and seizures may be present
- Full fontanelle
- Poor feeding
- Purpuric rash may be present
- Kernig's sign: Reflexive neck flexion and pain upon leg extension
- Brudzinski's sign: Reflexive flexion of legs upon neck flexion

Diagnosis

- History and physical exam is often suggestive of meningitis; however, no single symptom or sign is pathognomonic, especially in very young patients—fever and altered mental status should provoke suspicion of meningitis
- CBC may show leukocytosis (however, a normal WBC count does not exclude meningitis)
- Obtain blood and urine cultures
- Head CT should be obtained prior to LP if signs of elevated intracranial pressure, prolonged or focal seizure, focal neurologic signs, increased purpuric rash, GCS <13, or pupillary asymmetry/dilatation are present
- Lumbar puncture is often diagnostic
  - Record opening pressure, cell count, differential, glucose, protein, bacterial culture, PCR for viruses
  - CSF will show >5 WBCs, low glucose, high protein, or organisms on gram stain (gram stain may be negative)

Treatment

- Ensure adequate airway, breathing, and circulation
- Begin empiric IV antibiotics immediately (even before LP if necessary—within 1 hour of ED arrival is standard of care)
  - <8 weeks of age: Ampicillin (for *Listeria*) plus cefotaxime (vancomycin may also be added if suspect penicillin-resistant *S. pneumoniae*)
  - >8 weeks of age: Ceftriaxone or cefotaxime plus vancomycin
  - Rifampin may also be added
- Steroids are controversial: May decrease the risk of hearing loss in *H. influenzae* and *Neisseria* meningitis if given prior to antibiotics
- Chemoprophylaxis
  - *N. meningitidis*: Prophylaxis for all household, day care, and school contacts
  - *H. influenzae*: Prophylaxis for all household contacts, even if previously immunized
  - Meningococcal vaccine for college students and in endemic areas

Disposition

- All patients should be admitted if bacterial meningitis is suspected or etiology is unclear
- Fatal in up to 20% of pediatric cases
- Complications may be acute (e.g., seizure, brainstem herniation, SIADH) or chronic (e.g., deafness, weakness, seizure disorder, mental retardation)
- Patients already on antibiotics will have a more subtle presentation and less convincing CSF fluid studies
- Rapid onset with rash raises suspicion of *Neisseria meningitidis* meningitis
- Nonbacterial meningitis is generally a relatively benign viral disease that requires only supportive care, has a good prognosis, and may be discharged with close follow-up
- Herpes encephalitis has a poor prognosis

213. Seizures

Etiology & Pathophysiology

- Transient, involuntary alterations of consciousness, behavior, or motor activity due to excessive neuronal discharges
- Febrile seizures occur in previously healthy children 6 months to 5 years old without defined cause (e.g., intracranial infection)
  - Simple febrile seizure: A single generalized seizure of <15 minutes duration with no residual focal neurologic deficits
  - Complex febrile seizure: A febrile seizure lasting >15 minutes, >1 seizure in 24 hours, or seizure with focal neurologic features
- Neonatal seizures are more commonly due to an epilepsy syndrome or underlying disorder (e.g., infection, mass lesion)
- Breakthrough seizure: Seizure in a patient with known epilepsy
- Status epilepticus: Continuous seizure >30 minutes without recovery
- Causes of seizures include CNS infection, sepsis, anoxia, hypoglycemia, trauma, brain tumor, stroke, intoxication, abuse, encephalopathy, drug reaction, hereditary metabolic disorder

Differential Dx

- Syncope
- Drug withdrawal
- Congenital heart disease
- Myoclonus
- Movement disorders
- Breath-holding spells
- Tic disorder
- Hypoglycemia
- Infantile spasms
- Airway obstruction

Presentation

- Presenting signs in neonates and infants may be subtle (e.g., chewing, eye deviation, or apnea)
- Partial seizures: Brief movements of specific muscle groups (e.g., face, neck, or extremity movement; head turning; or eye deviations)
- Complex partial: Partial seizure with impairment of consciousness
- Tonic-Clonic: Generalized muscle jerks/spasms, loss of consciousnes
- Absence: Brief LOC (rarely >30 sec) without loss of postural tone
- Myoclonic: Brief, often symmetric, jerking causing loss of body tone
- Infantile spasms: <1 sec contractions of head, neck, and extremities

Diagnosis

- The history, including eyewitness accounts, will often define the type of seizure and narrow the differential
- Examination of the child may reveal genetic syndromes that predispose to seizures (e.g., hypopigmented areas and shagreen patches seen in tuberous sclerosis)
- Simple febrile seizure: No further testing necessary, unless CNS infection is a concern
- Non-febrile seizure or complex febrile seizure
  - Check glucose, electrolytes, CBC, liver and renal function, toxicology screen, and urinalysis
  - Consider head CT to rule out underlying cerebral pathology
  - Lumbar puncture if CNS infection is a concern
- Head CT scan should be performed in the ED on children who have had focal seizures, persistent focal neurologic findings, a history of trauma, and in all neonatal seizures
- Breakthrough seizures: Measure anticonvulsant levels
- EEG is not routinely performed in the ED

Treatment

- Treat underlying systemic causes and avoid substances (e.g., medications) that provoke seizures
- Febrile seizures: Manage the fever; anti-epileptic drug (AED) therapy is not required
- Neonatal seizures: Most are treated with AEDs
- Management of status epilepticus
  - Maintain airway, breathing, and circulation
  - IV glucose bolus as infants may rapidly develop hypoglycemia
  - Antiepileptic drugs should be administered if seizure activity persists longer than 3–5 minutes
  - Benzodiazepines (lorazepam/diazepam) are first line
  - Phenobarbital bolus is given soon after benzodiazepines
  - Fosphenytoin or phenytoin if seizures persist
  - If the above drugs fail, a pentobarbital coma can be instituted with EEG monitoring to prove CNS seizure activity is not continuing
- The need for long-term antiepileptic drug therapy should be reserved for a pediatric neurologist

Disposition

- Prognosis and risk of further seizures depends on etiology
- Simple febrile seizures: Discharge home with follow-up; excellent prognosis
- Patients with non-febrile motor seizures or complex febrile seizures are admitted for observation/workup
- Infantile spasms require admission and workup; they are associated with poor developmental outcome
- Absence seizures can be discharged without ED workup
- Less than half of first-time seizures will have a recurrence; however, after a second seizure, nearly 75% will develop epilepsy
- Prolonged status epilepticus may result in permanent neurologic impairment due to anoxia

214. Kawasaki's Disease

Etiology & Pathophysiology

- A systemic vasculitis of small and medium sized arteries, primarily involving mucous membranes, skin, lymph nodes, and coronary vessels
- Also known as "mucocutaneous lymph node syndrome"
- Etiology is unknown; possibly autoimmune, infectious, or toxic
- Age of onset peaks at 1–2 years; 80% are less than 4 years old
- Multiple organ systems may be involved
    - Coronary artery aneurysms are the most feared complication—may present as MI, cardiogenic shock, or sudden death
    - Other cardiac pathologies include myocarditis, pericarditis, valvulitis, and arrhythmia
    - CNS (aseptic meningitis, irritability)
    - GI (hepatitis, abdominal pain, acalculous cholecystitis)
    - Arthritis/arthralgias
    - Desquamation of palms/soles
    - Urethritis
    - Pneumonitis

Differential Dx

- Scarlet fever
- Staphylococcal scalded skin syndrome
- Toxic epidermal necrolysis
- Rocky Mountain spotted fever
- Toxic shock syndrome
- Leptospirosis
- Juvenile rheumatoid arthritis
- Polyarteritis nodosa
- Measles
- Drug reaction
- Erythema multiforme

Presentation

- An acute febrile phase for 1–2 weeks is followed by a 1–2 week subacute phase
- Acute phase: High fever, irritability, cervical adenitis, conjunctivitis, rash, mucous membrane changes, edema/erythema/pain of the hands and feet, desquamation in the diaper area, and occasionally abdominal pain and diarrhea
- Subacute phase: Resolving fever, desquamation of digits, and occasionally arthritis; coronary artery aneurysms may occur in 20% of untreated patients (5% of treated)

Diagnosis

- Diagnosis requires the presence of fever for at least 5 days plus 4 of 5 of the following criteria (not all criteria must be met before initiating therapy):
    - Bilateral conjunctivitis, usually bulbar
    - Cervical lymphadenopathy (>1.5 cm)
    - Non-vesicular rash, usually on the trunk
    - Mucous membrane changes, such as erythema, cracked lips, strawberry tongue, or palatal petechiae
    - Extremity changes, such as erythema of palms and soles, dorsal edema, or finger desquamation
- Laboratory evaluation
    - No diagnostic test is available
    - Acute phase: Increased ESR, WBC, and LFTs; mild normochromic anemia; sterile pyuria; CSF pleocytosis with mononuclear predominance
    - Subacute phase: Increase platelet count, declining ESR
- Obtain a baseline echocardiogram if Kawasaki's is suspected

Treatment

- IVIG is the mainstay of therapy: Treats the clinical syndrome and decreases the incidence of coronary artery aneurysm
- Aspirin, initially at high anti-inflammatory doses (100 mg/kg/day), is used to decrease vascular inflammation, prevent vascular thrombosis, and limit coronary artery aneurysm formation
- The use of steroids has not been proven helpful
- Active management of coronary thrombosis (such as thrombolytics) has no proven role

Disposition

- All patients with suspected Kawasaki's disease require admission
- Long-term sequelae may include coronary stenosis with cardiac ischemia if coronary aneurysms occur
- Treatment with IVIG and aspirin reduce the prevalence of coronary abnormalities from 20% to 2%

215. Viral Exanthems

Etiology & Pathophysiology

- Measles (Rubeola): Primary infection of nasopharynx followed by viremia and rash; incubation 10 days; affects preschool/school-aged children (adults may be susceptible due to waning immunity); >99% reduction of disease following childhood MMR immunization (most cases in US occur in individuals who recently entered the country)
- Mumps: Primarily causes parotitis; incubation 18 days; affects children ages 5–9; had been the greatest cause of aseptic meningitis prior to MMR vaccine; may result in permanent unilateral deafness
- Rubella ("German measles"): Prevalence increasing due to decreased vaccination rates (although there is no proven relationship of MMR vaccine to autism); incubation of 16 days
- Erythema infectiosum (5th disease): Parvovirus B19 infection; immune complex formation/deposition in joints and skin; ages 5–14
- Roseola: Most common viral exanthem; Herpesvirus 6 infection; affects children ages 6 months–5 years

Differential Dx

- Drug rash
- Infectious mononucleosis
- Scarlet fever
- Erythema multiforme
- Rocky Mountain spotted fever
- Mycoplasma pneumonia
- Disseminated gonococcus
- Tinea versicolor (fungus)
- Kawasaki's disease
- Insect bites
- Scabies
- Varicella (chicken pox)
- Influenza/parainfluenza virus
- Hand-Foot-Mouth disease

Presentation

- Measles: 3–5 day prodrome (high fever up to 41°C, cough, coryza, conjunctivitis), Koplik's spots (oral lesions), then rash
- Mumps: 1–2 day prodrome (low fevers, myalgias, HA, anorexia), followed by parotid/salivary swelling and ear pain
- Rubella: Prodrome (low fever, malaise, cough, coryza), arthralgias, adenopathy, rash
- Erythema infectiosum: Prodrome (malaise, low fever, sore throat) followed by rash
- Roseola: 4–5 day prodrome (high fever, vomiting, adenopathy), rash, may result in febrile seizures

Diagnosis

- Primarily clinical diagnoses based on characteristic rashes that follow the prodromal period
  - Measles: Maculopapular eruption lasting 5–7 days; typically begins on the face/head (behind ears and on forehead) and progresses to hands/feet; Koplik's spots are pathognomonic
  - Mumps: No characteristic rash
  - Rubella: Pink maculopapular erythematous rash develops on the face and moves downward to the trunk then extremities; petechiae may be present on soft palate; lasts about 3 days
  - Erythema infectiosum: "Slapped cheek" rash with bright red macular lesions occurs on the cheeks; perioral pallor may be present; rash spreads to extremities (palms and soles spared)
  - Roseola: Non-pruritic, erythematous, rose-colored, macular rash beginning on trunk that spreads peripherally; lasts 2–5 d
- Serologic testing (anti-IgM antibodies) may be used for diagnosis or confirmation of measles and mumps

Treatment

- Symptomatic therapy with fluids, rest, antihistamines, acetaminophen, and NSAIDs
- Do not use aspirin in children due to theoretical risk of Reye syndrome
- Measles, mumps, and rubella are largely prevented by administration of MMR vaccine (live vaccine which confers lifelong immunity, given in two doses at 12–15 months and then again at 4–6 years of age)
- Antibiotic agents may be used for secondary bacterial superinfection of skin lesions
- Vitamin A supplementation has been shown to decrease morbidity and mortality in measles and rubella in developing countries where vitamin A deficiency occurs (consider supplementation in immunodeficiencies, clinical evidence of vitamin A deficiency, malnutrition, and/or recent emigration to US)
- Immune compromised patients, including symptomatic HIV patients, who are exposed to measles should receive immune globulin within 6 days of exposure

Disposition

- Majority of patients are discharged
- Admit for serious complications
- Complications
  - Measles: Pneumonia or encephalitis
  - Mumps: Orchitis or meningoencephalitis
  - Rubella: TTP or encephalitis
  - Erythema infectiosum: Aplastic crisis
  - Roseola: Febrile seizures
- Infectious periods
  - Measles: 5 days after rash appears
  - Mumps: 9 days after parotitis onset
- Measles, mumps, and rubella should be reported to the Department of Health

216. Physical Assault of a Child (Child Abuse)

Etiology & Pathophysiology

- Physical or mental injury, sexual abuse, or negligent treatment of a child by a person responsible for the child's welfare
- Parental risk factors include social isolation, substance abuse, mental illness, poor parenting skills, and unrealistic expectation of child's developmental level
- Child risk factors include physical illness or disability, mental illness, and "difficult" temperament
- Situational risk factors may include financial and other stressors and concurrent domestic violence
- Shaken baby syndrome: Altered level of consciousness, intracerebral hemorrhage, and retinal hemorrhages (pathognomonic) in an abused infant; may have no external signs of abuse
- >1 million cases of child abuse per year with >1000 deaths
- Injuries may involve the dermatologic, CNS, genitourinary, or orthopedic systems

Differential Dx

- Dermatologic: Coagulation disorders, Mongolian spots, HSP, ITP, coin rubbing, connective tissue disease
- Orthopedic: Rickets, osteogenesis imperfecta, congenital syphilis, septic arthritis, infantile cortical hyperostosis
- Burn: Bullous disease, staph scalded skin syndrome
- CNS: Seizure disorder, SIDS, toxin exposure

Presentation

- Bruises and burns are the most common signs of physical abuse, especially if on unusual body areas (e.g., ears, face, abdomen, buttocks, genitals), in patterned shapes (e.g., circular for cigarette burns), covering many body areas, or in various stages of healing
- Fractures are most common in children <3 years of age and in older children with mental or physical handicaps (especially of the posterior rib, sternum, scapula, metaphyseal corner)
- Perineum may show signs of penetration, genital tract trauma, or sperm

Diagnosis

- Be aware of suspicious historical elements
  - History given by parents or patient does not match findings
  - Denial of trauma to the child
  - Child's development not compatible with injury mechanism (e.g., non-ambulatory patients rarely have bruises or fractures)
  - Delay in seeking care
  - Story of events changes
  - Child's and parents' stories are inconsistent
  - History of past injuries
  - History of violence or substance abuse in the home
- Laboratory studies may include pregnancy and STD testing, rape kit, CBC, coagulation studies (look for thrombocytopenia, or hypocoagulability), CT for suspected head trauma, abdominal CT, and toxicology screen
- Unexplained elevation of LFTs should raise a suspicion of abuse
- Children with head injury require an ophthalmologic examination to evaluate for retinal hemorrhages

Treatment

- Evaluation must begin by identifying and treating all immediate medical problems
- Prophylaxis for sexually transmitted diseases and pregnancy if indicated, with the consent of a responsible caretaker and the child
- Consider consultation with medical personnel who specialize in cases of suspected child abuse
- Report all cases of suspected or confirmed abuse to local child protective service and local law enforcement agencies to ensure the child's safety
- Provide support to child and caretakers throughout the medical evaluation
- After initial evaluation, provide referral for counseling and ongoing medical care as appropriate
- Maintain a professional, non-judgmental attitude towards all involved caretakers
- Pictures should be taken for documentation of injuries

Disposition

- Mandatory reporting: Physicians are required by law in all states to report to child welfare authorities any suspected cases of abuse (proof is not required—must report with any reasonable suspicion)
- Child protective services should evaluate the child/family before discharging the patient home
- Admit for further workup of injuries, unclear diagnosis, or to protect the child
- If there is any question at all about the child's safety, the child must be hospitalized until the state child welfare board can find a safe home environment
- Child may experience anxiety, mistrust, aggressive or withdrawn behavior, and low self-esteem as a result of abuse

Traumatic Emergencies

JEFFREY M. CATERINO, MD

217. General Approach to the Trauma Patient

Etiology & Pathophysiology

- The hallmark of trauma management is a systematic team approach between physicians, nurses, medics, X-ray technicians, and respiratory therapists
- Patient evaluation is a multi-step process which attempts to rapidly identify life-threatening injuries
    - Primary survey: Airway, breathing, circulation, disability (neurologic status), and exposure/environment (completely disrobe patient and maintain body temperature with warm blankets)
    - Secondary survey: Complete physical exam

Differential Dx

- Immediate life-threatening injuries may include:
- Airway: Obstruction
- Breathing: Tension or open pneumothorax, large hemo-thorax, flail chest
- Circulation: Massive hemor-rhage, pericardial tamponade
- Traumatic arrest (cardiac arrest following trauma with loss of pulses or blood pressure)

Presentation

- Airway: Assess ability to protect airway and for presence of obstruc-tion (e.g., foreign bodies, facial or neck trauma, soft tissue trauma)— airway is intact if the patient can talk
- Breathing: Assess breath sounds, chest wall movement, respiratory rate, tracheal position, and skin color (i.e., for cyanosis)
- Circulation: BP, pulses (quality and rate), skin color (pallor or gray skin signify hypovolemia), level of con-sciousness, ongoing bleeding
- Disability: Level of consciousness, pupillary response, response to verbal or painful stimuli

Diagnosis

- Steps in the resuscitation
- Preparation: Airway equipment, IV fluids, gown and gloves
- Triage: Identify the most severely ill patients; institute mass casualty protocols if appropriate
- Primary survey (ABCDE): Designed to identify and treat any imme-diately life-threatening injuries
- Resuscitation/treatment of life-threatening injuries
- Secondary survey: Head-to-toe physical evaluation with history of medical problems, medications, allergies, and so forth
- Adjunct examinations: May include chest and pelvis X-rays, lateral C-spine X-ray, Foley and NG tubes, FAST ultrasound or DPL, CT scans, and laboratory tests
- Post-resuscitation monitoring and re-evaluation
- C-spine precautions should be maintained throughout the resuscita-tion until the patient is stable enough to undergo required studies for radiologic and clinical clearance

Treatment

- IV access, supplemental O_2, and cardiac monitoring
- Protect C-spine (assume injury in any trauma patient)
- Airway: Indications for intubation include GCS <8, obstruction, inadequate breathing, or inability to protect airway; obtain surgi-cal airway if unable to intubate
- Breathing: Intubate for inadequate ventilation or oxygenation
    - Three-sided occlusive dressing for open pneumothorax
    - Needle decompression for tension pneumothorax
    - Chest tube for hemothorax or pneumothorax
- Circulation: Hypotension is considered to be due to blood loss and hypovolemia until proven otherwise
    - Establish 2 large bore IVs +/− central IV line
    - Control bleeding with direct pressure—bleeding may not be evident (e.g., into pelvis, retroperitoneum, or thigh)
    - Replace volume with bolus of warmed Ringer's lactate; infuse O^- blood if unresponsive to initial 2 liters of fluids
    - May require surgical control of bleeding
    - Immediate ED thoracotomy may be indicated for traumatic cardiac arrest

Disposition

- Indications for transfer to trauma center
    - Vital signs: GCS <14; RR <10 or >29; BP <90
    - Anatomy: Flail chest, two or more proximal long bone fractures, ampu-tation proximal to wrist/ankle, pene-trating injuries, CNS injury, limb paralysis, pelvic fracture, or trauma with associated burn injury
    - Mechanism of injury: Ejection, car versus pedestrian, death in same car, high speed accident or roll-over, >20 minutes extrication, fall >20 feet, severe motorcycle crash, explosion
    - Age <5 or >55, pregnancy, or seri-ous comorbid conditions
- Prognosis of traumatic arrest is poor (0% survival for blunt trauma, <10% survival for GSW, 20% survival for chest stab wounds)

218. Traumatic Brain Injury

Etiology & Pathophysiology

- Primary brain injury occurs at the time of trauma and is irreversible
- Secondary injury due to hypoperfusion (hypotension, increased ICP), hypoxia, hyperglycemia, or anemia occurs after the initial insult and is potentially reversible
- Concussion: Blunt trauma resulting in transient symptoms of vomiting, confusion, loss of consciousness, dizziness, or amnesia
- Intracranial hemorrhage: Bleeding into the epidural space, subdural space (acute or chronic), subarachnoid space, or intraparenchymal tissue
- Brain herniation: Increased intracranial pressure forces brain components from their compartments
- Diffuse axonal injury: Irreversible shearing of axons due to sudden deceleration, often due to motor vehicle accident or shaken baby
- Penetrating injury (usually GSW): Damage is due to physical path of the bullet plus associated concussive forces

Differential Dx

- Concussion
- Cerebral contusion
- Intracranial hemorrhage
- Diffuse axonal injury
- Laceration
- Skull fracture
- Anoxic encephalopathy
- Herniation
- C-spine/spinal cord injury
- Other causes of decreased mental status (e.g., drugs, alcohol, hypoglycemia, seizures)

Presentation

- Hemotympanum
- Battle's sign (mastoid ecchymosis)
- Raccoon eyes
- Signs of increased ICP: Cushing's reflex (HTN, bradycardia, hypopnea), decreasing level of consciousness, dilated pupils, posturing (decorticate or decerebrate)
- Pupils may be fixed and dilated
  - Unilateral suggests ipsilateral bleed with herniation
  - Bilateral suggests anoxic injury or bilateral herniation
- May present with headache, LOC, or other signs of intracranial hemorrhage

Diagnosis

- Glascow coma scale (eye opening, verbal response, motor response) is a simple and reproducible measure of mental status that provides information on clinical course, prognosis, and treatment decisions (e.g., intubate if GCS <9)
- Head CT is indicated in all patients with GCS ≤14 or any patient with loss of consciousness, seizure, vomiting, amnesia, focal neurologic findings, alcohol use, skull fracture, anticoagulant use, or subgaleal swelling
  - May show hemorrhage, contusion, swelling, midline shift or loss of sulci (due to increased intracranial pressure), or skull fractures
  - Concussion: Normal CT scan
  - Cerebral contusion: Intraparenchymal hyperdensity
  - Epidural hematoma: Convex hyperdensity
  - Subdural hematoma (acute): Concave hyperdensity
  - Subdural hematoma (chronic): Concave hypodensity
  - Traumatic subarachnoid: Blood in subarachnoid spaces

Treatment

- Rapid intervention is necessary to prevent secondary injury
- Airway/breathing: Intubate early to prevent hypoxia
  - Rapid sequence intubation: Pretreat with lidocaine and defasciculating paralytics to prevent increased ICP
  - Ketamine is contraindicated because it increases ICP
- Circulation: Aggressively restore volume to prevent hypotension (goal is mean arterial pressure of 90 mmHg); avoid vasopressors if possible due to vasoconstriction
- Treat elevated ICP only if symptomatic
  - Sedate patient and elevate head of bed 30°
  - Hyperventilation may be performed acutely to cause cerebral vasoconstriction thereby decreasing ICP, but should not be used routinely or for prolonged time
  - Mannitol for osmotic diuresis and free radical scavenging
  - Surgical decompression of deteriorating/herniating patients via trephination (burr hole) or ventriculostomy
- Intracranial bleeds require seizure prophylaxis and may require surgical drainage
- Depressed skull fracture may require surgical repair
- Penetrating trauma may require surgical exploration

Disposition

- Admit all patients with intracranial lesions or persistently decreased mental status
- Discharge patients with negative CT scan and baseline mental status
- Neurosurgical evaluation is required for any intracranial lesion
- Factors that increase mortality include anemia, hypotension, hypoxia, or hyperglycemia
  - One episode of SBP <90 doubles mortality
  - 40% mortality if initial GCS <9
- Concussions may result in a post-concussive syndrome (vague, persistent symptoms such as headache, dizziness, and poor concentration) for weeks to months

219. Spinal Cord Injury

Etiology & Pathophysiology

- Identify location of cord injury based on presenting neurologic dysfunction
- Document sensory and motor level of deficits and determine if lesion is complete or incomplete (i.e., some sensation or motor function below the lesion)
- Complete cord transection: Total loss of function below the lesion
- Anterior cord (hyperflexion) injury: Spinothalamic and corticospinal tract damage with ipsilateral motor and contralateral pain/temp dysfunction
- Central cord (hyperextension) injury: Central corticospinal tract damage resulting in upper extremity motor deficit
- Cauda equina syndrome: Lower extremity motor and sensory loss, bowel/bladder dysfunction, and "saddle" anesthesia
- Brown-Sequard (hemisection): Loss of ipsilateral motor function and proprioception with contralateral pain/temperature dysfunction

Differential Dx

- Blunt cord trauma (MVA, diving, athletics, falls, electrical injury, disc herniation)
- Penetrating cord trauma (bullet, knife)
- "Stinger" (transient brachial plexus palsy)
- Spinal cord injury without radiographic abnormality (SCIWORA) resulting in transient neurologic symptoms (common in children)
- Neurogenic shock

Presentation

- Note motor or sensory dysfunction—document the lowest nerve root providing good sensation and muscle strength >3/5
- Check reflexes (e.g., Babinski, DTRs, bulbocavernosus, cremasteric)
- Examine for cauda equina syndrome (e.g., perianal sensation, sphincter tone)
- May result in neurogenic shock in which loss of sympathetic tone causes unopposed parasympathetic activation, resulting in hypotension, bradycardia, peripheral vasodilation (warm, dry skin), and shock

Diagnosis

- Plain films in areas of spine tenderness may reveal fractures associated with cord injury
- Spine CT
  - Better sensitivity than plain films for evaluating bony structures
  - Indicated to further evaluate fractures identified on X-ray or if X-ray is negative but there is high clinical suspicion for vertebral fracture
- Spine MRI
  - Evaluates soft tissue structures, cord injury (e.g., inflammation, contusion, hemorrhage), cord compression, and acute herniated disc
  - Indicated for patients with neurologic deficits but non-diagnostic CT and X-rays
  - CT myelogram may be used in patients unable to undergo MRI

Treatment

- Airway
  - Immediate intubation for hypoxemia or hypercarbia
  - Protect C-spine with manual in-line stabilization
  - Succinylcholine is often used for neuromuscular blockade during intubation but may cause hyperkalemia following cord trauma (safe during the initial 24–48 hours)
- Circulation
  - Aggressively treat neurogenic shock to maintain mean arterial pressure >70 mmHg for adequate cord perfusion
  - Treat with IV fluids (lactated Ringer's or normal saline) and vasopressors
  - Atropine is used for symptomatic bradycardia
- IV methylprednisolone (30 mg/kg bolus followed by 5.4 mg/kg/hr × 24 hours) has been shown to improve neurologic outcome in acute *blunt* spinal cord trauma if infused within 8 hours of injury (inhibits free radical-induced lipid peroxidation)
- No benefit of steroids for penetrating cord injuries
- No other therapy has been shown to improve outcomes

Disposition

- Neurosurgical consultation in all spinal cord injuries
- Admit all spinal cord injuries to ICU
- Emergent surgical decompression is indicated if there is evidence of cord compression (i.e., radiologic evidence of bony fragments in spinal canal or cord impingement) or for retained foreign bodies in penetrating injuries
- Complete lesions have minimal recovery
- Incomplete lesions have better prognoses
- Increased risk of spinal cord injury in elderly or intoxicated patients and those with arthritis, cervical stenosis, osteoporosis, and metastatic disease

220. Maxillofacial Trauma

Etiology & Pathophysiology

- Often results from MVCs, penetrating trauma, sports, assaults, falls
- Bony anatomy includes the mandible (jawbone), zygoma (lateral arch of face), orbit (composed of 7 bones enclosing the globe—fractures may cause eye damage and blindness), and maxilla (midface bone)
- Maxillary fracture classification
  - LeFort I: Mobile hard palate and teeth due to a transverse fracture that separates the maxillary body from the pterygoid plate
  - LeFort II: Fracture of central palate and maxilla with mobile nose and palate
  - LeFort III: Fracture through the frontozygomatic suture, orbit, and nose/ethmoid, resulting in complete craniofacial dysjunction with mobile orbits, nose, and palate
- Scalp lacerations may result in exsanguination and death due to the scalp's rich vascular supply and should be addressed emergently

Differential Dx

- Fractures (frontal bone, orbit, nasal bone, zygoma, maxilla, mandible, naso-ethmoidal-orbit complex)
- Eye injury
  - Intrinsic eye injury (e.g., lens, retina, cornea)
  - Globe penetration or rupture
  - Optic nerve injury
  - Extraocular muscle injury
  - Lacrimal injury
- TMJ dislocation
- Nasal septal hematoma
- C-spine injury

Presentation

- Bony point tenderness
- Battle's sign (mastoid ecchymosis) suggests basilar skull fracture
- Raccoon eyes (orbital ecchymoses) suggests orbital fracture
- Nasal septal hematoma
- CSF rhinorrhea
- LeFort fracture: May have elongated face or unstable maxilla
- Mandible fracture: Malocclusion, positive tongue blade test (pain with twisting of the blade as the patient bites down)
- Orbital blowout fracture: Enophthalmos (sunken eye), infra-orbital anesthesia, diplopia, decreased extraocular movements

Diagnosis

- Complete vision assessment, extraocular muscle assessment, and eye exam are required in all patients
- CT scan is the gold standard to evaluate presence and extent of fractures and globe injuries
- Plain X-rays of face (3 views are required)
  - Not as sensitive as CT for facial fractures
  - May show fracture lines, asymmetry, air-fluid levels or complete lucency of sinuses (sinus fracture with bleeding into sinuses), or presence of soft tissue in the superior maxillary sinus (orbital herniation)
- Panoramic X-ray (Panorex) may be slightly more sensitive than CT scan to diagnose mandibular fractures; however, C-spine must be cleared and patient must be able to sit upright prior to obtaining this study
- MRI is occasionally used to visualize soft tissue (e.g., optic nerve entrapment)

Treatment

- Control of the airway is the most important concern—swelling/fractures may result in rapid airway deterioration
  - Pull jaw forward to open airway in mandible fractures
  - Nasotracheal intubation is contraindicated as cribriform plate disruption may allow the tube to pass intracranially
  - Surgical airway may be necessary
- Ice, analgesia, and direct pressure or nasal packing as needed
- Fracture management
  - LeFort: Open reduction with internal fixation (ORIF)
  - Orbital: ORIF if entrapped or compressed eye structures
  - Frontal bone: ORIF and antibiotics for depressed or posterior wall fractures (may extend intracranially)
  - Nasal bone and zygoma: Conservative management is generally sufficient; however, surgery may be necessary
  - Mandible fracture: ORIF for open fractures
  - TMJ dislocation: Reduction in the ED
  - Nasal septal hematoma: Drain hematoma and pack nose
- Scalp lacerations should be emergently secured by whip stitch or Raney clamps

Disposition

- Most facial injuries are not life-threatening; manage associated serious injuries prior to facial injuries
- Facial injury is the most common complaint in domestic violence
- Complications include blindness (especially in LeFort III), chronic pain, disfigurement, intracranial infection (frontal bone or ethmoidal fractures), and lacrimal duct damage
- Ophthalmology, ENT, OMFS, and/or plastic surgery consults may be necessary
- Admit patients with LeFort fractures, any eye injury, frontal bone fractures, ethmoidal fractures, or orbital disruption

221. Neck Trauma

Etiology & Pathophysiology

- Involved neck structures may include carotid/jugular/vertebral vessels, esophagus, pharynx, trachea, larynx, vertebrae, spinal cord
- Penetrating neck trauma is generally due to stab or gunshot wounds
  - Management decisions are based on the involved neck zone
  - Zone I: Clavicles to cricoid cartilage (may involve intrathoracic vascular structures)
  - Zone II: Cricoid cartilage to angle of the mandible
  - Zone III: From angle of the mandible to base of the skull
- Blunt trauma: may be due to MVA, "clothesline" injury (e.g., on motorcycle or snowmobile), direct blow, strangulation, hanging
  - Associated with vascular, esophageal, and laryngotracheal injury
  - Blunt vascular injury may cause carotid dissection or pseudoaneurysm formation with vessel thrombosis or occlusion
  - Strangulation may result in vertebral and spinal cord injury, soft tissue trauma, vascular injury, or airway occlusion

Differential Dx

- Vascular injury to the carotid or vertebral arteries or jugular vein (transection, dissection, or pseudoaneurysm)
- Nervous system injury (cranial nerves, spinal cord, or autonomic nerves)
- Esophageal injury/perforation
- Laryngotracheal injury (vocal cord damage, cartilage fracture, recurrent laryngeal nerve injury, complete laryngotracheal disruption)
- C-spine injury
- Intrathoracic injury

Presentation

- Airway injury: Dyspnea, stridor, hoarseness, hemoptysis, air bubbles from the wound, subcutaneous air, tracheal deviation
- Vascular injury: Active bleeding, decreased carotid pulse, neck bruit, neck hematoma (may compromise airway)
- Neurologic symptoms of carotid injury: Horner's syndrome, CVA/TIA with motor or sensory deficits
- Arterial or esophageal injuries may initially be asymptomatic
- Intrathoracic structures may be involved in lower neck trauma (e.g., subclavian vessels, lung)

Diagnosis

- CT scan or plain films are used to evaluate blunt neck trauma
  - Lateral neck X-ray may reveal foreign body or airway impingement
  - C-spine X-rays are indicated to clear the C-spine
  - Chest X-ray may reveal thoracic involvement (e.g., pneumo/hemothorax, pneumomediastinum)
  - Bronchoscopy or esophagoscopy may be required in blunt trauma
- Angiography is used to evaluate for vascular injury
  - Penetrating injury to Zones I or III require angiographic examination prior to operative exploration (due to the complex vascular anatomy of these zones)
  - Penetrating injuries to Zone II may be operatively explored or selectively managed with angiography, laryngo-tracheobronchoscopy, and esophagram/esophagoscopy

Treatment

- Control of airway may be extremely difficult due to distorted anatomy and ongoing bleeding—intubatation is indicated for any evidence of respiratory distress, large subcutaneous air, blood in the airway, or tracheal shift
- Control bleeding with direct pressure
- Immediate surgery is indicated if the patient is unstable or if there is obvious airway, esophageal, or vascular injury
- Penetrating neck trauma
  - Local repair if platysma muscle has not been penetrated
  - Imaging should be done before surgical exploration for Zones I and III injuries; Zone II injuries may undergo immediate surgical management
- Blunt neck trauma
  - Surgery often required for laryngeal or esophageal injury
  - Systemic anticoagulation is often indicated for vascular injuries to prevent clot formation and embolization
- Begin antibiotics in cases of suspected esophageal or pharyngeal injury (clindamycin, penicillin plus metronidazole, or penicillin/anti-penicillinase)

Disposition

- Admit all patients with penetrating neck injuries and all cases of symptomatic blunt neck trauma; however, blunt injuries may be asymptomatic despite significant pathology—consider observation in blunt injuries with significant mechanisms even in the presence of negative imaging
- Discharge is acceptable for blunt trauma patients who are asymptomatic with negative imaging, trivial mechanism of injury, and good follow-up
- Esophageal and arterial injuries may also initially be asymptomatic
- Missed esophageal injury may result in life-threatening infection of neck or mediastinum

222. Thoracic Trauma—Lung and Esophagus

Etiology & Pathophysiology

- Injuries result from blunt trauma (i.e., due to organ compression, direct trauma, or deceleration injury) or penetrating trauma
  - Pulmonary contusion: Blunt trauma results in direct lung damage with alveolar hemorrhage and edema
  - Pneumothorax (PTX): Air in the pleural space
  - Tension pneumothorax: PTX with hemodynamic instability resulting from increasing intrapleural pressure, mediastinal shift, and decreased venous return
  - Hemothorax: Blood in pleural space, often due to lung laceration
  - Flail chest: Multiple contiguous rib fractures resulting in free-floating ribs with paradoxical motion on respiration
  - Tracheobronchial injury: Laceration of the airway
  - Diaphragmatic injury: May be due to penetrating trauma or blunt rupture and may result in bowel herniation into thorax
  - Esophageal injury: May be iatrogenic or due to trauma

Differential Dx

- Pulmonary contusion/laceration
- Hemothorax/pneumothorax
- Tracheobronchial injury
- Diaphragmatic injury
- Air embolism
- Clavicle, sternum, rib fracture
- Flail chest
- Esophageal injury
- Pericardial tamponade
- Penetrating injury to heart
- Cardiac contusion
- Cardiac wall rupture
- Valvular rupture
- Aortic rupture or dissection

Presentation

- Lung contusion: Dyspnea, tachypnea, crackles, hemoptysis
- Tension PTX: Hypotension, tracheal deviation, absent breath sounds, hyperresonance, distended neck veins, high airway pressures
- Hemo/pneumothorax: Respiratory distress, decreased breath sounds
- Flail chest: Paradoxical motion of fractured ribs
- Tracheobronchial injury: Dyspnea, subcutaneous air, pneumothorax, pneumomediastinum
- Diaphragmatic injury: Dyspnea, abdominal pain, or asymptomatic
- Esophagus injury: Chest/neck pain, dysphagia, fever, subcutaneous air

Diagnosis

- Chest X-ray is the initial test obtained but has poor sensitivity
  - Pulmonary contusion: Patchy infiltrates
  - Pneumothorax: Thin, radiolucent pleural line; absent lung markings peripheral to the line (difficult to diagnose on supine film)
  - Tracheobronchial injury: Pneumomediastinum, cervical air
  - Diaphragmatic rupture: Bowel herniation into chest, elevated hemidiaphragm, may see NG tube in the chest or chest tube in the abdomen
  - Esophageal injury: Pneumomediastinum, wide mediastinum
  - May show fractures of ribs, sternum, clavicle, and scapula and sternoclavicular dislocation
- Chest CT will identify hemothorax, pneumothorax, pulmonary contusion or laceration, pneumomediastinum, and some cases of diaphragm injury
- Esophagram and/or esophagoscopy if suspect esophageal injury
- Bronchoscopy if suspect tracheobronchial injury

Treatment

- Resuscitation as necessary with IV fluids and blood
- Intubate for respiratory distress or hypoxemia
- Pulmonary contusion: Pain control, encourage deep breathing
- Pneumothorax: Insert chest tube if large or expanding
- Tension PTX: Immediate needle decompression, chest tube
- Open pneumothorax ("sucking chest wound"): Cover with a three-sided partially occlusive dressing, surgical repair
- Hemothorax: Insert chest tube or proceed to surgery if large, expanding, or persistently bleeding
- Pneumomediastinum: Identify source (e.g., esophageal or tracheobronchial injury) and treat appropriately
- Tracheobronchial injury: Surgical repair
- Diaphragmatic injury: Surgical repair
- Esophageal rupture: Broad-spectrum antibiotics and surgical repair

Disposition

- Admit all patients with intrathoracic injuries
- Tracheobronchial injuries result in high morbidity and mortality; may result in stricture, bronchopleural fistula, or death
- Diaphragmatic injury may allow bowel herniation into chest with resulting bowel ischemia and/or infarction (may present years after injury with bowel in thorax)
- Delay in diagnosis of esophageal injury may result in significant mortality due to mediastinitis (>50% mortality if repaired after 24 hours)

223. Thoracic Trauma—Heart and Great Vessels

Etiology & Pathophysiology

- Penetrating heart injuries generally occur by gunshot or knife wound
  - Result in shock, either due to hemorrhage or pericardial tamponade (sealed-off bleeding into the pericardial space impedes cardiac output)
  - Stab wounds are more likely to result in tamponade
- Blunt cardiac injury may occur secondary to high speed MVCs, crush injuries, falls, explosions, and athletics (e.g., baseball-to-chest trauma)
  - May result in cardiac contusion, wall/septal rupture, valve injury, pericardial injury/tamponade, or coronary artery damage
- Penetrating great vessel injury (laceration) may lead to hemothorax, tamponade, shock, and/or exsanguination
- Blunt great vessel injury is generally caused by a high speed MVC with rapid deceleration, most commonly resulting in aortic rupture or dissection—90% die at scene due to traumatic cardiac arrest

Differential Dx

- Pulmonary contusion/laceration
- Hemothorax
- Pneumothorax (may be tension)
- Tracheobronchial injury
- Diaphragmatic injury
- Clavicle, sternum, rib fracture
- Flail chest
- Esophageal injury
- Pericardial tamponade
- Penetrating heart/vessel injury
- Cardiac contusion
- Cardiac wall rupture
- Valvular rupture
- Aortic rupture or dissection

Presentation

- Penetrating heart injury will present with signs/symptoms of shock or with cardiac arrest
- Cardiac contusion: Tachycardia, chest pain, arrhythmias, chest wall ecchymosis
- Valvular injury: Heart murmur, hypotension, shock
- Cardiac tamponade: Hypotension, distended neck veins, pulsus paradoxus
- Aortic injury: Upper extremity hyper- or normotension with weak femoral pulses if aorta is injured in the most common location (distal to the left subclavian artery), interscapular murmur, hemothorax

Diagnosis

- Penetrating thoracic trauma involves heart until proven otherwise
- CXR is the initial test used but has poor sensitivity
  - Penetrating injuries: Hemothorax
  - Aortic injury: Mediastinal widening, obscured aortic knob, tracheal deviation, pleural cap (blood in lung apex)
  - Acute tamponade may have normal CXR because as little as 50–200 cc in pericardium may cause tamponade
- Echocardiogram in ED will show pericardial fluid/tamponade (formal cardiac echo is necessary to observe valvular injuries)
- Chest CT may show great vessel injury or aortic dissection
- Transesophageal echo or aortography may also be used to evaluate the aorta (if CT is negative)
- ECG may show ischemic changes, ectopy, or arrhythmia due to cardiac contusion or to ischemia from coronary artery injury
- Cardiac enzymes may be elevated due to ischemia or infarction resulting from hypotension, cardiac contusion, coronary occlusion/dissection, or aortic dissection into coronary vessels

Treatment

- All patients require resuscitation with IV fluids and blood
- Immediate ED thoracotomy for shock not responsive to fluid therapy, cardiac arrest, or impending arrest
- Penetrating heart injuries
  - If unable to perform ED thoracotomy, immediate pericardiocentesis may be used to evacuate possible cardiac tamponade
  - Proceed to surgery ASAP for thoracotomy and repair
- Blunt heart injuries
  - Treat rhythm or conduction disturbances per ACLS
  - Valve injuries should proceed to surgery once stabilized
- Penetrating vessel injury
  - IV fluids must be used cautiously to maintain SBP near 90—increasing blood pressures may cause rupture of formed clot and hemorrhage
  - All patients ultimately proceed to surgery
- Blunt aortic injury
  - Maintain SBP <120 with β-blockers and nitroprusside
  - Most patients will require surgery

Disposition

- All patients with intrathoracic injury should be admitted
- Penetrating trauma with no initial signs of life (i.e., in the field) has 2% survival
- Blunt trauma with no initial signs of life has 0% survival
- Blunt thoracic trauma with initial signs of life but ensuing cardiac arrest has 2% survival
- Penetrating injuries that present with shock have 30–50% survival
- Stab wounds have a better prognosis than gunshot wounds

224. Approach to Abdominal Trauma

Etiology & Pathophysiology

- Penetrating abdominal trauma
  - Most commonly due to stab or gunshot wounds (GSW)
  - May be associated with chest, diaphragmatic, or retroperitoneal injury
  - Liver and small bowel are the most likely damaged organs
  - Stab wounds may not penetrate the peritoneum and are often managed conservatively; however, GSWs nearly always require exploratory surgery to manage intraperitoneal injuries
- Blunt abdominal trauma
  - Most commonly due to motor vehicle crashes
  - Other causes include falls and assaults
  - Results from crush or deceleration injuries to solid organs (causing hemorrhage) or intestine (causing perforation and peritonitis)
  - Spleen and liver are the most frequently involved organs

Differential Dx

- Thoracic injury (lung, heart, or esophagus)
- Diaphragmatic injury
- Abdominal injury
  - Liver
  - Spleen
  - Bowel
  - Pancreas
  - Stomach
- Genitourinary injury
- Pelvic fracture
- Rib fracture

Presentation

- Normal physical exam does not reliably rule out intra-abdominal injury
- Note the presence of superficial wounds, abrasions, ecchymoses, or entrance/exit wounds
- Abdominal pain/tenderness
- Peritoneal signs may be present
- Kehr's sign: Left shoulder pain referred from splenic injury
- Small bowel injuries may be asymptomatic
- May present with shock due to blood loss: Hypotension, tachycardia, and poor peripheral perfusion

Diagnosis

- Focused assessment with sonography for trauma (FAST) ultrasound exam is a quick, non-invasive method to examine abdominal compartments and the pericardium for blood
  - Sensitive for hemoperitoneum and faster than DPL
  - Does not identify the specific cause of peritoneal bleeding
- Diagnostic peritoneal lavage (DPL) assesses for blood in the peritoneal cavity, but does not identify involved organ or evaluate retroperitoneum—considered positive in blunt trauma if 10 cc of gross blood or fluid lavage with >100,000 RBCs, >500 WBCs, fecal matter, or increased amylase
- Plain films are quick and cheap, but rarely helpful—CXR may reveal intrathoracic injury, free abdominal air, or ruptured diaphragm; pelvic X-ray may reveal pelvic fracture
- Abdominal CT is used only for stable patients
  - Unstable patients should proceed directly to surgery
  - Very sensitive for intra- and extra-abdominal injury, though less sensitive for bowel, pancreas, and diaphragmatic injuries

Treatment

- Unstable patients or those with clear signs of intra-abdominal injury (e.g., peritoneal signs on exam, diaphragmatic injury, abdominal free air, or evisceration) should immediately proceed to surgery
- Blunt trauma may be observed and managed non-operatively based on clinical status and the degree of injury seen on CT
- Penetrating trauma
  - Proceed to surgery under the above indications
  - Most GSWs require surgery due to the depth of penetration and frequent intraperitoneal involvement
  - Stab wounds may be explored locally in the ED (under sterile conditions) to determine peritoneal violation; if peritoneum is intact, patient may be sutured and discharged
  - Stab wounds proven to violate the peritoneum but without clinical signs of injury or evidence of bleeding on DPL may be managed conservatively
  - Stab wounds with intraperitoneal injury require surgery
  - Retained foreign bodies must be surgically removed

Disposition

- Penetrating trauma
  - Admission if surgery is required or for observation of asymptomatic intraperitoneal stab wounds
  - Discharge patients with superficial stab or gunshot wounds that do not violate the peritoneum
- Blunt trauma
  - Admit patients with identified injury
  - Patients without identified injury but with co-morbid conditions or with significant mechanisms of injury should be admitted for observation and serial CT scans
  - Discharge patients with negative CT and low risk of intra-abdominal injury
  - Patients may return to the ED with late presentation of bowel or pancreatic injury

225. Abdominal Trauma—Liver, Biliary, and Pancreas

Etiology & Pathophysiology

- Injuries may occur due to blunt or penetrating trauma
- Grade of liver injury is based on the extent of hematoma or laceration seen on CT
  - I: Subcapsular hematoma <10% surface area or a laceration <1 cm
  - II: Subcapsular hematoma 10–50% of liver surface area, intra-parenchymal hematoma <10 cm, or a laceration 1–3 cm
  - III: Subcapsular hematoma >50% of liver surface area, subcapsular hematoma with active bleeding, or a laceration >3 cm
  - IV: Intraparenchymal hematoma with active bleeding or a laceration of 25–75% of a hepatic lobe
  - V: Laceration >75% of a hepatic lobe or an IVC injury
  - VI: Hepatic avulsion (complete disruption of vascular supply)
- Pancreatic injury follows a similar classification scheme
- Biliary injury is difficult to diagnose by CT or physical exam

Differential Dx

- Liver injury
- Pancreatic injury
- Biliary tree injury
- Hollow viscus (e.g., stomach, intestine) injury
- Rib fracture
- Intrathoracic injury
- Pelvic fracture
- Genitourinary injury

Presentation

- Abdominal exam may be normal—patients may appear stable even with significant injury
- Abdominal pain, tenderness, guarding, rebound, and distension may be present
- Symptoms of significant blood loss or 3rd spacing include tachycardia, hypotension, diaphoresis, cool skin, mental status changes, shock
- Note any superficial wounds (ecchymosis, abrasions) on abdomen or thorax
- Biliary injuries are often asymptomatic—delayed symptoms include jaundice, ascites, and sepsis

Diagnosis

- Unstable patients or those with penetrating abdominal injuries with obvious peritoneal invasion should proceed directly to surgery without pausing for CT, DPL, or FAST ultrasound
- CXR is usually normal, but liver injury may be associated with lower rib fractures
- FAST ultrasound/DPL are quick, sensitive screening tests for intraperitoneal bleeding; however, they do not identify the specific bleeding organ
- Abdominal CT is indicated for stable patients with blunt injuries to identify the extent of liver injury; however, CT is less sensitive for early biliary or pancreatic injuries
- Angiography is used in stable patients to identify and embolize persistently bleeding hepatic vessels
- Pancreatic injury may cause elevated lipase (may be normal initially) and amylase (nonspecific in pancreatic trauma)
- Biliary injury often requires ERCP, HIDA scan, or surgical exploration for diagnosis

Treatment

- Unstable patients and those with penetrating liver injuries should undergo immediate exploratory laparotomy
- Blunt liver injuries
  - Most cases are managed conservatively
  - Indications for operative management include expanding hematoma, hemodynamic instability, multiple injuries, or poor physiologic reserve
  - Operative interventions include either laparotomy or angiography with embolization of bleeding vessels
  - Non-operatively managed patients require serial exams and vital signs, serial blood counts, and repeat CT scans
- Angiographic embolization may be used in stable patients with persistent bleeding, especially if the bleeding site is identified by a contrast blush on CT
- Biliary injuries require surgical repair
- Pancreatic injury is generally treated conservatively with no oral intake and with large volumes of fluid due to 3rd spacing of intravascular volume into the retroperitoneum

Disposition

- Admit all patients for either surgical intervention or observation
- 10% mortality in liver injuries
- Non-operative management of liver injuries may be complicated by delayed bleeding, missed injury, bile leakage, abscess, and sepsis
- Complications of pancreatic injury include pancreatitis, pseudocyst formation, pancreatico-duodenal fistula, and hemorrhage
- Due to difficulty of diagnosis, biliary injuries are often missed initially and may present later with jaundice, ascites, and sepsis

226. Abdominal Trauma—Spleen

Etiology & Pathophysiology

- Injury occurs due to both blunt and penetrating trauma
- Grading of splenic injury
  - I: Nonbleeding laceration <1 cm or subcapsular hematoma <10% of spleen surface area
  - II: Laceration 1–3 cm, subcapsular hematoma 10–50% of spleen surface area, or intraparenchymal bleed <5 cm in diameter
  - III: Laceration >3 cm, subcapsular hematoma >50% surface area, ruptured subcapsular hematoma, or intraparenchymal bleed >5 cm
  - IV: Laceration involving segmental vessels or a ruptured intraparenchymal hematoma
  - V: Completely shattered spleen or hilar injury with spleen devascularization

Differential Dx

- Liver injury
- Pancreatic injury
- Biliary tree injury
- Hollow viscus injury
- Rib fracture
- Intrathoracic injury
- Pelvic fracture
- Genitourinary injury

Presentation

- Splenic injury may present after only trivial trauma
- Patient may appear stable even with significant injury
- Left upper quadrant abdominal pain/tenderness (abdominal exam may be normal)
- Abdominal wall signs include ecchymosis, bullet holes, or "seat-belt sign"
- Kehr's sign: Left shoulder pain referred from spleen
- Symptoms of significant blood loss may include mental status changes, tachycardia, hypotension, cool skin, diaphoresis, and shock

Diagnosis

- Unstable patients require immediate surgical intervention without pausing for imaging studies
- Chest X-ray is generally normal; however, splenic injury may be associated with left lower rib fractures
- FAST ultrasound/DPL are very sensitive screening tests for intraperitoneal bleeding but do not identify the specific bleeding organ
- Abdominal CT is very sensitive for splenic injury and may identify associated injuries
- Angiography is used in stable patients to identify and embolize persistently bleeding vessels

Treatment

- Immediate surgical intervention is indicated for unstable patients or those with penetrating trauma and obvious intraperitoneal injury
  - Splenorrhaphy (splenic repair) is attempted first if the patient is stable
  - Total splenectomy is usually reserved for uncontrollable bleeding, grade IV–V injury, or significant associated injuries that preclude a lengthy surgical repair
- Penetrating trauma often results in intraperitoneal injury and requires immediate surgical intervention
- Blunt trauma is often managed non-operatively
  - Conservative management entails serial exams, vital signs, blood counts, and CT scans
  - Surgical management is indicated for high-grade splenic lesions, hypotension, persistent transfusion requirements, or poor physiologic reserve
  - Children with blunt injury are usually managed without surgery
  - Angiographic embolization of persistently bleeding vessels may be indicated in stable patients

Disposition

- All patients with splenic injury should be admitted (patients with significant injury may appear stable)
- Splenic injuries fail non-operative management at a greater rate than liver injuries
- Even simple grade I injuries may require embolization due to persistent bleeding
- Failure to diagnose splenic bleeding may result in delayed splenic rupture days to weeks post-trauma

227. Abdominal Trauma—Intestine

Etiology & Pathophysiology

- Small bowel and transverse colon are intraperitoneal organs; the duodenum, ascending and descending colon are retroperitoneal
- Duodenal trauma
  - Most cases are due to penetrating trauma
  - About 25% of cases are due to blunt trauma (i.e., abrupt deceleration or a direct blow)
  - May result in laceration, perforation, or duodenal wall hematoma
- Small bowel and colon trauma
  - Penetrating trauma: Small intestine is injured in >80% of gunshot wounds and 50% of stab wounds
  - Blunt trauma: Bowel is injured in 10% of blunt abdominal trauma, most commonly the sigmoid colon (e.g., due to MVA, bicycle handlebars, child abuse)
  - Bowel injuries may include perforation, wall hematoma, and disruption of vascular supply

Differential Dx

- Diaphragmatic injury
- Splenic injury
- Liver injury
- Biliary tract injury
- Pancreatic injury
- Mesenteric artery injury
- Intrathoracic injury

Presentation

- Abdominal pain, tenderness, guarding, rebound, and decreased bowel sounds may be present
- Retroperitoneal injuries (duodenum and ascending/descending colon) may result in back or flank pain, flank ecchymosis, or flank hematoma
- Gross blood may be present on rectal exam
- Delayed symptoms may include fever and other signs of infection, worsening pain, and peritoneal signs

Diagnosis

- Diagnostic peritoneal lavage may show bile, blood, or feces
  - Not specific for bowel injury—may be positive with other abdominal injuries that result in bleeding into the peritoneum
- FAST ultrasound will show free intraperitoneal fluid but is not sensitive for hollow viscus (i.e., stomach, intestine) injury
- Abdominal CT has limited sensitivity for bowel injuries
  - Duodenal injury may show wall hematoma, retroperitoneal air, or fluid between the kidney and the duodenum
  - Blunt intestinal injury may show free air, intraperitoneal fluid, bowel wall thickening, or mesenteric streaking
  - Penetrating intestinal injury may show free air or intraperitoneal fluid, but has extremely poor sensitivity
- Upright X-ray
  - Bowel perforation results in free air
  - Duodenal injury results in retroperitoneal air, air around the right kidney, or loss of psoas shadow
- Surgical exploration is often necessary to identify injury

Treatment

- Mild injuries can often be managed conservatively with bowel rest, nasogastric decompression, and parenteral nutrition
- Indications for exploratory laparotomy include any penetrating wound into the peritoneum, peritoneal signs, free air, high index of suspicion for bowel injury, hemodynamic instability, gross blood on rectal exam, positive FAST or DPL, impaled foreign body, or evisceration
- Severe duodenal lacerations require surgical repair
- Blunt intestinal injuries require exploratory laparotomy if there is evidence of perforation
- Penetrating intestinal injuries
  - Laparotomy is necessary if peritoneal violation is suspected or obvious
  - Observation alone is sufficient if only the anterior abdominal wall is involved
  - Observation of penetrating flank injuries should include triple contrast CT (oral, IV, rectal) in the management
- Broad-spectrum antibiotics should be administered in any patient undergoing surgery

Disposition

- Complications include gastric outlet obstruction, small bowel obstruction, peritonitis, sepsis, shock, and bowel necrosis
- Mortality is 10–30%, and may be higher if diagnosis is initially missed
- Admit all patients with duodenal or intestinal injuries
- Discharge is acceptable for GSWs or stab wounds that do not penetrate the peritoneal cavity

228. Genitourinary Trauma

Etiology & Pathophysiology

- GU injuries occur in up to 5% of trauma patients (increased incidence in children)
  - Kidney injuries account for 80% of GU trauma
  - Other injuries to bladder, urethra, ureter, penis, testicles, prostate
- Often associated with lumbar, sacral, and pelvic fractures
- Grading of renal injuries (via imaging or surgical exploration) is necessary for clinical management
  - Grade I: Contusion or subcapsular hematoma without laceration
  - Grade II: Laceration <1 cm or nonexpanding retroperitoneal hematoma
  - Grade III: Laceration >1 cm or collecting system rupture
  - Grade IV: Laceration extending to collecting system or a renal vascular injury (e.g., thrombosis, laceration)
  - Grade V: Shattered kidney or avulsed hilum

Differential Dx

- Kidney: Contusion (90% of kidney injuries), laceration, hematoma, vascular injury or thrombosis, rupture, avulsion
- Ureteral transection
- Bladder: Contusion, rupture
- Urethra: Partial or complete transection
- Penile or scrotal injuries
- Traumatic rupture of corpora cavernosa (penile fracture)

Presentation

- Clues to GU injury may include blood on undergarments, perineal hematoma or ecchymosis, buttock injury, poor rectal tone, abnormal prostate exam, rectal lacerations, or blood at penile meatus
- Kidney injury: Flank pain, tenderness or ecchymoses (renal vascular injury may be asymptomatic)
- Scrotal injury: Ecchymosis, testicular tenderness
- Urethral injury: Blood at penile meatus, high-riding prostate, penile or scrotal hematoma; may have associated pelvic fracture
- Testicular injury: Hematocele

Diagnosis

- Urinalysis results determine the need for further workup
  - Gross hematuria requires imaging studies and further workup
  - Microscopic hematuria (>5 RBC/hpf) requires further workup only in cases of rapid deceleration injury (due to risk of renal vascular injury), hypotension, penetrating injury, pelvic fractures, or a pediatric injury with >50 RBC/hpf
- CT scan with contrast will identify and grade renal injuries, renal vascular injury, and associated injuries
- Urethrogram (place catheter 2 cm into urethra and inject contrast): X-ray showing extravasation of contrast indicates urethral injury
- Cystogram (place contrast into bladder via Foley catheter): X-ray showing extravasation of contrast indicates bladder injury
- IV pyelogram will identify ureteral injuries but is seldom used
- Angiography is only used to rule out renal vascular injury if CT scan is not definitive
- X-rays may show pelvic or lumbar fracture, suggesting the possibility of associated GU injury

Treatment

- Do not place a Foley catheter until urethral injury has been ruled out by exam or appropriate studies
- Renal trauma
  - Grades I and II: Conservative management
  - Grades III and IV: Attempt non-operative management with serial blood counts, bed rest, and re-imaging
  - Nephrectomy may be necessary for penetrating injuries, uncontrolled hemorrhage, vascular injury, ruptured kidney (grade V injury), or large urinary extravasation
- Ureteral injuries: Require operative repair
- Bladder trauma: Intraperitoneal rupture requires surgery; extraperitoneal rupture may be observed with placement of Foley catheter and repeat cystograms to ensure healing
- Urethral injury: Drain bladder via suprapubic cystostomy or fluoroscopic Foley placement to allow healing of urethra; complete lacerations require surgical repair
- Testicular or penile injuries: Require surgical exploration and/or repair

Disposition

- In general, GU injuries are not immediately life threatening
- Consider discharge for patients with uncomplicated microscopic hematuria or grades I–II renal injuries
- Admit patients with grades II–V renal injuries and patients requiring operative management
- Upper urinary tract injuries may result in bleeding, delayed ureteral leakage with infection, urinoma, incontinence, fistula, or infected hematoma
- Urethral injury may result in stricture or fistula formation
- Patients with missed ureteral or renal pelvis injuries may present 1–2 weeks following trauma with pain, fever, or sepsis

229. Trauma in Special Populations

Etiology & Pathophysiology

- Trauma in pregnancy requires evaluation/care for mother and fetus
  - Even minor trauma may cause placental abruption and fetal death
  - Physiologic changes during pregnancy (20% increase in pulse, 20% decrease in blood pressure, and 50% increase in blood volume) may mask early signs of shock
  - Uterine blood flow is compromised before there is evidence of maternal hypotension
- Geriatric trauma
  - May not tolerate even minor injuries due to poor reserve
  - May not be able to appropriately increase heart rate due to medications (e.g., β-blockers) or heart disease
  - High risk of organ ischemia during hypovolemia
- Pediatric trauma is the leading cause of death in children >1 year old
  - Children have a large physiologic reserve; they may appear stable but then rapidly decompensate

Differential Dx

- Pregnancy: Preterm labor, placental abruption, premature rupture of membranes, fetal-maternal hemorrhage, uterine rupture, direct fetal injury, fetal distress
- Elderly: Increased risk of subdural hematoma, C-spine or great vessel injury, fractures, and ischemia secondary to blood loss
- Pediatric: Increased risk of intracranial injury

Presentation

- Pregnancy
  - Assess gestational age (fundus is at the umbilicus at 20 weeks)
  - Palpate uterus for tenderness or contractions
  - Pelvic exam to evaluate bleeding or amniotic membrane rupture
  - Assess fetus via fetal heart tones
- Elderly require frequent reassessment (can deteriorate rapidly); medical history and medications are important
- Pediatric shock or hypoxia may present as agitation, poor capillary refill, or tachycardia before hypotension is evident

Diagnosis

- Follow basic trauma guidelines for all patients
- Pregnancy
  - Rh status and Kleihauer-Betke assay (detects fetal-maternal blood mixing) to determine need for Rh immune globulin
  - Perform all necessary imaging while shielding abdomen/pelvis
  - External fetal monitoring in all patients looking for evidence of fetal distress (e.g., brady- or tachycardia, lack of heart rate variability, persistent or late decelerations); uterine contractions may indicate abruption
  - Obstetric ultrasound may not detect all injuries (especially uterine rupture or fetal-placental injuries)
- Elderly
  - Identify potential underlying cause of trauma (e.g., syncope, CVA/TIA, arrhythmia, aortic dissection, MI, AAA)
  - Use CT scans/X-rays liberally as exam may be unreliable
- Pediatric
  - Head CT scan may be necessary to rule out intracranial injury

Treatment

- Trauma in pregnancy
  - Stabilize mother first and involve obstetrics early
  - Place a wedge under right hip to roll uterus off the IVC
  - Administer Rh immune globulin to Rh-negative patients
  - Consider tocolysis versus delivery for preterm labor
  - Emergent C-section for fetal distress or abruption
  - Perform perimortem C-section within 5 minutes of maternal traumatic arrest; continue maternal resuscitation throughout
- Elderly trauma
  - Early use of invasive hemodynamic monitoring improves outcomes as volume management may be difficult due to co-morbidities (e.g., CHF)
  - Avoid hypoxia/hypoperfusion via volume resuscitation and transfusion
- Pediatric trauma
  - Airway anatomy is different than adult patients
  - BP alone does not reflect adequate resuscitation—clinical evidence of good peripheral perfusion must be present

Disposition

- Pregnancy
  - Admission is usually required
  - Discharge only after OB consultation and 4 hours of fetal monitoring without uterine irritability
  - Maternal surgery *does not* worsen fetal outcome
  - Consider domestic violence (present in up to 30% of cases)
  - Fetus may be in distress even if mother is stable
- Elderly
  - Higher mortality rates
  - Elder abuse in 5–15% of cases
  - Close follow-up after discharge
  - Minor injuries may cause significant morbidity
- Pediatric: Consider abuse; consider transfer to a pediatric trauma center

230. Burns

Etiology & Pathophysiology

- Thermal, electrical, or chemical injury resulting in damage to the skin barrier, inflammation and cellular damage/death, and systemic immunosuppression, predisposing to infection (especially by *Staphylococcus, Streptococcus,* and *Pseudomonas*)
- Loss of skin integrity results in increased insensible fluid losses, impaired thermoregulation, and increased risk of infection
- Fluid volume is rapidly lost both due to disrupted skin integrity and due to 3rd spacing into the interstitium of damaged tissues—adequate fluid resuscitation is essential
- Smoke inhalation injury is often associated with burns, resulting in acute lung injury with bronchospasm, airway and airspace edema, pneumonitis, and eventually ARDS; inhalation may also result in carbon monoxide or hydrogen cyanide poisoning
- Facial burns, singed nose hair or eyebrows, voice changes, and carbonaceous sputum suggest upper airway injury

Differential Dx

- Thermal burn
- Chemical burn
  - Acids—cause coagulation necrosis, which limits the depth of penetration
  - Alkali (e.g., lye, lime, cement)—cause liquefaction necrosis, resulting in deep penetration with systemic effects
  - Metals
- Electrical burn (including lightning)
- Child abuse
- Scalded skin syndrome

Presentation

- 1st degree (e.g., sunburn)
  - Superficial epidermal burn
  - Erythema, pain, no blistering/scar
- 2nd degree (partial thickness)
  - Dermis is involved
  - Pain, redness, and blistering
  - Deeper 2nd degree burns result in destruction of hair follicles and sebaceous glands but *do not* cause pain (due to dead nerve endings)
- 3rd degree (full thickness)
  - White pearly appearance due to absent blood flow
  - Visible thrombosed vessels are pathognomonic
  - Do not cause pain
- 4th degree: Burn of muscle or bone

Diagnosis

- Estimate burn size by "rule of 9s" (% of total body surface area — TBSA) to guide therapy and need for transfer to burn center
  - Each arm 9% –Anterior torso 18% –Head/neck 9%
  - Each leg 18% –Posterior torso 18% –Perineum 1%
- Percentages of TBSA in children are different than in adults
- Minor burn: <15% TBSA (<10% in children/elderly)
- Moderate burn: 15–25% TBSA (10–20% in children/elderly)
- Major burn: >25% TBSA (>20% in children/elderly), full-thickness burns covering >10% TBSA, burns in areas that may cause cosmetic or functional problems (e.g., hand, face, perineum, or circumferential burns), or other complications (e.g., inhalation injury, deep tissue damage due to electric burns)
- Labs may include CBC, electrolytes, renal function, ABG, carboxyhemoglobin level, alcohol and toxicology screens
- CXR for inhalation injury may show pulmonary edema or ARDS
- Burn wound infection is diagnosed by wound culture or biopsy that demonstrates $>10^5$ organisms

Treatment

- Airway edema may compromise breathing—intubate if significant facial or neck burns or for respiratory distress
- Aggressive fluid administration to replace insensible losses is the most important aspect of resuscitation
  - Continually reassess adequacy of fluids by monitoring blood pressure, urine output, and peripheral perfusion (central venous pressure monitoring may be useful)
  - Parkland formula (adults): Infuse crystalloid at 4 cc/kg/% TBSA over the first 24 hours, with ½ in the first 8 hours
  - Children: Parkland formula plus hourly maintenance rate
- Administer IV antibiotics and tetanus prophylaxis
- Pain control with IV narcotics
- Minor burns
  - NSAIDs or narcotics for pain
  - Debride dead tissue but leave blisters intact
  - Apply non-adherent dry gauze to skin twice a day and clean wound during each dressing change
  - Apply topical antimicrobials (e.g., silver sulfadiazine—avoid use on face as may bleach skin)

Disposition

- 1st degree burns heal within a week
- Superficial 2nd degree heal in 1–3 wks
- Deep 2nd degree and 3rd degree often require skin grafting to prevent scarring
- Complications include infection, inhalation injury, carbon monoxide or cyanide poisoning, hypothermia, and eschar formation
- Admit to specialized burn unit patients with smoke inhalation, electrical burns, >20% of body surface involved, or severe burns to hands, feet, face, or perineum
- Discharge minor burns with follow-up in 24–48 hours
- 50% of deaths due to inhalation injury
- Emergent escharotomy in patients with constrictions caused by circumferential burns (neck, thorax, extremity)

Orthopedic Trauma

CAROLYN S. DUTTON, MD
ADEMOLA O. ADEWALE, MD
MELISSA McCLANE, DO
AMAR J. SHAH, MD, MS

231. General Approach to Orthopedic Injuries

Etiology & Pathophysiology

- Fractures may be traumatic, stress-related (i.e., overuse injuries), or patho-logic (e.g., secondary to existing weakness of bone due to tumor or osteoporosis)
- Obtain a detailed history of the type of injury, direction of force, and any attempts in the field to manually reduce or immobilize the affected area
- History of osteoporosis, Paget's disease, chronic steroid use, or end stage renal disease increases fracture risk
- Early complications include tendon injury, infection from open wounds, compartment syndrome, hemorrhage, or neurovascular deficit
- Late complications include malunion, nonunion, delayed union, avascular necrosis, arthritis, neurovascular deficits, osteomyelitis, and pulmonary embolus

Differential Dx

- Septic arthritis
- Rheumatoid arthritis
- Osteoarthritis
- Crystalline arthritis (e.g., gout, pseudogout)
- Fracture
- Dislocation
- Subluxation
- Sprain
- Ligament tear
- Tendon rupture

Presentation

- Assess for neurovascular compro-mise (e.g., examine distal pulses, observe capillary refill, and check for sensory deficits)
- Inspect for deformity, obvious bleeding, open wounds, foreign bodies, swelling, and discoloration
- Palpate for bony crepitus
- If no gross bony abnormality is present, evaluate active and passive range of motion
- Check function and stability of ligaments and tendons

Diagnosis

- X-rays should always include at least 2 views (may also require additional specialized views) of the involved bones and must visualize a joint above and below the suspected injury
- Strain: A muscular or soft tissue injury (usually due to overuse)
- Sprain: A ligamentous injury
- Dislocation/subluxation: Complete/partial loss of contact between two articulating surfaces
- Fracture characteristics
  - Location: Metaphysis, diaphysis, or epiphysis
  - Type: Comminuted (>2 fragments), transverse, oblique, spiral
  - Angulation: Direction (dorsal or volar) and magnitude (in degrees) of the distal fragment
  - Rotation
  - Displacement: Quantify based on % the fragments are offset
  - Shortening or impaction
  - Joint involvement
  - Open (any break in skin) versus closed

Treatment

- General fracture management: Immobilize the affected area (including the joint above and below the injury), analgesia (NSAIDs and/or narcotics), ice, compression, and elevation
- Perform frequent neurovascular checks, particularly before and after any movement or reduction
- Immobilization is usually accomplished with a plaster splint and ace bandage wrap (early circumferential casting may compromise blood supply)
- Buddy splinting by taping an injured digit to an adjacent digit is appropriate in some cases
- Dislocations, rotational deformities, and angulation deformities should be reduced under sedation to the approximate anatomic position
- Obtain radiographs before and after reduction
- Open fractures require anti-staphylococcal antibiotics

Disposition

- Orthopedics consultation is required for open fractures, irreducible fractures or dislocations, compartment syndrome, uncontrollable hemorrhage, or any neurovascular deficits
- Most patients are discharged home with immobilization, ice, elevation, NSAIDs/analgesics, and close orthope-dic follow-up
- Open fractures carry risk of infection and osteomyelitis
- Patients should be instructed to return to the ED if they have any decreased sensation, intractable pain, or impaired circulation

232. Pediatric Fractures

Etiology & Pathophysiology

- Anatomy of long bones: Diaphysis (shaft), metaphysis, physis (growth plate), and epiphysis (bone distal to growth plate)
- Fractures often occur at the physis, which is the weakest component
- Ligament injuries are uncommon—the physis is weaker than the ligaments and thus generally fractures before a ligament tears
- Salter-Harris classification of physeal fractures
  - Type I: Fracture through the physis only (X-rays are often normal)
  - Type II (most common): Fracture through the physis that extends across the metaphysis
  - Type III: Fracture through the physis, across the epiphysis, and into the joint
  - Type IV: Fracture involving the metaphysis, physis, and epiphysis
  - Type V: Crush injury of the physis (often misdiagnosed as a Type I injury)

Differential Dx

- Physeal growth plate fracture
- Supracondylar fracture
- Dislocation
- Sprain
- Slipped capital femoral epiphysis
- Malignancy
- Brodie abscess
- Infectious arthritis
- Osteomyelitis
- Juvenile arthritis
- Rheumatic fever
- Legg-Calve-Perthes disease
- Osgood-Schlatter syndrome

Presentation

- Pain, tenderness, and swelling
- Refusal to use the extremity or to bear weight
- Ecchymosis
- Tenderness over any physis (even with negative X-rays) is presumptively diagnosed as a Salter-Harris Type I fracture
- Pediatric bones (more so than adult bones) are more likely to deform without breaking
- Radial head subluxation (Nursemaid's elbow) classically presents with the arm held in flexion and pronation

Diagnosis

- Plain X-rays may reveal diaphyseal, metaphyseal, and Salter-Harris fractures (except Type I)
- Fracture types
  - Complete (most common): Both sides of cortex are disrupted—may be spiral, transverse, oblique, or comminuted
  - Buckle: Incomplete disruption of the cortex, resulting in compression and bulging deformity of the cortex
  - Greenstick: Unilateral cortical fracture with bending of the opposite cortex
  - Plastic deformity: Stress on the bone results in a bowing or bending deformity while the cortex remains intact
  - Toddler's fracture: Oblique distal tibia fracture in infants
- Other pediatric injuries include radial head subluxation, transient hip tenosynovitis (hip pain following URI), Legg-Calve-Perthes (avascular necrosis of femoral head), Osgood-Schlatter (apophysitis caused by repetitive traction to the tibial tuberosity), slipped capital femoral epiphysis (groin or hip pain in a teen)

Treatment

- Analgesia with NSAIDs and narcotics
- Avoid oral intake until the need for fracture reduction with conscious sedation is determined
- Reduction should be attempted for all displaced fractures—complicated physeal or articular fractures may require orthopedic reduction
- Splinting to immobilize the joint above and below the fracture
- Salter-Harris Types III, IV, and V fractures require orthopedics consult in the ED or soon thereafter
- Salter-Harris Types I and II may be discharged home after splinting
- Open fractures require tetanus immunization, anti-staphylococcal antibiotics, and orthopedic consultation
- Displaced epiphyseal fractures, intra-articular fractures, open fractures, or fractures unable to be reduced appropriately in the ED will often require open reduction with internal fixation

Disposition

- All pediatric fractures should receive prompt orthopedic follow-up
- Maintain a high index of suspicion for child abuse
- Return to the ED if child complains of numbness, tingling, cold extremity, worsening pain, or bluish skin
- Obtain follow-up X-rays 10–14 days after injury to identify Salter I fractures
- Complications include non-union, deformity, and growth arrest
- Salter-Harris fracture outcomes
  - I, II: Good healing, normal growth
  - III, IV: Increased risk of growth disruption
  - V: Growth complications are common

233. Cervical Spine Fractures

Etiology & Pathophysiology

- See associated "Neck Pain" entry
- The cervical spine has 7 vertebrae, each consisting of a body, an arch encompassing the spinal cord, and posterior elements (spinous processes and facets)
- 50% of vertebral injuries are due to motor vehicle accidents, 20% are due to falls, 15% are sports-related, and 15% are due to weapons/violence
- Up to 50% of C-spine fractures have associated neurologic injury
- Classified based on the mechanism of injury and stability of the fracture
- Fracture stability dictates treatment and need for urgent neurosurgical consultation; C1 and C2 fractures are generally less stable (due to less ligamentous and muscular support in the upper neck)

Differential Dx

- Cervical strain ("whiplash")
- Disc herniation
- Atlanto-occipital dislocation
- Atlanto-axial dislocation
- Vertebral subluxation
- Vertebral fracture
- Ligament sprain
- Unilateral facet dislocation
- Facet dislocation
- Hangman's fracture
- Posterior neural arch fracture
- Jefferson's fracture

Presentation

- Odontoid fracture may result in a feeling of impending doom
- Atlanto-occipital/atlanto-axial dislocation: Severe instability at C1/2 due to ligamentous disruption
- Teardrop fracture: Fragmental loss of antero-inferior vertebral body
- Clay shoveler's fracture: Avulsion of a C5-7 spinous process
- Hangman's fracture: Unstable bilateral C2 pedicle fracture
- Jefferson's fracture: Burst fracture of the C1 ring due to axial loading
- Burst fracture: Comminuted vertebral body fracture; fragments may intrude into the spinal cord (high risk of neurologic deficit)

Diagnosis

- Imaging is indicated if the clinical presentation reveals neck stiffness or pain, muscle spasm, tenderness to palpation, or neurologic symptoms (e.g., weakness, numbness, paresthesias, abnormal DTRs)
- X-rays include AP, lateral, open-mouth, and oblique views
- CT scan to visualize bony structures is indicated to better characterize a fracture or if plain films are inadequate
- MRI will evaluate ligaments, soft tissue, and spinal cord compression
- If plain films are normal but the patient still complains of pain or tenderness, further workup is institution-dependent
  - Some institutions obtain a CT scan and flexion-extension films (however, this may not rule out all ligamentous injuries)
  - Some discharge the patient in a hard C-collar with spine follow-up in 5–7 days—if pain has resolved at that time, the collar is removed; if not, a MRI is ordered
  - Some immediately order a MRI

Treatment

- Patients with suspected injury must remain immobilized until clinically or radiographically cleared of injury
  - Resuscitation should take place with cervical spine precautions, including in-line stabilization for intubation
  - If the patient is awake, oriented, cooperative, has no history of alcohol ingestion or distracting injuries, and denies neck pain or tenderness, the spine can be cleared clinically (i.e., without radiographic evidence)
- All fractures require neurosurgical/orthopedic evaluation
- Stable injuries can generally be treated with hard collar immobilization and analgesics
  - Stable injuries include unilateral facet dislocation, wedge and clay shoveler's fractures, Type 1 odontoid fractures
- Unstable lesions require reduction, surgery, or halo brace
  - Unstable injuries include bilateral facet/atlanto-occipital dislocations, subluxation injuries, burst fractures, Type 2 odontoid fractures, teardrop fractures, posterior neural arch fractures, Hangman's and Jefferson's fractures
- Follow protocols for spinal cord injury (including IV steroids) if any neurologic deficit is detected on exam

Disposition

- Due to the significant risk of morbidity and mortality associated with missed spinal fractures, obtain spine consultation if necessary
- Emergent surgery is required for any evidence of cord compression
- Patients with unstable fractures should be admitted; some stable fractures may be discharged in a hard collar after spine consultation

234. Shoulder Dislocations and Fractures

Etiology & Pathophysiology

- See "Shoulder Pain and Soft Tissue Injuries" for further discussion
- Acute bony injuries include sternoclavicular dislocation, acromioclavicular dislocation ("separated shoulder"), glenohumeral (shoulder) dislocation, and proximal humeral fractures
- Sternoclavicular dislocations are very rare; however, posterior dislocation is a life-threatening orthopedic emergency
- Acromioclavicular dislocations (separation) usually occur secondary to trauma; severity depends on the degree of acromioclavicular and coracoclavicular ligament damage; complications include osteoarthritis and impingement syndrome
- Glenohumeral joint is the most frequently dislocated joint in the body; anterior in 95% of cases, posterior (5%), inferior (luxatio erecta), or superior
- Proximal humerus fractures may be caused by trauma and/or osteoporosis; axillary artery and nerve are at risk

Differential Dx

- Impingement syndrome
- Calcific tendonitis
- Adhesive capsulitis
- Subacromial bursitis
- Rotator cuff tendonitis/tear
- Bicipital tendonitis
- Osteoarthritis
- Acute axillary vein thrombosis
- Thoracic outlet syndrome
- Brachial plexus injury
- Septic arthritis
- Referred pain from MI, cholecystitis, splenic injury
- Malignancy (e.g., apical lung)

Presentation

- Decreased range of motion
- Pain with movement
- Tenderness
- Crepitus
- Acromioclavicular injuries range from tenderness to obvious clavicular displacement
- Glenohumeral dislocation
  - Anterior: Arm held in abduction and external rotation with prominent acromion and loss of deltoid contour
  - Posterior: Arm held in adduction and internal rotation
  - Inferior: Fixed hyperadduction
  - Superior: Humeral head displaced superiorly, arm adducted

Diagnosis

- Perform a complete neurovascular exam
- Pre- and post-reduction X-rays on all suspected dislocations
- Scapular fracture requires AP and axillary views
- Glenohumeral dislocation: AP, axillary, and scapular Y X-rays may show displaced humeral head, associated fractures, Hill-Sachs deformity (compression fracture of the humeral head secondary to impact against the glenoid rim), or Bankhart's lesion (avulsion of the anterior-inferior glenoid labrum)
- AC dislocation: X-ray shows joint space widening with possible inferior, superior, or posterior displacement of the distal clavicle
- Proximal humerus injuries: X-ray may show a fracture or inferior pseudosubluxation of the humerus
- MRI/CT may be used on outpatient basis to further evaluate bony and soft tissue pathology or complex fractures; however, these have limited utility in the ED

Treatment

- Reduction (if necessary), ice, sling immobilization, and NSAIDs are indicated for most acute shoulder injuries
- Sternoclavicular dislocation: Anterior dislocations may be reduced in the ED; posterior dislocations are orthopedic emergencies requiring surgical reduction
- Acromioclavicular injury: Conservative management; serious injuries (e.g., displaced distal clavicle) may require ORIF
- Glenohumeral dislocation: ED reduction with IV sedation
  - Anterior reduction techniques: Liedelmeyer (start with arm adducted and elbow at 90°, then externally rotate); modified Hippocratic (as above, but add traction and counter-traction using sheets wrapped around patient); Stimson (hanging weight on arm with patient prone); Milch (forward extension and abduction of arm, then extend arm over head and pull)
  - Posterior: Longitudinal traction with humerus abduction
  - Superior/inferior: Generally require surgical reduction
- Humeral head fracture: Immobilize with sling and swathe; ORIF for comminuted (fragmented) fractures

Disposition

- Trauma/acute pain may limit evaluation of soft tissues
- Neurovascular exam is required pre- and post-reduction; emergent orthopedics evaluation is required for any neurovascular problem
- Majority of patients may be discharged
- Arrange orthopedic follow-up for all fractures or dislocations
- Delay in diagnosis or treatment significantly worsens prognosis
- Complications include rotator cuff tear, chronic pain or weakness, labrum tear, fracture, adhesive capsulitis, recurrent dislocation, brachial plexus injury, axillary nerve or artery injury
- Early mobilization of the joint is required to prevent adhesive capsulitis

235. Shoulder Pain and Soft Tissue Injury

Etiology & Pathophysiology

- See "Shoulder Dislocations and Fractures" for further discussion
- Acute cases are due to trauma (e.g., forced hyperabduction) or excessive demands; most chronic cases are due to overuse
- Impingement syndrome: Progressive degeneration and inflammation of the subacromial contents (rotator cuff and subacromial bursa) in part due to compression between the acromion and humerus, potentially resulting in rotator cuff tear
- Rotator cuff tear may occur acutely (secondary to trauma) or, more commonly, due to a relatively mild insult on a chronically degenerative cuff (e.g., reaching overhead)
- Adhesive capsulitis: Thickened, scarred joint capsule and "frozen shoulder" due to prolonged post-injury or post-surgery immobilization
- Calcific tendonitis: Deposition of calcium crystals in the rotator cuff with resulting inflammation and severe pain

Differential Dx

- AC joint injury
- Shoulder dislocations
- Humeral fracture
- Clavicle fracture
- Scapular fracture
- Bicipital tendonitis
- Osteoarthritis
- Acute axillary vein thrombosis
- Thoracic outlet syndrome
- Brachial plexus injury
- Septic arthritis
- Referred pain from MI, cholecystitis, splenic injury
- Malignancy (e.g., apical lung)

Presentation

- Subacromial bursitis: Aching, deep pain that worsens with activity and improves with rest; minimal tenderness; intact strength
- Rotator cuff tendonitis: Night pain, tenderness at cuff insertion, decreased ROM, mild weakness, pain with abduction
- Rotator cuff tear: Weakness, pain, inability to fully abduct arm
- Calcific tendonitis: Acute onset of pain at rest and with motion
- Adhesive capsulitis: Diffuse pain with significantly decreased ROM
- Biceps tendonitis: Pain at insertion, painful elbow flexion/supination

Diagnosis

- Focused history and physical exam: Note weakness, disuse atrophy of shoulder muscles, palpable crepitus, or pain with limited range of motion
- X-rays (AP, axillary, and scapular Y views) may show acromial osteophytes and joint degeneration in impingement syndromes and calcium deposits in calcific tendonitis
- X-ray or CT scan may identify chronic, degenerative arthritis
- Shoulder MRI evaluates the anatomy of the rotator cuff and associated soft tissue; may differentiate partial from complete tears

Treatment

- Slings may be used for comfort but early range of motion (24–48 hrs) is necessary to prevent adhesive capsulitis
- Conservative therapy is beneficial for most cases of shoulder pain: Rest, ice, NSAIDs, and opioid narcotics as necessary
- Subacromial cortisone injection if other anti-inflammatory methods fail; however, multiple injections are discouraged due to the development of tissue atrophy
- Physical therapy is generally the mainstay of treatment
  - Conditioning and strengthening
  - Progressive range of motion exercises for adhesive capsulitis
- Full thickness rotator cuff tears may require surgical repair
- Adhesive capsulitis may require surgical lysis of adhesions

Disposition

- Most patients may be discharged with orthopedic follow-up in 7–14 days
- Patients with suspected acute rotator cuff or biceps tendon tears require prompt evaluation by an orthopedic surgeon (retraction of muscles may occur within 1–2 weeks)

236. Arm and Elbow Injuries

Etiology & Pathophysiology

- The elbow joint is formed by the radius, ulna, and distal humerus
- Injuries frequently result from falling on an outstretched hand
- Associated nerve injury (axillary, radial, ulnar, median) is common
- The elbow is the 3rd most commonly dislocated large joint; posterior dislocation is most common
- Radial head fracture is the most common fracture
- Humeral fractures are classified by location on the bone
- Epicondylitis is a degeneration of the tendinous insertion at the lateral or medial epicondyles
    - Lateral (tennis elbow) epicondylitis: Due to extensor muscle overuse (results in pain with pronation and wrist dorsiflexion)
    - Medial (golfer's elbow) epicondylitis: Due to flexor muscle overuse (results in decreased grip strength and pain with pronation or wrist flexion)

Differential Dx

- Elbow dislocation
- Humeral fracture
- Bicipital tendonitis
- Biceps tendon rupture
- Epicondylitis
- Triceps tendon rupture
- Olecranon fracture
- Radial head subluxation (Nursemaid's elbow)
- Glenohumeral dislocation
- Bone tumor or cyst
- Rotator cuff injury
- Overuse injury
- Adhesive capsulitis

Presentation

- Arm held in a fixed position
- Pain
- Paresthesias
- Bony point tenderness
- Crepitus on palpation
- Swelling and ecchymosis
- Limited range of motion
- Neurovascular compromise (e.g., coolness, pallor, loss of distal pulses) may occur
- Pain with wrist flexion may indicate a medial condyle fracture
- Pain with pronation/supination may indicate a radial head fracture

Diagnosis

- Standard X-rays include AP and lateral views
    - Anterior humeral line should intersect with the anterior middle third of the capitellum
    - Radial-capitellar line should be present
    - Any visible posterior fat pad or an enlarged anterior fat pad is evidence of joint effusion
- Common fractures (listed proximal to distal)
    - Humeral shaft (may be associated with radial nerve injury)
    - Supracondylar (the most common elbow fracture in children)
    - Intracondylar (common in the elderly)
    - Capitellum (often associated with radial head fracture)
    - Epicondylar (may occur from repetitive stress in a child)
    - Radial head (the most common elbow fracture in adults)
    - Olecranon (may be associated with ulnar nerve injury)
- Dislocations may be posterior (90%) or anterior; 20% have an associated ulnar or median nerve injury

Treatment

- General principles of fracture management include immobilization, analgesia, NSAIDs, and elevation
- Antibiotics and tetanus boosters for open injuries
- Immediate anatomic reduction is required in cases of neurovascular compromise
- Nondisplaced fractures should be immobilized with the elbow flexed at 90°
- Displaced or intra-articular fractures usually require ORIF
- Nondisplaced radial head fractures require early range of motion (within 24–48 hours)
- Joint aspiration may afford pain relief if effusion is present
- Epicondylitis is treated with rest, NSAIDs, physical therapy, and improved athletic technique
- Elbow dislocation requires reduction (place traction-countertraction on arm and forearm; then press downward on the proximal forearm while flexing the elbow); follow with splint immobilization

Disposition

- Close orthopedic follow-up is recommended
- High-risk injuries include any intra-articular fracture, neurovascular compromise, crush injuries, difficult anatomic reductions, supracondylar fractures, and medial condylar fractures
- High-risk injuries warrant immediate orthopedic consultation and possible hospital admission
- Complications include arthritis, avascular necrosis, malunion, nonunion, cubitus varus or valgus, permanent neurologic deficit, adhesive capsulitis, and contracture deformity

237. Wrist and Forearm Injuries

Etiology & Pathophysiology

- Wrist injuries account for nearly 10% of ED visits
- The eight carpal bones are held in alignment by a series of ligaments and cartilaginous connective tissue; disruption of these connections results in carpal instability or dislocation
- The most common mechanism of injury is a fall on the outstretched hand (FOOSH)
- The most commonly fractured carpal bone is the scaphoid
- FOOSH involves significant force transmitted through the entire extremity; therefore, a careful history and exam of the entire arm is necessary to detect associated secondary injuries
- Other mechanisms include direct blows, crush injuries, fall on a volarly angulated wrist, and severe twisting motions of the wrist or forearm

Differential Dx

- Contusion
- Scaphoid, lunate, or other carpal fracture
- Lunate or perilunate dislocation
- Smith's or Colles' fracture
- Radial or ulnar styloid fracture
- Ligament sprain
- Overuse injury
- Bone or ganglion cyst
- Distal radioulnar joint dislocation
- Radial head subluxation
- Carpal tunnel syndrome
- Compartment syndrome

Presentation

- Pain and swelling
- Decreased range of motion
- Angulation
- Foreshortening of wrist or forearm
- Crepitus on palpation
- Bony point tenderness
- Snuffbox tenderness or pain with axial loading of the thumb suggests scaphoid fracture
- Lunate fossa tenderness suggests lunate fracture
- Fractures may result in few visible signs of injury
- Vascular injury may present with decreased distal pulses, extremity discoloration, or coolness

Diagnosis

- Standard X-rays include PA, lateral, and oblique views
- Ligament injury: Increased space between bones, disruption of carpal arcuate lines, and bony rotation
- Perilunate dislocation: Capitate displaced posteriorly to lunate
- Lunate dislocation: Lunate displaced volarly off the radius ("spilled tea cup" sign)
- Carpal fractures may require additional films (e.g., scaphoid view)
- Distal radius fractures include Colles' fracture (dorsal displacement and angulation with "dinner fork" deformity), Smith's fracture (volar displacement and angulation), Barton's fracture (intra-articular fracture with carpal dislocation), and Chauffeur's fracture (intra-articular radial styloid fracture)
- Radioulnar dislocation: Ligament tear associated with distal radius fracture (X-ray shows loss of radioulnar overlap)
- Galeazzi's fracture: Fracture of the distal radial shaft with radioulnar dislocation
- Monteggia's fx: Proximal ulnar fx with radial head dislocation

Treatment

- General fracture care includes immobilization, analgesia, rest, ice, and elevation
- Reduce displaced fractures and dislocations
- Immobilization of radial fractures is accomplished via a sugar tong splint (immobilizes wrist and elbow) to prevent radial movement with pronation/supination
- Open fractures require antibiotics (cover skin flora) and tetanus prophylaxis
- Carpal fractures often have normal X-rays; thus, the need for splinting should be based on clinical exam (i.e., if patient has point tenderness, treat as if a fracture is present by splinting and ensure close orthopedic follow-up)
- ORIF may be necessary for carpal dislocations, Colles' fracture, Smith's fracture, Barton's fracture, Monteggia's fracture, and Galeazzi's fracture

Disposition

- There can be significant long-term morbidity with missed or improperly treated fractures; therefore, these patients require close follow-up with orthopedics
- Admission is generally required for open fractures, neurovascular injury, compartment syndrome, and ORIF
- Patients should be instructed to return to the ED if discoloration, numbness, tingling, worsening pain, fever, or erythema occurs, suggesting neurovascular compromise
- Complications may include chronic arthritis, carpal instability, avascular necrosis (especially scaphoid, lunate, and capitate), nonunion or malunion, decreased grip strength, and nerve injury

238. Metacarpal Injuries

Etiology & Pathophysiology

- The hand is the most commonly fractured part of the body
- The most frequently fractured bone in the hand is the 5th metacarpal
- Fractures occur due to direct blows, axial loading, or crush injuries
- Classification of metacarpal injuries
  - Thumb metacarpal versus 2nd–5th metacarpals
  - Intra-articular versus extra-articular
  - Anatomic location (head, neck, shaft, or base)
  - Type of shaft fracture (transverse, oblique, spiral, or comminuted)
- 1st (thumb), 4th, and 5th metacarpals have some mobility, allowing for bone deformity without compromise of hand function
- 2nd and 3rd metacarpals are fixed—minimal angulation may result in decreased hand function
- Distinguish simple dorsal MCP joint dislocations versus complex volar dislocations (metacarpal head ruptures through the volar plate, becomes trapped, and requires ORIF)

Differential Dx

- Fracture
- Dislocation
- Subluxation
- Ligamentous sprain
- Ligamentous tear
- Rheumatoid arthritis
- Abscess
- Osteoarthritis
- Gout
- Septic arthritis

Presentation

- Pain with movement
- Swelling
- Crepitus on palpation
- Angulation deformity
- Malalignment of fingers when a fist is made (scissoring) indicates rotational deformity (normally all flexed fingers should point towards the scaphoid)
- Interphalangeal joint laxity indicates sprain or tear of the ulnar or radial collateral ligaments
- Dislocations generally present with a hyperextended finger—position of the metacarpal head determines simple versus complex dislocation

Diagnosis

- X-rays should include AP, lateral, and oblique views
  - Bennett's fracture: Intra-articular fracture at the base of the 1st metacarpal with subluxation of the carpometacarpal joint (proximal fragment remains attached to the trapezium, distal fragment is pulled laterally by tendon attachments); caused by an axial load on the thumb (e.g., closed-fist injury)
  - Rolando's fracture: Comminuted intra-articular fracture at the base of the 1st metacarpal; also caused by an axial load on the thumb
  - Reverse Bennett's fracture: Intra-articular fracture at the base of the fifth metacarpal
  - Boxer's fracture: Fracture of the neck of the 5th metacarpal
- Open wounds may be contaminated by skin flora (e.g., *Staphylococcus*) and/or oral flora (i.e., due to bite wound)
- Obtain X-rays prior to repair of open wounds to rule out a foreign body

Treatment

- General fracture management: Rest, ice, elevation, analgesia
- Reduce as necessary and obtain post-reduction radiographs
- Immobilize fractures in the "safe position" with ulnar or radial gutter or thumb spica splints
- Any rotational deformity or shortening >3 mm requires ORIF
- Metacarpal angulation deformities may require ORIF if angulation exceeds the acceptable level
  - 2nd–3rd neck fractures: 15° of angulation is acceptable
  - 4th neck fracture: 30° of angulation is acceptable
  - 5th neck fracture: 40° of angulation is acceptable
  - 2nd–3rd shaft fractures: No angulation allowed
  - 4th shaft fracture: 10° of angulation is acceptable
  - 5th shaft fracture: 20° of angulation is acceptable
  - 1st (thumb) fractures: 20–30° of angulation is acceptable
- Bennett's and Rolando's fractures are unstable fractures and require ORIF
- Administer antibiotics to cover skin flora (e.g., cephalexin) in open injuries; modify antibiotic coverage for oral flora (e.g., amoxicillin plus clavulanic acid) in bite wounds

Disposition

- All hand fractures should receive close orthopedic follow-up
- Immediate orthopedic consultation for any suspected tendon injury
- Reductions are difficult to maintain in place, even with splinting—obtain ED orthopedic consult or close outpatient follow-up
- Open wounds may require surgical debridement
- Complications may include loss of hand power, painful/weak grip, extensor tendon injury, arthritis, scarring of associated muscles, and infection
- Any wound over the MCP joint is a bite wound (closed-fist injury or "fight bite") until proven otherwise

239. Finger Injuries

Etiology & Pathophysiology

- Joints of the finger include the distal interphalangeal (DIP), proximal interphalangeal (PIP), and metacarpal phalangeal (MCP) joints
- 15–30% of hand fractures involve the phalanges
- The majority of phalangeal fractures are stable and non-displaced
- Mechanisms of injury include axial loading (proximal phalanx fracture or dislocation), crush injury or direct blow (comminuted and transverse fractures), twisting injury (oblique and spiral fractures), and forced thumb abduction (ulnar collateral ligament or [UCL] tear)

Differential Dx

- Ligament sprain
- Subluxation
- Dislocation
- Volar plate rupture
- Ulnar collateral ligament tear
- Radial collateral ligament tear
- Tendon laceration
- Fracture
- Trigger finger
- Gout, pseudogout
- Septic arthritis
- Rheumatoid arthritis
- Osteoarthritis

Presentation

- Pain with movement
- Swelling or discoloration
- Crepitus on palpation
- Test for tendon involvement
  - Weakness to resisted flexion/extension or inability to fully flex/extend the finger
  - Weak or absent thumb adduction, abduction, or opposition
- Malalignment of fingers when a fist is made (scissoring) indicates rotational deformity (all flexed fingers should point towards the scaphoid)

Diagnosis

- X-rays should include AP, lateral, and oblique views of the involved fingers
  - Some angulation of fractures is acceptable, but rotation on X-ray or scissoring on exam is unacceptable and may result in functional limitation
  - Tuft fracture is a comminuted fracture of the distal phalanx, often due to crush injuries and associated with nail bed injury
- Differentiate tendon and ligament injuries from fractures
  - Extensor tendon injuries: Mallet finger (avulsion of the dorsal extensor tendon at the distal phalanx, resulting in a flexion deformity), swan neck deformity (flexed DIP and MCP with extended PIP), and Boutonniere deformity (extended DIP and MCP with flexed PIP)
  - Flexor tendon injuries: Inability to flex DIP suggests injury to the profundus tendon; inability to flex PIP suggests injury to the superficialis tendon
  - Gamekeeper's thumb: Tear of thumb UCL due to radial stress

Treatment

- Protection, rest, ice, elevation, and analgesia
- Procedural analgesia (i.e., digital nerve block) may be necessary to allow for a thorough exam
- Perform closed reduction on all dislocations and displaced, rotated, or angulated fractures
- Explore open wounds and repair lacerations
- Fractures are generally treated by immobilization
  - Stable transverse fracture: Buddy tape +/− splint
  - Distal phalanx fracture: Immobilize DIP in full extension
  - Middle/proximal phalanx fracture: Gutter or volar splint
  - Gamekeeper's thumb: Thumb spica (complete tear results in >40° of laxity, requiring surgical correction)
  - Indications for surgery include inability to maintain alignment, any rotational deformity, complete ligamentous or tendon disruption, irreducible dislocation, some intra-articular fractures, and some open wounds
- Mallet finger: Dorsal splint in extension
- Nail bed injuries: In the presence of a significant subungual hematoma, consider trephination or nail removal in order to repair a presumed nail bed laceration

Disposition

- Discharge simple wounds and fractures with close follow-up
- Orthopedic follow-up is required within 24 hours for any rotational deformity, spiral fracture, displaced intra-articular fracture, tendon or ligament injury, fracture with bone or skin loss, or open fracture
- Complications include nonunion, malunion, arthritis, finger or nail deformity, loss of function, and compartment syndrome
- Re-implantation of finger amputations is attempted if they are proximal to the DIP joint, involving multiple digits, in children, or a thumb amputation

240. Pelvic Injuries

Etiology & Pathophysiology

- The pelvis has a ring structure comprised of two innominate bones (each with an ilium, ischium, and pubis) and the sacrum; anteriorly they are attached by ligaments at the pubic symphysis; posteriorly they are attached by ligaments between the sacrum and pelvic bones
- Integrity of the pelvic ring is necessary for pelvic stability—single breaks are generally stable; double breaks in the ring are unstable
- Due to a rich vascular supply of venous plexuses and arterial vessels, hemorrhage is the primary cause of death in pelvic fractures (up to 6 L of blood may be lost into the retroperitoneal and pelvic spaces)
- Lumbar and sacral nerve plexuses are at risk during pelvic fractures
- Pelvic fractures may result in bladder rupture or urethral injury
- Mechanisms of injury include MVA or motorcycle accident, pedestrian vs automobile, industrial crush accident, fall from height

Differential Dx

Presentation

- Pelvic or perineal edema
- Ecchymoses
- Obvious pelvic deformity
- Pain/instability with pressure on the pelvis
- Destot's sign: Hematoma above the inguinal ligament or on the scrotum
- Earle's sign: Hematoma or bony point tenderness on rectal exam
- Roux's sign: Decreased distance between the greater trochanter and pubic spine (versus other side)
- Signs of genitourinary injury may be present (e.g., hematuria, blood at urethral meatus, high-riding prostate)

Diagnosis

- Physical exam may be more reliable than a single plain X-ray to identify pelvic fractures in awake, cooperative patients
- X-rays: AP trauma view will show most significant fractures; lateral, acetabular (Judet), or inlet/outlet views may be added
- CT scan is indicated if plain films are unclear and/or to identify the extent of fractures; may also show retroperitoneal hemorrhage
- Unstable fractures occur with two or more breaks in pelvic ring
  - Straddle fracture: Fracture of all 4 pubic rami
  - Bucket handle fracture (due to lateral compression): Fracture of pubic rami with SI joint dislocation or sacral fracture
  - Open book fracture (due to AP compression): Separation of the pubic symphysis > 8 mm and possible SI joint disruption
  - Malgaigne fracture (due to vertical shear): Fracture and vertical displacement of pubic rami, the ipsilateral sacrum, and/or the SI joint

Treatment

- All pelvic fractures require orthopedic consultation
- Stable fractures: Bed rest, pain control, early weight bearing
- Unstable fractures: Generally require ORIF
- Control hemorrhage as necessary
  - Avoid unnecessary patient movement as this may cause further vessel damage and increase bleeding
  - Rapid administration of IV fluids (normal saline or LR) and blood products if hypotension occurs
  - Consider further intervention (e.g., fixation or embolization) after 3 L of IV fluids and 5–7 units of blood have been infused without adequate response
  - Pneumatic anti-shock garments may stabilize fractures and decrease further bleeding
  - Angiography with selective arterial embolization is indicated for persistent hypotension (does not affect venous bleeding)
  - Internal surgical fixation
  - External fixation may be used to prevent further injury and vessel damage in some hemodynamically unstable patients who are unable to tolerate internal fixation

Disposition

- All patients should be admitted
- Look for associated extremity and intra-abdominal injuries
- Overall mortality may be as high as 25% due to associated injuries, hemorrhage (more common in unstable fractures due to greater risk of intrusion into the vasculature), and long-term sequelae
- Complications may include hemorrhage, urologic injury (urethral rupture, bladder injury), acetabular/hip joint injury, fat embolism, ARDS, wound infection/sepsis, and pulmonary embolus

241. Hip and Femur Injuries

Etiology & Pathophysiology

- The hip is a ball and socket joint composed of the head of the femur and the acetabulum of the pelvis
- Mechanism of injury depends on age
  - Young patients: MVC, fall from height, gunshot wound
  - Elderly: Spontaneous fracture secondary to osteoporosis, minimal trauma, or falls
- Fractures of acetabulum or femoral head, neck, or shaft may occur
- Hip is at risk of dislocation due to its relatively weak posterior fibrous capsule (often associated with fractures)
  - Posterior (90%): Usually due to high impact against a flexed hip
  - Anterior: Forced abduction or blow to back while hip is flexed
- Trochanteric bursitis: Inflammation of the hip bursa due to trauma, gout, infections, or overuse
- Blood supply to femoral head is tenuous—high risk of avascular necrosis of the hip following injuries

Differential Dx

- Contusion
- Pelvic fracture
- Acetabular fracture
- Femur fracture
- Pathologic fracture (secondary to tumor or osteomyelitis)
- Dislocation
- Trochanteric bursitis
- Iliotibial band pain
- Septic joint

Presentation

- Inability to stand or walk
- Unilateral hip pain/tenderness
- Limited range of motion
- Hip fracture: Shortened leg; flexed, abducted, and externally rotated
- Posterior dislocation: Shortened, immobile leg; flexed, adducted, and internally rotated
- Anterior dislocation: Leg is immobile; abducted, flexed, and externally rotated
- Femoral shaft fracture: Swelling, ecchymoses; leg may be shortened with obvious deformity; may have decreased blood pressure
- Bursitis: Superficial tenderness, able to bear weight

Diagnosis

- Fractures are described by location, displacement, and angulation
- Obtain AP and lateral hip X-rays plus an AP view of the pelvis
- Common X-ray patterns may indicate fractures
  - Cortical disruption/displacement
  - Shenton's line (a smooth line that can be traced along the inner femur and obturator foramen) may be disrupted in fractures
  - Disruption of the normal S-curve and reverse S-curve along the femoral head and neck
  - Disrupted trabecular patterns from femoral shaft to head
- Consider CT, bone scan, or MRI to evaluate for pathologic fractures in patients with persistent pain but negative X-rays
- Joint aspiration may be necessary to rule out a septic joint

Treatment

- Pain management with IV narcotics or femoral nerve block
- Neurovascular deficits (e.g., diminished pulses) require immediate angiography or surgical exploration
- Consult orthopedics for all hip/femur fractures
  - Most fractures require ORIF or hip replacement
  - Femoral shaft fracture: Stabilize in the ED with traction and support blood pressure with blood and fluids (significant hemorrhage into the thigh may occur); open fractures require IV antibiotics and emergent surgical debridement and fixation
- Dislocations require immediate reduction, usually with conscious sedation
  - Posterior (Allis maneuver): In-line traction, flex hip, and externally rotate
  - Anterior: In-line traction, flex and internally rotate hip, then abduct
  - Following reduction, immobilize limb and obtain X-rays
- Bursitis: NSAIDs, rest, ice

Disposition

- Admission and orthopedics consult for all hip and femoral fractures
- Complications include avascular necrosis of femoral head (especially following femoral neck fractures), degenerative arthritis, chronic joint instability, sciatic nerve injury (especially in posterior dislocations), femoral artery injury
- Hip injuries in trauma are often associated with intra-abdominal and urologic injuries
- Compare films of dislocations before and after reduction for associated acetabular and femoral fractures
- Always consider elder and child abuse as a possible cause

242. Knee Injuries

Etiology & Pathophysiology

- A diarthrodial joint with patellofemoral and tibiofemoral articulation
- High risk of neurovascular injury (popliteal artery and nerve) following posterior knee dislocations
- Stability depends on ligamentous integrity—ligament damage ranges from strained to completely torn
  - Anterior cruciate (ACL): Provides anterior stability; commonly injured by flexion and rotation during deceleration
  - Posterior cruciate (PCL): Provides posterior stability; injured by a strong anterior force on a flexed knee (e.g., "dashboard injury")
  - Medial (MCL) and lateral (LCL) collateral ligaments: Injured by lateral or medial forces to the knee (MCL is more often injured)
- Medial and lateral menisci cushion the tibiofemoral joint
- Bursa: Synovial collections which may become inflamed—pre-patellar (housemaid knee), infrapatellar, and Baker's (popliteal) cyst
- Assume knee dislocation in any unstable knee

Differential Dx

- Ligament strain/tear (ACL, PCL, MCL, LCL)
- Knee dislocation
- Patellar fracture
- Femur fracture
- Tibial plateau fracture
- Patellar dislocation
- Chondromalacia patellae
- Meniscal injury
- Bursitis
- Infective arthritis
- Osteochondritis dissecans
- Iliotibial band syndrome
- Compartment syndrome

Presentation

- Inability to walk/bear weight
- Decreased range of motion
- Decreased strength
- Swelling, ecchymosis
- Joint or bony tenderness
- Joint effusion/hemarthrosis (patellar ballottement, fluid wave)
- Laterally displaced patella (dislocation)
- Knee "clicking," "locking," or "giving way" (meniscal injury)
- Inability to extend leg (patellar tendon rupture)
- Joint pain, swelling, redness, and warmth (bursitis)

Diagnosis

- Mechanism of injury is the best predictor of type of injury
- X-rays may include AP, lateral, and sunrise (patella) views; may reveal fractures of the patella, distal femur, tibia (plateau, spine, subcondylar, or shaft), or fibula
- Ligament injury may be indicated by joint laxity
  - Leg extension (patellar tendon)
  - Lachman's (ACL): Flex knee 30° and pull tibia anteriorly
  - Anterior drawer (ACL): Flex knee 90° and pull tibia anteriorly
  - Posterior drawer (PCL): Flex knee 90° and push tibia posterior
  - Collateral stress (MCL, LCL): Flex knee 30° and apply varus (LCL) and valgus (MCL) stress to lower leg
- McMurray's test (flex/extend knee while externally/internally rotating the lower leg—positive test elicits clicking and/or pain over medial or lateral joint line) and Apley's compression test (externally/internally rotate lower leg while applying compressive pressure) may identify meniscus injury
- CT scan or MRI may further evaluate injury

Treatment

- Joint aspiration may be necessary to relieve pain from tense effusions and/or rule out infection
- Ligamentous and meniscal injuries generally only require conservative therapy acutely (e.g., knee immobilizer, ice, elevate, pain control, compression bandage, and crutches) with semi-urgent orthopedic follow-up
  - Surgery may be necessary
  - Risk of popliteal artery injury with PCL injury
- Patellar dislocation: Reduce patella by extending leg and pushing the patella into place; immobilize and use crutches
- Knee dislocation: Usually spontaneously reduces on own; however, reduce immediately if present in the ED
  - Associated with ACL and PCL rupture
  - Arterial injury in 40% of cases (caution: 10% of vascular injuries have normal pulses)
- Consider angiography to evaluate vascular structures in all patients with dislocations, PCL tears, or decreased peripheral pulses
- Fractures: Apply long leg splint; may require ORIF

Disposition

- Knee dislocations are orthopedic emergencies that must be admitted for serial neurovascular exams and/or angiography
- PCL injury with joint instability should also be admitted due to high risk of arterial injury
- Distal femur, tibia, and some patellar fractures should be admitted for ORIF
- Most ligamentous injuries can be treated with outpatient orthopedic referral to determine the need for surgery
- Complications of knee injury include DVT, arterial injury, nerve injury, compartment syndrome (in fractures and dislocations), chronic degenerative arthritis

243. Ankle Injuries

Etiology & Pathophysiology

- Ankle joint is composed of the tibia, fibula, and talus
  - Mortise: The joint space
  - Plafond: The distal tibia or ceiling of the joint
- Three groups of stabilizing ligaments
  - Laterally: Anterior and posterior talo-fibular ligaments (ATFL and PTFL) and calcaneo-fibular ligament (CFL) limit ankle inversion and prevent lateral subluxation of the talus
  - Medially: Deltoid ligaments limit eversion and talar subluxation
  - Antero-posterior: Tibio-fibular ligaments limit bony displacement
- The direction of injury suggests injured structures (e.g., an inversion injury will cause lateral ligamentous injury)

Differential Dx

- Ankle sprain
- High ankle sprain (syndesmosis injury of the anterior/posterior tibio-fibular ligaments)
- Fracture
- Ankle dislocation
- Achilles tendon rupture (due to forced dorsiflexion)
- Peroneal tendon injuries (anterior subluxation of the tendon due to excess dorsiflexion)

Presentation

- Ecchymosis, tenderness, swelling
- Anterior drawer: Tests the ATFL (apply posterior force to the tibia while drawing the heel forward—positive if subluxation is greater than on the uninjured side)
- Talar tilt (inversion stress test): Tests ATFL and CFL (plantar flex and invert/evert the foot)
- Squeeze test: Tests the tibio-fibular syndesmosis (positive test is ankle pain upon squeezing of proximal lower leg)
- Thompson test: Tests the Achilles tendon (intact tendon should cause plantar flexion when squeezed)

Diagnosis

- X-rays: AP, lateral, and mortise views
- Ottawa ankle rules determine the need for X-rays in acute injury
  - Unable to walk more than 4 steps
  - Bony tenderness on posterior edge or tip of either malleolus
  - Foot X-ray is indicated for tenderness at the 5th metatarsal head or navicular
- Fractures include
  - Unimalleolar fracture of the lateral or medial malleolus
  - Bi- and tri-malleolar fractures
  - Plafond fracture: Fracture of anterior tibia
  - Pilon fracture: Comminuted high-energy distal tibial fracture
  - Maisonneuve fracture: Proximal fibula fracture, disruption of the interosseous membrane, and either a medial malleolus fracture or a rupture of the deltoid ligament
  - Osteochondritis dissecans: Subacute or chronic talar dome defect that results from a partially treated or untreated osteochondral fracture; may be missed on initial X-rays

Treatment

- General injury management: Rest, ice, elevation, compression dressing, pain control (NSAIDs +/− narcotics), and crutches as needed
- Ligament sprains: Range from grade 1 (tenderness only) to grade 3 (significant joint instability on ligament testing)—splinting and orthopedic referral for higher grade sprains
  - ATFL is the most commonly injured ankle ligament
- Ankle dislocation: Immediate reduction and orthopedics consultation
- Achilles rupture: Splint foot in neutral position or plantar flexion, avoid weight bearing, and ensure close follow-up
- Fracture management
  - Stable fractures should be splinted with orthopedic follow-up
  - Open fractures require tetanus immunization, IV antibiotics, and urgent orthopedic consultation
  - Unstable fractures or any joint disruption/widening require ORIF (e.g., bi- and tri-malleolar, plafond, pilon, and Maissoneuve fractures)

Disposition

- Potential exists for serious morbidity from unrecognized fractures
- Persistent pain >2 weeks mandates repeat X-rays or CT scans to look for missed fractures or newly visible talar dome osteochondral fractures
- Ensure adequate orthopedics or sports medicine follow-up for fractures

244. Foot Injuries

Etiology & Pathophysiology

- The foot can be divided into the hindfoot (calcaneus and talus), midfoot (navicular, cuboid, and cuneiforms), and forefoot (metatarsals and phalanges)
- Subtalar joint: Articulation of the inferior talus and calcaneus, allowing hindfoot inversion and eversion
- Chopart's joint: Connects the hindfoot to the midfoot, allowing forefoot adduction and abduction
- Lisfranc's joint: Connects the midfoot to the forefoot
- Mechanisms of injury:
    - High energy (e.g., MVC, fall) injuries may result in calcaneal and talar fractures and Lisfranc's joint dislocations; lumbar spine fracture may occur secondary to transmitted forces
    - Crush or twist injuries may result in midfoot or forefoot fracture
    - Overuse injuries may result in metatarsal stress fractures

Differential Dx

- Fracture
- Dislocation
- Puncture wound
- Turf toe (tear in the capsule of the 1st metatarsophalangeal joint at the metatarsal neck)
- Tarsal tunnel syndrome (entrapment of the posterior tibial nerve beneath the medial flexor retinaculum)
- Plantar fasciitis (inflammation of plantar fascia due to overuse)
- Compartment syndrome
- Achilles tendon rupture

Presentation

- Tenderness, pain, swelling, ecchymoses, deformity
- Metatarsal fracture: Pain with axial load
- Calcaneal fracture: Severe heel pain
- Talar fracture: Ankle swelling, pain
- Lisfranc's injury: Pain with forefoot pronation or abduction
- Plantar fasciitis: Pain in the arch or heel with tender fascia; increased pain upon arising and with toe dorsiflexion
- Tarsal tunnel syndrome: Medial paresthesias and pain radiating to the heel and calf; worse at night

Diagnosis

- Assess neurovascular status (e.g., posterior tibial and dorsalis pedal pulses, gross sensation)
- X-rays include AP, lateral, oblique, and calcaneal views
    - Ottawa foot rules: X-ray is indicated if the cuboid or base of the 5th metatarsal is tender
- Common fractures
    - March fracture: Stress fracture of the 2nd and 3rd metatarsals
    - Jones fracture: Transverse fracture at base of the 5th metatarsal
    - Nutcracker fracture: Fracture of the cuboid when crushed between the metatarsals
- Dislocations (often have associated fractures)
    - Lisfranc's: Fracture around the tarso-metatarsal joint (Lisfranc's joint) associated with dislocation of the joint; most commonly involves a fracture of the 2nd metatarsal; X-ray shows malalignment of metatarsals with their respective tarsal bones
    - Metatarsophalangeal: Due to dorsal toe hyperextension

Treatment

- General injury management: Rest, ice, elevation, NSAIDs
- Fracture management
    - ORIF is generally required for displaced or open fractures
    - Calcaneal and talar fractures should be manually reduced; many will require ORIF
    - Metatarsal fractures: Non-displaced fractures of 1st–4th metatarsal should be immobilized; 5th metatarsal fracture or displaced 1st metatarsal fracture requires ORIF
    - Splinting is sufficient for midfoot fractures
    - Buddy taping is sufficient for phalangeal fractures
- Dislocation management
    - Prompt reduction of subtalar and Lisfranc's joint dislocations in the ED; most will require ORIF
    - Metatarsophalangeal and intraphalangeal joints may be manually reduced in the ED
- Tarsal tunnel syndrome: Rest, ice, NSAIDs; may require orthotics and/or surgery
- Plantar fasciitis: NSAIDs, rest, stretching exercises, orthotics

Disposition

- Orthopedic follow-up for all fractures
- Admit patients with multiple fractures or associated injuries
- Hindfoot (talus and calcaneus) fractures are usually admitted due to associated injuries and need for ORIF
- Talus fractures are associated with a high risk of avascular necrosis, chronic ankle pain, peroneal tendon dislocation, and arthritis
- Complications include nonunion or delayed union, chronic arthritis, neurovascular injury, and skin infections
- Bone scan may be obtained as an outpatient in cases of suspected occult fractures or other bony lesions (e.g., osteomyelitis, osteosarcoma)

245. Compartment Syndrome

Etiology & Pathophysiology

- A limb-threatening condition caused by increased pressure in a closed anatomic space, resulting in decreased perfusion as tissue pressure exceeds perfusion pressure
- Compartments have a fixed volume; extraneous constriction or introduction of excess fluid increases pressure in the compartment, thereby decreasing perfusion and ultimately resulting in tissue hypoxia, anaerobic metabolism, and ischemic necrosis
- May occur in any compartment; especially common in the hand, forearm, upper arm, abdomen, and lower extremity
- Etiologies include trauma (e.g., fractures, crush injuries), edema (e.g., nephrotic syndrome, envenomation, burns), coagulopathies, external compression (e.g., MAST trousers, casts, and prolonged compression from falls)

Differential Dx

- Arterial injury
- Peripheral nerve injury
- Rhabdomyolysis
- Cellulitis
- Deep venous thrombosis
- Thrombophlebitis
- Gas gangrene
- Necrotizing fasciitis
- Snakebite
- Jellyfish envenomation
- Ruptured Baker's cyst

Presentation

- Pain (especially with passive stretch)
    - Intense pain out of proportion to exam
    - May occur at rest
    - Exacerbated by movement, touch, elevation, or muscle stretch
- Paresthesias (due to nerve ischemia)
- Pallor
- Pressure (palpable tenseness in the affected compartment)
- Pulselessness may be a late finding—since compartment syndrome is a disorder of the microvasculature, the major vessels are frequently not affected
- 2-point discrimination is the best method to test nerve compression (do not use pinprick as pain fibers are the last to be compromised)

Diagnosis

- History and clinical suspicion should prompt diagnostic tests—physical exam is not reliable enough to rule out the diagnosis
- Intracompartment pressure measurement should be performed if the diagnosis is suspected
    - Pressure >20 mmHg is abnormal
    - Pressure >30 mmHg may require fasciotomy
- Serum creatinine phosphokinase (CPK), myoglobin, and urine myoglobin should be evaluated to rule out rhabdomyolysis
- Urine toxicology screen may help define the etiology but is not helpful in patient treatment
- Coagulation studies (PT/PTT) to rule out suspected coagulopathies
- X-ray may show gas due to infection or other abnormalities in the affected extremity
- Ultrasound may be used to rule out DVT but will not diagnose compartment syndrome

Treatment

- Keep extremities level with the body (extremity elevation decreases limb mean arterial pressure without affecting intra-compartmental pressure, further decreasing perfusion)
- IV hydration and supplemental O_2
- Serial exams and pressure measurements
- Fasciotomy is the definitive therapy
    - Indicated for intracompartmental pressure >30–45 mmHg

Disposition

- Admission and surgical consultation for all patients with compartment syndrome
- Complications
    - Tissue damage: Irreversible tissue death can occur in 4–12 hours, depending on the tissue type and compartment pressures
    - Ischemic muscle contractures can develop after prolonged ischemia
    - Amputation is indicated to prevent gangrene if fasciotomy is not performed prior to muscle death
    - Myoglobinuria occurs after reperfusion of the damaged tissue following fasciotomy
    - Death may occur secondary to infections or cardiac arrhythmias (due to hyperkalemia from tissue death)

274

246. Neck Pain

Etiology & Pathophysiology

- See associated "Cervical Spine Fractures" entry
- Etiologies include trauma (e.g., MVA, falls, diving accidents), mechanical disorders (e.g., degenerative and/or herniated disc, spondylosis, and spinal stenosis), and inflammatory diseases (rheumatoid arthritis, spondyloarthropathy, infection)
- Cervical muscle strain/sprain: Soft tissue injury of the C-spine without associated neurological symptoms
- Spondylosis: Compression of nerve roots or the spinal cord due to degenerative arthritis of the vertebral disc with formation of osteophytes and narrowing of the spinal canal or neural foramina
- Disc disease: Neck pain with or without radicular neurologic symptoms caused by a degenerative or herniated disc
- Rheumatoid arthritis of the neck may result in unstable atlantoaxial subluxation following even minor trauma

Differential Dx

- Muscle spasm/torticollis
- Arthritis (e.g., osteoarthritis, rheumatoid, psoriatic, ankylosing spondylitis)
- Cervical disc disease
- Tension headache
- Meningitis
- Subarachnoid hemorrhage
- Thoracic outlet syndrome
- Brachial plexus injury
- Tumor (e.g., apical lung tumor)
- Osteomyelitis
- Myocardial ischemia
- Carotid dissection

Presentation

- Radicular symptoms (due to nerve root compression) may include paresthesias, weakness, and decreased sensation
- Spinal cord compression causes weakness, paralysis, sensory symptoms, and bowel/bladder dysfunction
- Fever may be present in cases of infection
- Spondylosis causes increased pain with flexion
- Disc disease causes increased pain with neck extension

Diagnosis

- Plain films (5–7 views) are indicated in trauma with localized spinal tenderness, in the presence of any neurologic signs, and in patients at risk for tumor or compression fracture
    - May show spondylosis with degeneration and osteophytes
    - Flexion/extension views may show ligamentous injury
    - Generally will not show soft tissue injuries
- Neck CT to visualize bony structures is indicated to better characterize a fracture or if plain films are inadequate
- Head CT followed by lumbar puncture may be necessary to rule out intracranial hemorrhage and meningitis
- Emergent neck MRI is indicated in cases of suspected spinal cord compression or epidural abscess
- Outpatient MRI may be indicated to evaluate for nerve root compression or other persistent injuries
- CBC and ESR if suspect inflammatory processes (e.g. rheumatoid arthritis, ankylosis spondylitis, epidural abscess)
- EKG/cardiac enzymes if suspect myocardial ischemia

Treatment

- 90% of cases are self-limited
- Rest, ice, soft collar, NSAIDs, narcotics, and antispasmodic agents as necessary for symptomatic relief
- Trauma: Immobilize with hard collar until fracture and ligamentous instability has been ruled out
- Trauma with neurologic signs raises the possibility of cord compression; obtain emergent MRI and begin IV steroids within 8 hours of injury (in blunt trauma)
- Institute appropriate therapy for rheumatoid arthritis in consultation with the patient's rheumatologist
- Treat infectious causes (e.g., osteomyelitis, epidural abscess, meningitis) with IV antibiotics

Disposition

- Admit patients with progressive neurologic symptoms, possible serious conditions (e.g., MI), and those who need further workup to rule out severe pathology (e.g., MRI for epidural abscess)
- Follow trauma protocols in cases of trauma or acute neck injury
- Greater than 90% of cases of neck pain are self-limited

247. Low Back Pain

Etiology & Pathophysiology

- 2nd most common causes of doctor visits—up to 90% of the population will experience back pain (#1 cause of disability)
    - Arthritic: Osteoarthritis/degenerative joint (or disc) disease, rheumatoid arthritis, spondyloarthropathies
    - Mechanical: Disk/facet disease, spondylolisthesis, fractures
    - Postural: Osteoporosis, poor posture (excessive demands of back musculature to support weight causes lactic acid buildup and pain)
    - Myofascial: Muscle/ligament strain, fascial tension, fibromyalgia
    - Other serious causes include spinal stenosis, cauda equina syndrome, infection (e.g., osteomyelitis or epidural abscess), and malignancy (especially prostate, breast, lung metastases or myeloma)
- Red flags that may signal a serious cause of LBP (imaging should be strongly considered in these cases): Age >50 or <20, trauma, fever, abnormal neuro exam, worse pain at night/rest, known malignancy, immunosuppression, bowel/bladder dysfunction, anticoagulation

Differential Dx

- Muscle/ligament strain
- Disc herniation/DDD
- Malignancy (prostate, breast, lung metastases; myeloma)
- Compression fracture
- Spinal stenosis
- Nerve entrapment syndrome
- Vertebral osteomyelitis
- Epidural abscess/hematoma
- Sacroiliac joint disease
- Spondyloarthropathy
- Herpes zoster
- Referred pain from AAA, PUD, pancreatitis, renal colic, endocarditis, and others

Presentation

- Pain may be limited to back/buttock or radiate down the leg
- Pain plus fever suggests infection
- Disc herniation with nerve root impingement: Radicular pain/weakness that worsens with standing and flexion
- Spinal stenosis: Pseudoclaudication (burning pain upon walking short distances), pain with extension; sitting decreases pain
- Cauda equina/cord compression: Urinary/fecal retention or incontinence, decreased sensation, saddle/medial thigh anesthesia, hyperreflexia, upgoing Babinski and/or weakness

Diagnosis

- History and physical are the most important diagnostic tools
    - L4: ↓ knee extension, patellar reflex, medial knee sensation
    - L5: ↓ great toe extension and sensation at 1st dorsal web space
    - S1: ↓ plantar flexion, 5th toe sensation, and ankle reflex
    - Straight leg raise (pain below knee suggests disc herniation)
- Emergent imaging (MRI or CT myelogram) is indicated in patients with evidence of cord compression, red flag symptoms, or suspicion of epidural abscess or osteomyelitis
    - MRI is the study-of-choice: Visualizes soft tissue and spinal canal; can rule out epidural abscess, osteomyelitis, cord compression, cauda equina syndrome, nerve root compression
    - CT will only visualize bone (obtain CT myelogram to visualize cord/canal in patients unable to undergo MRI)
    - Plain X-ray may reveal compression spondylolisthesis, fractures, osteomyelitis, metastases, or ankylosing spondylitis
- ESR elevation is very sensitive for vertebral osteomyelitis, epidural abscess, and metastases

Treatment

- Conservative treatment is sufficient for patients without red flag symptoms
    - Return to activity as soon as possible; rest has not been shown to improve recovery
    - Acetaminophen, NSAIDs, opioids, and muscle relaxants
    - Educate patient on proper back biomechanics/ergonomics
    - Physical therapy: Pain relief modalities (e.g., ice, heat, ultrasound), stretching, strengthening, aerobic conditioning, relaxation
    - Surgery may be considered in cases of refractory disease, large neurologic deficits, unbearable pain, or significant functional limitations
- Acute trauma with neurologic symptoms requires immediate high-dose IV steroids (see "Spinal Cord Injury" entry)
- Cauda equina syndrome: High-dose IV steroids and may require immediate surgical decompression
- Epidural abscess: IV antibiotics and usually requires immediate surgical drainage/decompression (some are managed without surgery)
- Vertebral osteomyelitis: IV antibiotics

Disposition

- Neurosurgery/orthopedic consult for cord compression, compression fractures, epidural abscess, spinal stenosis with nerve impingement, or acute cauda equina syndrome from any cause
- Admit patients with symptoms of infection, cord compression, cauda equina syndrome, compression fracture, intractable pain, or inability to ambulate
- Patients with chronic back pain without neurologic manifestation can be safely discharged home with medications and appropriate follow-up
- Most patients (those without red flag symptoms) will improve within 4–6 weeks without any specific treatment
- Precise diagnosis is often not determined

Analgesia and Sedation

R. MARK SUMMERS, MD

248. Acute Pain Management

Etiology & Pathophysiology

- Pain is a sensation produced by noxious stimulation of the terminal branches of nerve fibers
- Acute pain is the most common presenting symptom in the ED; usually has an identifiable cause and remits as the etiology resolves
- Chronic pain may have no specific etiology and is generally difficult to localize, quantify, and treat
- Somatic pain involves skin, subcutaneous tissue, or bones; usually well-localized and described
- Visceral pain arises from internal organs which share segmental innervation with somatic structures; may be localized or referred
- Neurogenic pain is usually described as "shooting," "burning," "tingling," or "crushing" and presents in a nerve or dermatome distribution (e.g., sciatica, diabetic neuropathy, or RSD)
- Psychogenic pain is poorly defined and rarely corresponds to dermatomes

Differential Dx

- Acute pain
- Chronic pain
  - Tolerance to existing pain medications
  - New lesions/pathology (e.g., new metastases, intestinal obstruction)
- Malingering (feigning of illness for secondary gain)
- Drug seeking

Presentation

- History: Perception of pain is variable and affected by age, co-existing conditions, previous experiences, cultural differences
- Pain description (PQRST)
  - Provocative/palliative factors
  - Quality
  - Region/radiation
  - Severity
  - Temporal duration
- Assess severity by numeric scale (1–10), visual scale, or faces scale
- Categorize pain as acute vs chronic; moderate vs severe; real vs suspect
- Children may display pain in different ways than adults (e.g., crying, grimacing, not eating)

Diagnosis

- Diagnostic workup is directed at the cause of the pain; occasionally no specific etiology can be discerned
- There is no definitive test for malingering; diagnosis by exclusion of identifiable pathology and clinical judgment [the presence of an underlying factor (e.g., disability claim) does not preclude real pain]
- Drug seekers are difficult patients to manage; may have extensive knowledge of pain medications; may be flattering, seductive, manipulative, or may try to control the interview; may have a history of multiple visits for ill-defined pain—advise the patient of your concerns in a non-judgmental manner, offer non-narcotic alternatives, and advise the patient that his or her pain will require an outpatient workup
- Drug abusers can and do have real pain and usually require higher doses of medications for pain control

Treatment

- NSAIDs are anti-inflammatory, analgesic, and antipyretic agents; side effects include GI upset/ulceration and renal insufficiency (COX-2 specific inhibitors have fewer GI side effects than traditional NSAIDs but may cause hypertension and edema)
- Acetaminophen is an analgesic and antipyretic with minimal side effects; liver toxicity may occur in overdoses
- Aspirin is an anti-inflammatory but offers less analgesia than most NSAIDs; side effects include GI ulceration, bleeding, and renal insufficiency
- Opioid analgesics are first line agents for moderate to severe pain; side effects include respiratory depression, nausea/vomiting, sedation, constipation, tolerance, and potential for abuse and addiction
- Tramadol has opioid-like effects but is not addictive
- Adjuvant therapy to decrease the need for opiates may include muscle relaxants, antidepressants, anticonvulsants, biofeedback, and acupuncture/acupressure

Disposition

- All patients have a right to assessment and treatment of pain
- Do not avoid treating pain due to fears of masking illness or confusing the diagnosis
- Combine medications (e.g., acetaminophen plus NSAIDs) to decrease required opioid dosages
- Administer dosages on a regular schedule for better pain control
- Use NSAIDs for inflammation
- Consider pain center referral in cases of chronic pain
- Elderly patients are more likely to suffer side effects of medications
- There is a very low risk of narcotic addiction if used for short courses

249. Conscious Sedation

Etiology & Pathophysiology

- Definitions
  - Sedation: A state of decreased environmental awareness
  - Light sedation: Sedation with minimal decrease in level of consciousness; the patient responds to stimulation and maintains protective reflexes
  - Deep sedation: Marked decrease in level of consciousness with loss of airway protective reflexes (but adequate respiratory effort)
  - General anesthesia: Sensory, mental, reflex, and motor (including respiratory) blockade
- Conscious sedation is a light sedation with analgesia often used in the ED to minimize patient discomfort while performing painful procedures, studies, or examinations
- Complications of conscious sedation include medication side effects, hypoxia, respiratory depression, aspiration, hypotension, and need for intubation

Differential Dx

- Indications for conscious sedation include
  - Wound debridement
  - Chest tube placement
  - Incision and drainage
  - Laceration repair
  - Fracture/joint reduction
  - Cardioversion
  - Diagnostic studies (e.g., CT scan in children)
  - Difficult examinations (e.g., pelvic exam in children)

Presentation

- History: Focus on major medical and co-morbid problems, experiences with sedation or anesthesia, medications, allergies, and most recent oral intake
- Physical exam: Evaluate for possible difficult airway
- Continually assess the patient's level of consciousness by evaluating ability to respond to verbal commands (e.g., "thumbs up")

Diagnosis

- Confirm availability of resuscitation equipment (e.g., bag-valve mask, intubation equipment) and sedation reversal agents
- Monitor vital signs, spontaneous respirations, and O_2 saturation (consider reversal of sedation if hypoxemia occurs)
- Choice of agents depends on the individual patient and the procedure being performed
  - Anxiolysis (e.g., imaging procedures in children): Consider midazolam or ketamine
  - Painful procedures (e.g., fracture/dislocation reduction, laceration repair, minor procedures, gynecologic exam in children): Consider fentanyl plus midazolam; ketamine; or etomidate
- Medications should be given in small, incremental doses to allow titration to desired levels of analgesia and sedation
- Continue monitoring until consciousness has returned to normal

Treatment

- Fentanyl (provides analgesia): Onset in 90 seconds, lasts 20–30 minutes; side effects include respiratory depression, hypotension, truncal rigidity, and seizures
- Ketamine (provides analgesia, anesthesia, and amnesia): Onset in 60 seconds, lasts 15 minutes; side effects include hypotension, increased ICP, emergence phenomena, and increased secretions
- Midazolam (provides anxiolysis, sedation, and amnesia): Onset in 1–3 minutes (IV) or 10–20 minutes (IM), lasts 30–120 minutes; side effects include respiratory depression and hypotension
- Propofol (provides sedation): Onset <5 minutes, lasts 5–10 minutes; causes respiratory depression and hypotension
- Etomidate (provides amnesia and sedation): Onset 30 seconds, lasts 10 minutes; causes N/V, myoclonic jerks
- Reversal agents include naloxone (reverses effects of opioids) and flumazenil (reverses effects of benzodiazepines)

Disposition

- Following conscious sedation, patients should be observed until they are no longer at risk for cardiorespiratory depression
- Discharge criteria include stable cardiovascular and respiratory function; baseline cognitive, mental status, and motor function; and a responsible adult to accompany the patient home (the patient may not drive or participate in activities requiring optimal mental functioning for 24 hours)
- Admit patients who are unable to ambulate or who lack a responsible accompanying adult (ICU admission if intubation is required)

250. Rapid Sequence Intubation

Etiology & Pathophysiology

- Rapid sequence intubation (RSI) is the cornerstone of emergency airway management—a technique for providing optimal intubation conditions while minimizing the risk of gastric content aspiration in patients who may have a full stomach
- Endotracheal intubation is performed with nearly simultaneous administration of sedation (induction) and a neuromuscular blocking agent—goal is to rapidly sedate and paralyze the patient and intubate *without* assisted bag-mask positive pressure ventilation (which may dilate the stomach and increase the risk of aspiration)
- RSI should only be performed if emergent intubation is necessary, the patient may have a full stomach, the intubation is predicted to be successful, and ventilation is predicted to be successful by alternate means if the intubation fails

Differential Dx

- Indications for RSI
  - Failure to maintain airway or protect from aspiration (e.g., head injury, seizures, or decreased consciousness)
  - Combative behavior
  - Failure of ventilation (hypercarbia) or oxygenation
  - Expected worsening of clinical course (e.g., multi-trauma patient, impending shock)
  - Expected difficult airway
  - Massive facial trauma

Presentation

- Assess airway patency (ability to speak, presence of upper airway obstructions, stridor)
- Test gag reflex or ability to swallow
- Assess ability to speak and follow instructions
- Clinically assess ventilation and oxygenation (pulse oximetry, consider ABG)
- Consider short-term prognosis in light of other injuries
- Examine mouth and neck for signs of trauma or airway swelling

Diagnosis

- Preparation: Ensure that all needed items are available (IV, oxygen, monitor, suction, endotracheal tube, laryngoscope); assess airway; draw medications
- Pre-oxygenation: 100% O_2 for five minutes results in adequate oxygen stores to permit 3–5 minutes of apnea before desaturation ensues (children and obese patients desaturate quicker); avoid active bag-valve-mask ventilation if possible, or give 4 vital capacity breaths if necessary
- Pre-treatment: Lidocaine prevents elevated ICP; vecuronium reduces muscle fasciculations caused by succinylcholine
- Paralysis with induction: Administer a potent sedative agent concurrently with a neuromuscular blocker
- Protection/positioning: Sniffing position; apply cricoid pressure
- Placement: Place ET tube under direct visualization and confirm placement by auscultation, end tidal CO_2, and X-ray
- Post-intubation management: Secure tube, provide long-term paralysis and sedation, and initiate mechanical ventilation

Treatment

- Induction agents
  - Thiopental (a barbiturate sedative/hypnotic): Onset 30 seconds, lasts 5 minutes; will not elevate ICP
  - Midazolam and other benzodiazepines (sedation, amnesia, hypnosis but not analgesia): Onset 1–2 min, last 30 min
  - Ketamine (provides dissociative amnesia plus analgesia): Onset 1 minute, lasts 5 minutes; may increase secretions and ICP, and may cause emergence phenomena
  - Etomidate (hypnotic/sedative, no analgesia): Onset <1 minute, lasts 20 minutes; will not elevate ICP
- Neuromuscular blocking agents (NMBA)
  - Succinylcholine is a depolarizing NMB with rapid onset (<60 sec) and short duration (6 min); side effects include fasciculations (pretreat with vecuronium), hyperkalemia (e.g., in crush injury, burns, MS, or ALS), trismus, malignant hyperthermia, prolonged neuromuscular blockade, bradycardia (pretreat with atropine in children)
  - Vecuronium and rocuronium are non-depolarizing agents with longer time of onset and longer duration of action but fewer side effects than succinylcholine

Disposition

- Adjunctive drugs may include atropine (to prevent succinylcholine-induced bradycardia in children less than age 6), lidocaine (may be cerebroprotective by blunting increases in ICP), and non-depolarizing NMBAs (used in very low doses prior to succinylcholine to prevent fasciculations)
- Complications (success rate is >99%) may include unrecognized esophageal intubation, aspiration, inability to intubate, hypotension, and drug complications
- Techniques for the difficult airway include laryngeal mask airway or Combitube, fiberoptic intubation, lighted stylet intubation, or surgical airway (e.g., cricothyroidotomy or transtracheal jet ventilation)

Index

Index

Index

Index

Index

Index

Index

Index

Index

Index

Index

Index

Index

Index

Index

Index

Index

Index

Index

Index

Index

Index

Protozoa infections, 120
Pruritus ani, as differential diagnosis for anorectal disorders, 51
Pseudohemoptysis, as differential diagnosis for hemoptysis, 36
Pseudohyperkalemia, as differential diagnosis for hyperkalemia, 105
Pseudohypoparathyroidism, as differential diagnosis for hypocalcemia, 106
Pseudomonas, 99
  in bacterial meningitis, 238
  in pediatric epiglottitis, 230
  in UTIs, 95
Pseudomonas aeruginosa
  in otitis media, 156
  in pediatric pneumonia, 231
Pseudo-obstruction, as differential diagnosis for bowel obstruction, 46
Pseudoseizure, as differential diagnosis for seizures, 82
Pseudotumor cerebri, as differential diagnosis for migraine headache, 77
Psittacosis, as differential diagnosis for tick-borne illnesses, 118
Psoriasis, 142, 143
Psoriatic arthritis, as differential diagnosis
  for neck pain, 275
  for rheumatoid arthritis (RA), 136
Psychiatric emergencies, 206–210
Psychogenic chest pain, as differential diagnosis for chest pain, 10
Psychogenic polydipsia, as differential diagnosis for hyponatremia, 102
Psychosis, as differential diagnosis
  for altered mental status, 76
  for encephalitis, 84
  for hyperthyroidism/thyroid storm, 71
  for hypoglycemia, 68
  for mood disorders, 207
  for tricyclic antidepressant overdose, 167
Pulmonary agents, 201
Pulmonary anthrax, 118, 203
Pulmonary contusion/laceration, as differential diagnosis
  for heart and great vessel trauma, 250
  for lung and esophagus trauma, 249
Pulmonary edema, acute, 28
Pulmonary edema, as differential diagnosis
  for acute renal failure, 92
  for cardiomyopathy, 18
Pulmonary effusion, as differential diagnosis for pleural effusion, 34
Pulmonary embolus (PE), 35
Pulmonary embolus (PE), as differential diagnosis
  for acute aortic dissection, 21
  for acute respiratory failure, 27
  for adrenal insufficiency/crisis, 73
  for anaphylaxis, 132
  for asthma, 29
  for cardiac arrest, 2
  for cardiomyopathy, 18
  for chest pain, 10
  for complications of pregnancy, 216
  for COPD exacerbation, 30
  for dyspnea, 26
  for esophageal perforation, 42

  for GERD/esophagitis, 43
  for heart failure, 17
  for heat-related illness, 188
  for hematologic/infectious oncologic emergency, 64
  for hemoptysis, 36
  for panic disorder, 208
  for pericardial disease, 20
  for pleural effusion, 34
  for pneumonia, 31
  for pneumothorax (PTX), 33
  for respiratory alkalosis, 110
  for ST-elevation MI, 11
  for unstable angina and non ST-elevation MI, 12
Pulmonary emergencies, 26–36
Pulmonary HTN, as differential diagnosis for dyspnea, 26
Pulmonary infection, as differential diagnosis for chemical weapons, 201
Pulmonary sequestration, as differential diagnosis for pediatric pneumonia, 231
Puncture wounds, 146
Pyelonephritis, as differential diagnosis
  for appendicitis, 48, 237
  for complications of pregnancy, 216
  for diverticular disease, 50
  for ectopic pregnancy, 217
  for gallbladder disease, 56
  for nephrolithiasis, 94
  for ovarian pathologies, 215
  for pediatric fever without source, 224
  for PID, 214
  for sepsis, 112
Pyloric atresia, as differential diagnosis for pyloric stenosis, 234
Pyloric stenosis, 234
Pyloric stenosis, as differential diagnosis
  for intussusception, 236
  for pediatric gastroenteritis, 235

"Q-wave" myocardial infarction. *See* ST-elevation MI

Rabies, 123
Rabies, as differential diagnosis for tetanus, 121
Radial head subluxation, as differential diagnosis
  for arm and elbow injuries, 265
  for wrist and forearm injuries, 266
Radiation colitis, as differential diagnosis for inflammatory bowel disease (IBD), 49
Radiation esophagitis, as differential diagnosis for caustic ingestions, 182
Radiation exposure, 193
Rape, 222
Rapid sequence intubation (RSI), 280
Reactive airway disease, as differential diagnosis for pediatric pneumonia, 231
Rectal cancer, as differential diagnosis for anorectal disorders, 51
Rectal foreign body, as differential diagnosis for anorectal disorders, 51
Rectal prolapse, as differential diagnosis for anorectal disorders, 51
Red eye, 148
Red eye, as differential diagnosis for glaucoma, 151

Index

Index

Index

Index

Index

Index

Index

Index